MADNESS, BUREAUCRACY AND GENDER IN MUMBAI, INDIA

MADNESS, BUREAUCRACY AND GENDER IN MUMBAI, INDIA

Narratives from a Psychiatric Hospital

Annika Strauss

berghahn
NEW YORK • OXFORD
www.berghahnbooks.com

First published in 2023 by
Berghahn Books
www.berghahnbooks.com

Library of Congress Cataloging-in-Publication Data

Names: Strauss, Annika, author.
Title: Madness, bureaucracy and gender in Mumbai, India : narratives from a psychiatric hospital / Annika Strauss.
Description: [New York] : Berghahn Books, 2023. | Includes bibliographical references and index.
Identifiers: LCCN 2023016591 (print) | LCCN 2023016592 (ebook) | ISBN 9781805390688 (hardback) | ISBN 9781805390695 (ebook)
Subjects: LCSH: Psychiatric hospital care—India—Mumbai—Case studies. | Psychiatric hospitals—Administration—India—Mumbai—Case studies.
Classification: LCC RC451.I6 S77 2023 (print) | LCC RC451.I6 (ebook) | DDC 362.2/10954792—dc23/eng/20230703
LC record available at https://lccn.loc.gov/2023016591
LC ebook record available at https://lccn.loc.gov/2023016592

British Library Cataloguing in Publication Data

A catalogue record for this book is available from the British Library

ISBN 978-1-80539-068-8 hardback
ISBN 978-1-80539-369-6 epub
ISBN 978-1-80539-069-5 web pdf

https://dog.org/10.3167/9781805390688

ILLUSTRATIONS

Map

Figures

CONTENTS

Tables

ACKNOWLEDGEMENTS

I am deeply indebted to the people whom I encountered at my research sites and who told me their stories and shared their views and thoughts with me. Without you this book would not exist! Special thanks go to Rini Fernandes, Dhaval Joshi and Akshay Bapat for their help, fruitful collaboration and the many inspiring discussions and insightful conversations. I also want to thank Shashi Shinde, Kaveri Dadhich, Mansha Singh and Anand Manarkattu – thank you for your assistance, emotional support and companionship!

I thank the Deutscher Akademischer Austauschdienst (DAAD) for financially facilitating my research in Mumbai, India from May 2011 until February 2012. Thanks to the TATA Institute of Social Sciences (TISS), Mumbai for hosting me. Thanks also to my supervisor Prof. Dr Katy Y. Gandevia (School of Social Work, Centre for Health and Mental Health, TISS) for her indispensable advice and guidance in the field. Further, I thank Prof. Dr Helene Basu (Department for Social Anthropology, Westfälische Wilhelms-Universität Münster (WWU)) for unconditionally supporting me in this endeavour.

I want to thank the Department for Social Anthropology/WWU for discussing drafts of chapters and conceptual ideas with me. Finally, I want to thank Heike Timmen, Pablo Holwitt, Ankita Karode, Helmar Kurz, Mrinal Pande, Anna Stern, Thomas Hajduk, Constantina Rokos and Natalie Gies-Powroznik for reading and commenting on separate chapters. Thank you all for your critical yet supportive comments! I am also thankful to my colleagues and friends Julia Koch, Markus Schleiter, Marion Linska and Thomas Stodulka, whose ideas inspired my work and who offered comments, encouragement and criticism. I also thank the whole staff and several BA and MA students at the Department for Social Anthropology, WWU for their warm support and fruitful discussions in the corridor and in the classroom. Special thanks go to Anthony Mason, Tom Bonnington and Marion Berghahn for their support, and the two anonymous reviewers for their suggestions on the manuscript as a whole. Finally, thanks to Keara Hagerty and to Sarah Sibley for their help within the final stages of preparing the manuscript and with copy-editing.

Last but not least, I want to thank my family, my parents, Bernhard, Christian and all my dear friends for their love and support and for not getting tired of encouraging me to hang on and for waiting patiently for me to finish this project and become social and a companion again.

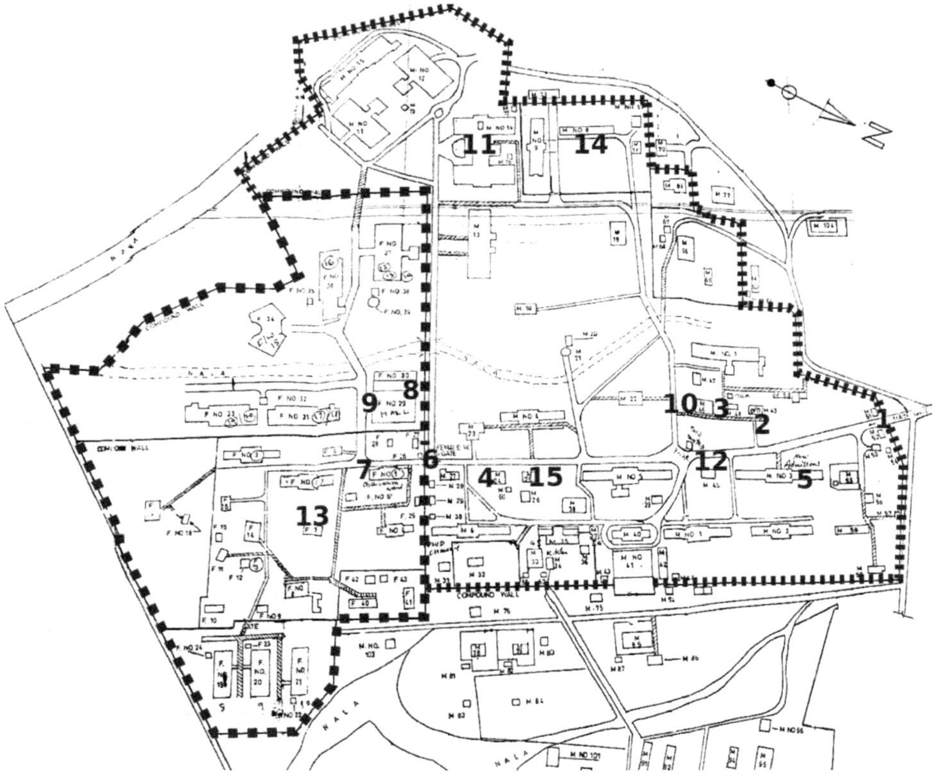

Map 0.1. Ground plan of the psychiatric hospital Asha in Mumbai, India.

Map Legend

The hospital buildings are divided into a male unit (front) and a female unit (back).

1. Main Gate
2. Outpatient Department (OPD)
3. Admission Office
4. The superintendent's (Dr Shukla's) Office
5. Admission Ward (Male)
6. Gate to Female Unit
7. Admission Ward (Female)
8. The Recreation Hall (Temple/Mandir)
9. Visiting Room (Female)
10. Visiting Room (Male)
11. Occupational Therapy Department (Male)
12. Social Workers' Office
13. Occupational Therapy Department (Female)
14. Criminal Ward (Male)
15. Psychiatrists' and Medical Officers' Room

INTRODUCTION

INDIAN PSYCHIATRIC SPACES AND 'MAD' NARRATIVES

In 2009 the *Mumbai Mirror* repeatedly reported cases of physical abuse in a huge psychiatric hospital in north Mumbai, the capital of the Indian state of Maharashtra. The article cited families that were worried about relatives who were admitted to the hospital, which I will call 'Asha'[1] in the following. Discussions in public but also among mental health professionals revolved around the bad conditions at Asha – a lack of hygiene, the poor quality of food, corruption and patients' regular corporal punishment by the hospital staff. In the same year, I accompanied two students of social work who were completing their field internship at Asha.[2] We met each other at the local university, the Tata Institute of Social Sciences, which I was affiliated to during my research endeavours. Mahi and Akash became my friends during the five years I carried out research in diverse mental health institutions in and around Mumbai. Both had a very critical and pessimistic view of the 'mental asylum'. Mahi and Akash told me about patients who had been there for decades, having been abandoned by their families. They spoke about roadside destitutes who neither spoke the local language Marathi nor any Hindi and were admitted against their will – some of them apparently deemed wrongly to have mental issues. They said attendants would take bribes from families who want to enter a ward to visit a relative under treatment. And they generally suspected that the staff were not really interested in taking good care of the patients but rather in the regular payment of their salary, which was guaranteed by occupying a government job. They also showed me around the hospital site. Together with

Mahi, I visited the high security cubicles in the admission ward in the female unit. Here patients who were violent or had tried to run away were locked up. In one of these cubicles, a woman lay on the floor, her breasts naked and exposed to the public. Her hair was cut ultrashort, and she seemed to have a mental disability. When Mahi asked her if something had happened, she did not respond and continued to lie on the floor motionlessly and to stare dead ahead. In the next dorm room, women were sleeping on nothing more than thin mats that were spread out on the floor. No beds were provided to the patients in this ward. The students' narratives and my impressions resonated with the media's representation of the hospital, which was rather unflattering during these years.

When I returned to Mumbai in 2011, Asha had undergone a remarkable change: the wards had been freshly painted, and plants and flowers decorated the spaces between the well-maintained pathways that connected the various hospital buildings. Garden swings and benches invited patients to take a seat and have a chat outside the wards. The hospital appeared far more inviting and welcoming than the last time I visited the place. Later I came to know that the current superintendent was the driving force behind these changes. In December 2009, the superintendent of Asha was suspended, and the new superintendent, Dr Praveen Shukla, took over. Dr Shukla promoted an image campaign that aimed at changing the grim picture Asha was associated with. I carried out extensive fieldwork at Asha between May and October 2011. During these five months, I used to spend at least three to four days in the hospital every week. I met up with Dr Shukla repeatedly during my research and discussed manifold issues concerning mental illnesses, psychiatry in India and everyday life in Asha. From November 2011 until February 2012, I continued my research in the psychiatric ward of a private hospital in southern Mumbai. However, this mental health institution is not discussed in more detail, although I draw on the material at times in order to illustrate or contextualize an issue tackled in this work. In 2013, 2014 and 2015, I travelled to Mumbai predominantly for work purposes and academic collaborations, which nevertheless enabled me to follow up on my research interests concerning mental health care in India. During my stays, I met up with friends and also several of my informants from the field.

These were predominantly mental health professionals but also two patients, Sarika and Ajay, whom I met for the first time in 2011 at Asha and whose stories I would follow up until 2014. Additionally, I discussed my material with people working in the mental health sector and other students and carried out several expert interviews that enhanced my understanding of themes that turned out to be pivotal in this ethnography: the production of psychiatric, bureaucratic, 'mad', gendered and queer narratives in the context of Indian psychiatric practice and the global mental health discourse.

The Bureaucratic and Biomedical Management of 'Madness'

The practices and self-representation of public hospitals are moulded according to the ideal of 'modern bureaucratic organizations' (Zaman 2005: 10). Two socio-historical aspects are worth taking into consideration here: psychiatric hospitals are institutions of the state, obliged to provide care for its citizens. At the same time, they are biomedical institutions that follow certain models of disease and population management that emerged in the first half of the twentieth century in industrial countries. The classification of medical diseases and psychiatric disorders and the generation of diagnostic and statistical manuals were products of the rising domain of 'public health' (Jutel 2011: 15). Psychiatric, allopathic medicine was introduced by the British colonial regime at the beginning of the twentieth century (Mills 2001), and its wide dissemination was possible mainly through its indigenization (Mukharji 2009). The introduction of psychiatric treatment was preceded by 'the emergence and functioning of science as a form of cultural authority' (Fabrega 2009: 563) in most colonial parts of India in the second half of the nineteenth century. In this context, the modern concept of disease and the growth of biomedical theory and practice was consolidated (ibid.: 563). In 1835, colonial authorities implemented Western medical education that was (and still is) conducted exclusively in English (ibid.: 567). This was the first time in the Indian context that the treatment of 'psychiatric diseases' was spatially secluded from the treatment of other illnesses. In 1858, the first Lunacy Act was passed by the colonial regime. The establishment of so called 'lunatic asylums' at the end of the nineteenth century was determined by European ideas and concepts of 'madness'. To protect the general population from the 'mad men and women', the asylums were built outside the cities and fenced off from their surroundings by huge stone walls. Similar to mental health establishments in Europe, the focus was mainly on the management and detention of social disorder rather than the treatment and cure of individual illnesses. Initially, mental health institutions established by the British in India only admitted 'one's own' people and 'privileged' Indians – that is, those employed by or affiliated to the colonial power – before the mental asylums finally also became accessible to the common Indian population (Ernst 1991). In the following decades, again analogous to the development of the psychiatric profession in the West, 'mental hospitals' generally developed more and more into medical institutions run and supervised by medical staff (Sharma 2004: 27f.). Nevertheless, in 1946 the Bhore Committee – a delegation that carried out a study to evaluate India's mental health care system – criticized 'mental hospitals', which still rather served the purpose of detaining patients than treating psychiatric diseases (Ganju 2000: 395). Finally, in 1987, after several failed attempts, the Indian Mental Health Act was passed to improve the quality of hospitals and strengthen the rights of psychiatric patients. At the beginning of the 1980s, the National Mental Health Programme (NMHP) was launched to implement the delivery of psychiatric services at the community level via the District Mental Health Programme (DMHP) (Gandevia 1993; Kapur 2004). Despite these initiatives, only minor changes occurred regarding the conditions in governmental mental health institutions. The allopathic psychiatric system to this day is perceived as suffering from an 'acute shortage of mental health professionals' (Bayetti, Jadhav and Jain 2019: 133), with approximately four thousand psychiatrists available for the entire country (equivalent to 0.301 psychiatrists per one million patients). Additionally, allopathic psychiatry remains an urban phenomenon, with most psychiatrists operating in major cities and towns. These also host the majority of state-sponsored services and academic research facilities, which are usually integrated into general hospitals' psychiatric departments and medical schools (ibid., see Wig and Awasthi 2004). The colonial system of former mental asylums, comprising forty-two institutions (Ganju 2000: 399), is supplemented by private clinics that can only be afforded by middle and elite-class clients (Kala 2004). The restricted availability of psychiatric services, particularly in the rural regions, is one of the reasons why a major portion of the population makes use of traditional institutions for treating *pāgal* (mad) persons. Additionally, a mental illness, a psychiatric diagnosis and admission to a psychiatric hospital is more stigmatizing than, for example, being possessed by a *bhūt* (spirit) and its treatment in a temple. Therefore, the act of admitting someone to a psychiatric hospital is often seen as the last and least desirable option, after a family has already unsuccessfully tried other options like traditional healing, Yoga, Unani, Siddha, Ayurveda or Homeopathy.

Asha was established on seventy-five acres of land, which was donated by a wealthy Mumbaikar family to the British regime. Its construction was completed in 1901, and the number of beds gradually increased from two hundred to 1,850. The outpatient department started in 1983 (source: hospital report 2011). Inpatients are admitted to separate units for male and female patients (see Map 0.1). The female wards are secluded by an additional wall from the publicly accessible part of the hospital in which the male wards are also located. Everybody who wants to enter the female unit has to pass through a gate and sign into a logbook. Except for doctors, no males are allowed in the female unit. This spatial organization resembles that of a traditional Hindu house (Khare 1976). The room where visitors are received and entertained can be found at the front. The kitchen, which is commonly occupied by the women of the household in India, is located at the back of the hospital and is usually not accessible to visitors. Both units comprise the following wards: an 'admission ward', a 'sick ward', a 'TB (tuberculosis) ward', an 'epileptic ward', and several so called 'chronic wards'. In the latter, patients are admitted who suffer from a long-term mental illness or who are not accepted back by their families after treatment. In the male unit, one also finds a designated 'old age ward' (which is Ward 17 in the female unit) and a 'criminal ward'. The latter accommodates patients who either committed a crime during an acute phase of their mental illness or who fell ill during their stay in prison. Long-term patients mentioned that in former times patients who behaved violently, had suicidal tendencies, or misbehaved in any way were brought to the criminal ward and put into isolation cells. There is no equivalent to a criminal ward in the female unit; during my time at Asha a female patient who killed her daughter during a psychotic phase was admitted to the admission ward, guarded by three female police officers.

In May 2011 when I started my research, there were 700 male and 693 female inpatients at Asha (total: 1,393).[3] Overall, 633 male patients were admitted to the hospital between January and May 2011. This was almost double the number of female patients (349) who were admitted during this period. Nunley (1992: 96) points out that while in American psychiatric institutions women are numerically over-represented, there are two times more men than women under psychiatric treatment in Indian medical institutions. Vindhya et al. (2012: 168) observe that while these numerical differences prevail in public psychiatric institutions, they become smaller in private hospitals. They conclude from these observations that women, especially from rural and poor economic backgrounds, have limited access to psychiatric treatment (Davar 1999: 154ff.).

While fewer women are admitted to the hospital, they tend to stay for a longer time, if they are brought in for psychiatric treatment (see Table 0.1). Indeed, it is more likely for a woman not to leave Asha ever again and to die there than for a male patient. The percentage of patients, male as well as female, admitted by

Table 0.1. Length of stay in correlation to patients' sex.

Length of stay	Male	Female	Total
Up to 3 months	290	172	462
Up to 6 months	79	46	125
6 to 12 months	82	46	128
1 to 2 years	63	69	132
2 to 5 years	48	94	142
5 to 10 years	48	94	142
10 to 20 years	41	98	139
Above 20 years	49	74	123
Total	700	693	1,393

a 'reception order' (RO) was around 40 per cent. The majority of patients, though, were admitted by a 'detention order' (DO), picked up by the police because they were wandering the streets or acting violently towards others. Only a minority (between 1–2 per cent) of patients were 'voluntary boarders' (VB), which formally denotes that they agreed to be admitted and treated in the psychiatric hospital and signed the admission papers themselves in addition to one of their relatives.

In the outpatient department (OPD), people collect medications, let a family member be re-examined or extend the 'leave of absence' (LOA) card of a formerly admitted patient. It is also the first stop in the hospital if a family seeks to admit a patient. Information boards on the walls outline every step of the admission and discharge procedure. Yet another board in the OPD waiting area informs that giving and taking bribes is considered a crime. The text on the board states that at Asha all charges comply with government regulations and in any case of reported corruption – for example, hospital staff who demand amounts exceeding the regular fees – the anti-corruption department bureau should be contacted immediately. In 2008–9, a total of 29,836 patients with their relatives visited the outpatient department.

When Asha was evaluated as part of the National Human Rights Commission Project Report on Quality Assurance in Mental Health, published in 1999 (Nagaraja and Murthy 2008), its overall rating was perceived as 'poor'. The report criticized the condition of some of the buildings and the overcrowding of wards, which led to many patients having to sleep on the floor, and that short stay and open wards were missing. Additionally, hygiene standards were found to be low. The report mentioned further that 'staff burnout' was common and that staff, particularly in the lower ranks, were transferred to the psychiatric hospital as a kind of 'punishment'. There were also vacant posts for clinical psychologists, and staff urgently needed to be sensitized to the needs and rights of people with mental health issues. The number of involuntary admissions was found to be too high. Finally, the report mentioned that psychosocial intervention and rehab services would have to be improved, which included psycho-education, individual counselling of the family and vocational rehab. In 2008, almost ten years after the first review, governmental psychiatric hospitals were evaluated again.

Regarding the follow-up report, Asha had improved in regard to certain aspects, such as new utensils for the kitchen and the addition of trollies to transport cooking pots to the wards. The hospital had also marginally reduced its official bed numbers from 1,880 to 1,850 and had 'significantly' reduced its (formerly exceeded) occupancy (from 2,000 to 1,253). A separate ward for 'the criminally mentally ill' had been established, and outpatient geriatric mental health services were offered (at that time, no outpatient service or old age ward existed). Regarding the other shortcomings previously mentioned, though, no significant change was recorded. The majority of admissions still occurred through courts and were therefore deemed as 'involuntary'. Again, staff numbers were noted as inadequate, even if the hospital was ranked at the upper end regarding the educational status of its professional staff compared to other state-run mental health hospitals. At least three psychiatric social workers were employed at Asha in 2008, while in twelve out of thirty-two evaluated hospitals not even one psychiatric social worker was present. The report further mentioned that nineteen of the hospitals had not employed a single psychiatric nurse during the last decade. However, the overall situation in hospitals located in Maharashtra was declared as better, with many nurses having received psychiatric training at the National Institute of Mental Health and Neurosciences (NIMHANS). In general, though, even if some improvements had occurred during the previous decade, the conditions in the four government-run hospitals in Maharashtra were still described as 'horrible' and 'shocking', according to the Bombay High Court. An article in the *Times of India* from 17 October 2007 described 'governmental mental hospitals' as places 'worse than jails'.

At the time I spoke to the superintendent, Dr Shukla, during an official interview in September 2011, he had been in charge of Asha for over a year and a half. His efforts in networking to make the hospital appear more open to outsiders and to establish partnerships with NGOs meant the tone of media reports about Asha had changed remarkably. Articles in the local newspapers reported that Dr Shukla had proposed changing the hospital's name from 'Asha Mental Hospital' to a more clinical-sounding one like 'Institute of Behavioural Science' or 'Institute of Psychiatry' in order to change the perception of public mental hospitals and decrease the stigma attached to them. The press also reported the superintendent's endeavour to train and educate the hospital staff on the particular needs of psychiatric patients. Another planned measure was the construction of a 'family ward' in which families could stay and accompany a family member for the length of their psychiatric treatment. The superintendent shared his vision of the inclusion of families not just as a moral support but to help train them in regard to handling 'a patient's emotions and behaviour later at home'. The education of families and so called 'lay counsellors' is a recent strategy adopted by NGOs, mental health professionals and activists to address the pressing shortage of qualified staff in the mental health sector (H. Basu 2018: 127f.). Another newspaper article reported plans to establish an additional hospital wing and rehabilitation centre that would include a college for the training of doctors and nursing staff. Dr Shukla imagined the project as a public-private partnership in offering potential investors a plot of land for the construction of their private hospitals or medical centres. Yet another article published during my time at Asha announced that the hospital planned to set up particular vocational training as part of occupational therapy and to train patients in making incense sticks and eco-friendly Ganesha statues[4] in order to sell these products under their brand name. The superintendent and the Maharashtrian health minister were mentioned as being the driving force behind these innovations and improvements in the hospital.

All these developments and initiatives took place in the context of the so called global mental health movement and the endeavour to 'modernize' Indian psychiatry (H. Basu 2009, 2010a; Davar 2014). In August 2001, in Tamil Nadu, twenty-five people who stayed near a *dargāh*, a Sufi healing shrine, where they sought treatment, were killed during a fire (the so called 'Erwadi tragedy'). The 'incident set off widespread alarm among some citizens' groups and professional sectors about modernizing mental health care and complying with international human rights standards' (Davar 2014: 266). The developments at Asha furthermore stood in the context of the emergence of the expanding private (mental) health sector from the early 1990s. Public-private collaborations, as put forward by Dr Shukla, are supported by a national health policy that sees such partnerships as a viable option to enhance health service delivery to underserved populations (Barua 2005; Davar 2012).

In this work, I understand public psychiatric institutions and their tendency to classify and treat people according to certain administrative and medical categories as typical 'bureaucratic organizations'. Don Handelman (1978: 16) argues that the idea of bureaucracy constitutes a 'mode of framing experiences' that particularly underlies Western and scientific thought. Bureaucracy as an administrative framework and by its systemic taxonomy produces social categories and things that constitute a certain social reality or domain to interact within. Discussing bureaucracy in relation to the modern state, Handelman understands bureaucracy as an instrument of modelling that works in a foreseen, controlled way. He understands the life in modern states as 'put together by organizations that are quite aware of their own systemic premises' (1998: 79) and constitute what he calls 'hegemony over transformational work': modern states engage in 'predictive modelling', which transforms the values of information they process.

Psychiatry resembles this systematic understanding in its approach to illness and its treatment. Biomedicine relies on a systemic classification of diseases and a causal-mechanistic interpretation of the human body. It treats 'disorders', whose identification in the diagnostic process implies the existence of an 'order' or status quo concerning a perceived healthy mind or social behaviour that has to be re-established to effect a cure. Psychiatric institutions that are embedded in a bureaucratic state apparatus and the public mental health system are therefore associated with a 'predictive modelling' function. Their approach stands in stark contrast to a 'transformative healing' process, which is often identified by medical anthropologists as the central mechanism of ritual healing approaches (see e.g. Hinton and Kirmayer 2017). Ironically, their stress on order, regulations and a systemic approach did not prevent bureaucratic institutions from being associated with 'madness' or sending people 'mad'. Think, for example, of the eighth task that Asterix has to master in the film *Les douze travaux d'Astérix* (1976), written and directed by René Goscinny and Albert Uderzo: 'Find permit A-38 in the place that sends you mad', a mind-numbing multistorey building founded on bureaucracy and staffed by unhelpful people who direct all their clients to other similarly unhelpful people elsewhere in the building.

Social anthropologists, among other social scientists, try to understand the inhuman and indifferent social spheres that bureaucratic organizations so often seem to produce and govern. Michael Herzfeld (1993) in his analysis of Greek and Western bureaucracy in general asks: 'How and why can political entities that celebrate the rights of individuals and small groups so often seem cruelly selective in applying those rights? Indifference to the plight of individuals and groups often coexists with democratic and egalitarian ideals' (ibid.: 1). Herzfeld draws a grim picture of bureaucracy and associates it with ineptitude and callous oppression by the nation-state against its citizens. According to Herzfeld, the bureaucrats' religion is nationalism, and he outlines how bureaucratic responses to disorder are ways of dealing with symbolic pollution. Similarly to Herzfeld, we can ask in the case of public psychiatric hospitals in India how it is possible that in medical institutions, which are supposed to help and serve people as public services, people are often not cared for but neglected, maltreated or even killed? When it comes to understanding individual behaviour, social practices, interaction and encounters, approaches like Herzfeld's that equate bureaucracy with nationalism and focus on the analysis of symbols and language necessarily remain on a rather superficial level. The political scientist Michael Lipsky (1980) argues that 'to understand how and why these [bureaucratic] organizations often perform contrary to their own rules and goals, we need to know how the rules are experienced by workers in the organization and to what other pressures they are subject' (ibid.: xi). Additionally, Akhil Gupta (2012) criticizes that 'most analyses of the state reinforce its unitary and purposive qualities, even when its power is criticized' (ibid.: 44). In contrast to these approaches, he refrains from treating the state as a unitary organization acting with a singular intention but sees it as characterized 'by various levels that pull in different directions' (ibid.: 47) and unintended outcomes that 'are systematically produced by the friction between agendas, bureaus, levels, and spaces that make up the state' (ibid.: 47). Dr Shukla faced this kind of friction when he tried to realize his visions and imaginations concerning Asha. The much-requested staff training, which was authorized by the state public health department at the beginning of 2011, could not be implemented because the government demanded it be conducted by 'experts' from outside the hospital. The superintendent struggled with these regulations, feeling that his own skills and expertise in the field were questioned, but he asked the government functionaries to hire anybody they thought would be appropriate to carry out the task. When I talked to Dr Shukla nine months later, there was still no progress or decision taken on this matter, and therefore the staff training was still pending. Another pending issue concerned the family ward and planned health care centre, the conceptualization of which he had initiated when he was appointed as Asha's medical superintendent the first time in 2004/5. Around this time, he took care of the basic planning in calling an architect and sending the architectural plan to the respective government office for approval. The approbation of the project took another five years. At the time of our conversation, the superintendent hoped the ward would be almost finished in another nine months. However, almost four years later, in 2015, I came across an article announcing that the family ward was soon to be established on the hospital premises. Meanwhile, the superintendent had changed again. Dr Shukla had obviously left his project unfinished once again and entrusted his follower with its completion.

Gupta replaces the notion of a bureaucracy as the rationalization of power in a disciplinary society with the idea that it is 'shot through with contingency and barely controlled chaos' (ibid.: 14). He does not perceive 'the production of arbitrariness' as peculiar to Indian bureaucracy, though, but denotes it as a feature of any complex bureaucratic organization. Additionally, not all outcomes of the administrative system are arbitrary, but some forms of discrimination are consistent, systematic and institutionalized. And, therefore, cultural capital tremendously helps in navigating bureaucratic structures in public hospitals (ibid.: 25). Bureaucratic procedures like the admission process can be accelerated remarkably if one has a contact at the hospital. An equally effective alternative is to pay an agent, of whom plenty wait for customers near the hospital gate, for their assistance in completing the necessary paperwork. Furthermore, giving *bakshīs* (a tip) to attendants or helpers to look after a patient is common practice at Asha (see Zaman 2005: 126). To be familiar with a bureaucratic habitus and its routines equips one with negotiating power within the institution. This encompasses language (Marathi, Hindi and/or English), reading and writing, navigating bureaucratic hierarchies and possessing or at least knowing how to get hold of relevant documents. Eventually, the mere familiarity with bureaucratic categories – that is, knowing one's age and birth date[5] – constitutes important cultural capital (Shamgar-Handelman and Handelman 1991).

The survivors of the Erwadi tragedy were admitted to the government mental health hospital in Chennai. Unfortunately, they did not enjoy much better conditions or receive better treatment than in the Muslim shrine. Indian media, which just shortly before had harshly criticized the 'cruelty' of traditional healing methods, now also discussed the problem of the outdated and obsolete institution of the 'mental asylum' (H. Basu 2009: 32f.). As a consequence of these events, the Indian Supreme Court passed several regulations that aimed at the reformation of Indian mental health services that many mental health professionals had so long called for. At the same time, religious healing sites became a contested and controversial topic, with the Supreme Court ordering 'a comprehensive awareness campaign' that was supposed to educate particularly the population in rural regions about the fact 'that mental patients should be sent to doctors and not to religious places such as Temples or Dargahs' (Agarwal 2004: 512). Since Indian Independence, a number of nongovernmental organizations (NGOs) have emerged that are also active in the mental health sector (Patel and Thara 2003; Patel and Varghese 2004). By their practices, the NGOs construct both religious healing and mental asylums as relics of the past, the latter of which are perceived as less complex but nevertheless outdated and something that should be abolished (H. Basu 2018: 120). These archaic practices have to be put aside in order for India to become a 'modern' and secular society that is built on the clear demarcation between religious salvation and psychiatric treatment that operates according to up-to-date scientific and psychological knowledge (ibid. 2010). Nevertheless, some activists bring up the question of whether modern biomedical practice too – and particularly private psychiatric services – needs to be controlled by the state more fiercely in order to protect its users. The topic was also taken up by the media on, for example, the popular talk show *Satyamev Jayate* (Truth Prevails), which was directed and presented by the famous Bollywood actor and director Aamir Khan. In one episode, he discussed biomedical malpractices in India's health system such as the administering of unnecessary or risky treatments and surgery (Satyamev Jayate 2012). During my own research, I was repeatedly confronted with the families' and patients' fear that private psychiatrists predominantly practise in accordance with their own (financial) interests and not for the well-being of their clients. This leads to a contrastive public image of mental health services. The huge and asylum-like public psychiatric hospitals are known for their scarce resources and lack of manpower but are nevertheless considered more reliable and less prone to exploiting clients financially. They have the reputation of being spaces of slow-working bureaucracy, leisure and corruption. In contrast, private institutions are often suspected of engaging in money-making practices and therefore of prescribing treatment that is unnecessary or even harmful to their patients.

Finally, a notable characteristic of Indian psychiatry is its heavy reliance on psychotropic drugs, with psychosocial interventions and therapies less developed, practised and even absent in many institutions (Nunley 1996; Jain and Jadhav 2009; Ecks and Basu 2009, 2014; Ecks 2014: 149). One reason may be the lay conception of biomedicine as a powerful, fast-acting and effective medicine, which a patient thus expects to receive (Nichter 1980). Psychiatrists bolster these conceptions and even stress the unique characteristics of biomedicine during interactions with their patients, something which is additionally fuelled by an experienced rivalry with other doctors and non-allopathic approaches like Ayurveda or ritual healing (Nunley 1996). Indian mental health professionals orient themselves towards the needs and expectations of the community, patients and their families in the context of markets and policies and make recourse to the conceptual tools and strategies that are part of national and global mental health discourses (Weiss et al. 2001). Earlier Indian mental health policies emphasized 'access to services and community participation with a focus on serious mental disorders' (Jain and Jadhav 2009: 63). More recent policies, though, advocate the provision and distribution of psychotropic medication while remaining unclear about the role of community participation, integration of mental health with primary care and psychosocial interventions (ibid.: 65). Furthermore, the government's neoliberal approach to the pharmaceutical industry in a highly competitive marketplace together with a poor regulation of drug companies' practices and marketing techniques allow pharmaceutical representatives to develop close 'working relationships' with medical professionals and students across all medical specialities (Bayetti, Jadhav and Jain 2019: 157). Consequently, Indian psychiatric culture relies heavily on pharmaceutical treatments, maybe more than in most other parts of the world, and this has become 'an essential part of being a psychiatrist' (ibid.: 138). Bayetti, Jadhav and Jain (2019) suggest that under the current lack of resources in the Indian mental health system a heavy reliance on biomedical psychiatry and psychotropics 'allows for the best possible compromise between *time-efficiency* and *treatment-efficacy*' (ibid.: 155) and enables professionals in OPDs to see and treat what is a vast number of patients. At Asha around 150 patients are seen every day during the OPD opening hours from 9.00 AM until 3.00 PM, which amounts to around thirty thousand each year.

Social Anthropology and Psychiatry: Cultural Allies and Alienated Opponents

Social anthropology and the psy-sciences have much in common when it comes to their historical origin and epistemological approach. Early anthropological and psychiatric authors shared many ideas and attitudes concerning the 'psychology of primitive man' (Skultans 2007: 101; see Freud 1960; Levy-Bruhl 1966). Both sciences actively construct and reproduce the other by translating people's behaviour, words and suffering into symbolic categories (Van Dongen 2000: 124). This gives rise to an asymmetrical relationship between psychiatrist/social anthropologist and the other: while the latter's behaviour and mental health is questioned, the moral order of the former is rarely under scrutiny (ibid.: 132). In the medical sciences as well as in social anthropology, the potential misuse of power was met with similar methodological measures. Ethical codes were supposed to prevent anything similar to the abhorrent medical experiments in Nazi Germany during the Second World War from happening again (Bell 2014) and evolved out of confronting its colonial past in social anthropology.

Both disciplines, psychiatry as well as social anthropology, assume that it is possible to understand the other by empathy and to a certain extent also by reflecting on and interpreting its limits (Van Dongen 2000: 124; Skultans 2007: 107; Kirmayer 2008). Medical anthropology's fascination for narratives, which reach 'out to reality' and in the process create 'a new social and personal reality which obscures it' (Skultans 2000: 96), is shared by psychoanalysis and talking therapies. Both disciplines draw on the rich meanings that are carried by the narrative form in their analytical writings and professional practices. Finally, the preoccupation with the 'abnormal' in a cultural comparative perspective once provided a fruitful basis for interdisciplinary collaboration between psychiatry, social anthropology and psychoanalysis (Jenkins 2015: 7; Hollan 2016).

In the following decades, though, a fundamental reorientation in the disciplines and therewith a diverging understanding and complication of the term 'culture' caused a disciplinary alienation prevalent to this today. Vieda Skultans traces one reason for the mistrust social anthropologists developed concerning psychology and psychiatry to Émile Durkheim's analysis of the origin of religious thought, which led to a 'reappraisal of concepts of mental health and illness as culturally grounded categories whose intelligibility depends upon a proper identification of their social roots rather than the identification of the behaviour to which they refer' (Skultans 2007: 103). Suddenly psychiatry itself became 'the other'. Psychiatry's own 'culture', its historical origins, the politics of its nosologies, its clinical engagement with its subjects and its understanding of 'culture' became the subject of social anthropological studies (Littlewood 2000: 67). The anthropological gaze excavated diverse facets of early psychiatry's ethnocentrism and shed light on the racist assumptions some psychoanalytic and psychiatric concepts were built on (Skultans 2007: 98). Under particular scrutiny was a psychiatric category that came into being in the 1950s, the so called 'culture-bound syndromes' (Littlewood 2000: 77; see Jadhav 2004). In contrast to the contemporary psychiatric perspective, social anthropologists propose that all illnesses and human responses to them are socioculturally determined and that human action is constitutive of biology as well (Littlewood 2000: 85). Janis Jenkins (2015: 4ff.) criticizes psychiatry for its tendency to reduce the locus of disorder to a biochemical 'substrate' rather than trying to grasp it in terms of a person's lived experience. Overall, it seems that the once 'cultural allies' have become 'alienated opponents' (Skultans 2007: 110).

By embracing the analytic concept of 'psychiatric culture', I attempt to develop an approach to the understanding of psychiatric practice that refrains from framing biomedicine, the psy-sciences or 'Western culture' as an immoral opponent in this work. The term 'culture' I understand as 'an orientation to being-in-the-world that is dynamically created and re-created in the process of social interaction and historical context' (Jenkins 2015: 9). This 'orientation to being-in-the-world' is constitutive for subjectivities, experiences and social realities. Several authors who influenced and shaped the field of medical anthropology have shown how culture informs body techniques (Mauss 1973), postures, styles and tastes (Bourdieu 2002), the expression and communication of distress (Nichter 1981), the performance of suffering and healing (Csordas 1990; Wilce 1995) and the creation of scientific knowledge (Latour and Woolgar 1986; Berger and Luckmann 1990 [1966]). Further, socioculturally created entities react to and act upon (Latour 2010) and can even make up people (Hacking 2007). Nevertheless, 'culture' always remains an abstract and analytical term that denotes a process or potential of meaning-making rather than a concrete, material or social object. Culture cannot be observed, measured or quantified as a materialized entity. Nor are people, things or symbols carriers of cultural meanings. Culture's meaning-making effects, created by certain 'causal powers' that enfold through an interplay between social and material entities, can be recognized as patterns and structures in social institutions, discourses, bodies, behaviour, language, perception and practices (Elder-Vass 2012). Medical anthropologists understand culture as a 'meaning-generating context' (Van Dongen 2000: 135; see Van Dijk 1998) that fundamentally shapes everything from risk/vulnerability factors to course and outcome of an illness but also serves as an important 'therapeutic tool' (Van Dongen 2000: 135) in itself. In this work, I draw on Laurence J. Kirmayer's (2006) understanding of culture as a dynamic system in which stories reshape people's perception of the world, drive individual action, imbue every action with meaning and at the same time act self-reflexively and change the frames of interpretation and understanding. This understanding of culture emphasizes 'the dynamically constructed and contested nature of lived experience and the social world' (ibid.: 133), builds on a conceptualization of the self as a narrative construction and frames a human's psychology as 'competing and conflicting stories of the self' (ibid.: 132).

As a critical scientific approach, social anthropology, and medical anthropology in particular, has the potential to problematize psychiatries as cultural organizations with diverse sociocultural and political practices. 'Local psychiatric cultures' are constituted by embodied institutional roles, social interactions, relationships and practices that shape the organizational everyday life (Caudill 1958; Fengler and Fengler 1984; Nunley 1992). Psychiatric institutions rely on certain ideologies that structure relationships within them and direct the behaviour of people towards certain organizational goals (Rhodes 1991; Young 1993; Strauss 2011). Talal Asad (1979) suggests understanding dominant ideologies structuring interactions in organizations as essential meanings that became authoritative under specific historical circumstances. Hospital cultures evolve in sociocultural and political contexts; they are not static but a product of a daily ongoing process of negotiation (Strauss et al. 1963; Long, Hunter and Van der Geest 2008).

Nevertheless, not all voices and perspectives within an organizational structure have an equal value and weight and therefore the same possibility to be heard or have the imaginations uttered by them realized (Graeber 2015: 45). Particularly in psychiatric organizations the voices of patients tend to be muted and their 'mad' speech and bodies are fiercely controlled by institutional practices (H. Basu 2009). What psychiatric patients speak about is often perceived as bizarre, unintelligible or nonsense and therefore is excluded from the discourse of sanity (Van Dongen 2004). Patients' bodies, movements and their speech are controlled or cut off in order to 'treat' and reshape them in a socially acceptable manner. The meaning of the term 'patient' is – not coincidentally one would suppose – twofold here. The term 'patient' denotes somebody who receives treatment from any kind of health care provider. Etymologically it is derived from the meaning for 'the one who suffers and endures' (from Latin *patientem* = bearing, supporting, suffering, enduring, permitting). This can be understood as somebody suffering from an illness or injury in a clinical sense. Additionally, the term 'patient' signifies somebody who is passively affected and acted upon. This is the case when somebody is 'treated' in a clinical institution, which includes being objectified by the 'medical gaze' (Foucault 1994).

Psychiatric patients are persons systematically acted upon, subordinated by forces that we might, theoretically, understand as 'structurally violent'. Akhil Gupta (2012) defines violence as occurring 'in any situation in which some people are unable to achieve their capabilities to their full potential, and almost certainly if they are unable to do so to the same extent as others' (ibid.: 20). Violence is structural when 'it is impossible to identify a single actor who commits the violence' and 'the violence is impersonal, built into the structure of power' (ibid.). Nevertheless, being a 'psychiatric patient' never eliminates agency – the capacity of the individual to actively exercise control over or at least influence how to live their life, even if subordinated by a local social system (Sieler 2014: 323). To gain an insight into social structures of power, Judith Okely (1991) proposes focusing on moments of individual resistance to subordination. In every organization, where ideological order categorizes, normalizes and stresses coherency, we find things and people resisting dominant meaning-making processes. Many of the anecdotes and case studies presented in the following chapters are about 'deviant' personalities, alien social moments and particularly aberrant narratives. Psychiatric patients make use of their voice and actively engage in meaning-making, borrowing terms and symbols from their surroundings and often drawing on the same meaning systems and notions of culture as psychiatry does (Lucas 2004). Furthermore, 'mad' narratives often implicitly criticize and sometimes even inverse dominant organizational discourses and challenge stereotypes and social norms. The focus on individual, defiant speech can provide social anthropologists with an understanding of normative forces at work in organizations and reveal 'cracks of contentment' (Okely 1991: 7). These are caused by atypical individuals who are nevertheless defined by the structures they resist. However, the existence of these cracks indicates that the given order is not the only one imaginable, unstable and not everlasting and that other social realities are possible and their realization may be just around the corner.

Narratives from Psychiatry

The ethnographer presents their insights gained from the analysis and interpretation of collected fieldwork material in the form of an ethnographic narrative. John van Maanen (1995) designates ethnography as a 'storytelling institution' that follows 'specific compositional practices . . . to fashion a cultural portrait' (ibid.: 5). The concept of a 'narrative ethnography' (Tedlock 1991: 69) gave rise to a reflexive approach, and Barbara Tedlock argues that the ethnographic stories we tell are always at least twofold: one strand engages with the researcher's experiences and the methodologies applied and another portrays the people encountered in the field and tries to grasp their experiences. The representation of the other as well as the ethnographer's self is what constitutes an ethnographic narrative.

A narrative is always both 'a mode of reasoning and a mode of representation' (Richardson 1995: 200). It is necessarily reductive and fragmentary, and therefore lived experience is always richer than a story told about it (Gay y Blasco and Wardle 2009: 9f.). The American psychologist Jerome Bruner (1991) understands narratives as being 'instrument[s] of mind in the construction of reality' (ibid.: 5). One central feature in the human organization of experience into temporally meaningful episodes is what Richardson (1995) calls 'narrative reasoning': 'the type of reasoning that understands the whole by the integration of its parts' (ibid.: 201). The latter stands in stark contrast to 'empiricist reasoning', which is 'the type of reasoning that "proves" statements' (ibid.). The narrative form is an inevitable cultural and communicative tool in social practices of meaning-making, explanation and persuasion. It is made use of by social anthropologists as well as by their informants. In the following, I frame the narrative ethnographic approach employed in this work to give meaning to patients', their families' and hospital staff narratives as well as to my, the researcher's, experiences.

Narrative Analysis in Medical Anthropology

The so called 'lifeworld' approach equipped social anthropology to understand individual experience and subjectivity as constitutive in itself, beyond its function as giving access to culture and meaning patterns. Skultans and Cox (2000) state that narratives and life stories are of such an interest for medical anthropology because they 'both provide a bridge which spans the earlier Enlightenment dualism of the individual and society and a means of accessing experience which would otherwise remain embedded in the body and beyond reach' (ibid.: 21). However, narratives cannot be considered as a congruent report of experiences and emotions. They are better understood as 'experiences put into words' in order to communicate them. The relation between experience and language is a problematic one, and if we can even access somebody's experience at all remains highly questionable. Nevertheless, narratives can inform us about how individuals speak about their (illness) experiences, construct and understand bodily symptoms and illustrate how social forces shape their experiences or even enable them (Kleinman 1989). Identifying cultural patterns and motives in narratives, particularly in stories and myths, has a long tradition in social anthropology, especially in structuralist approaches. Claude Lévi-Strauss (1997) and his identification of certain 'mythemes' is one example. The structuralist approach predominantly stressed and elaborated on the universal elements of stories and tales, their collective meanings and the social structures they refer to. In contrast, Nigel Rapport (2004), for example, focuses on the personal, private and fluid meanings of his informants' narratives. The sociocultural construction of reality oscillates between individual meaning-making and sociocultural themes, symbols and conventions. People make meaning of and think about the world by means of social principles and cognitive elements they learn and borrow from their sociocultural environment. Narrative analysis has to take into account both of these fundamental functions: the sociocultural as well as the psychological dimension of narratives. It has to acknowledge a narrative's function for its teller as well as for the audience – context constitutes one of the key elements in narrative analysis (Cortazzi 2013: 385ff.). In the following, I understand narratives as social events and as products of social entities and the causal powers and mechanisms the latter entail (Elder-Vass 2012). Furthermore, narratives themselves can be considered a part of social entities, for example, of organizations like psychiatric hospitals. In order to explain social events and the causal powers and mechanisms that produce them, the concrete phenomena that need explanation have to be identified and the explicit circumstances of their production clarified. Therefore, in order to adequately understand narratives as social events and to grasp their ontology, one must accurately contextualize them. This includes reflection on the situation in which they were produced and our own roles in their production; for example, as an interviewer or conversational partner (Csordas et al. 2010).

Psychiatric Diagnosis as a Mirror of Cultural Metanarratives

Arthur Kleinman (1977) successfully questioned the idea that the phenomenology of psychiatric disorders varies minimally across cultures and probed the social meaning and the clinical ambiguity of psychiatric diagnostic categories. His approach was taken up by numerous medical and transcultural psychiatric anthropologists in the following decades (Gaines 1992; Nuckolls 1992; Young 1993). While neighbouring disciplines like sociology and philosophy took up similar constructionist approaches to understand the 'sociology of diagnosis' (Hacking 1986; Jutel 2011), publications in the medical sciences and psychiatry are largely ignorant of these findings (with a few exceptions – see Jutel and Dew 2014). Psychiatry in its efforts to develop an international nosology and standardized approaches to diagnosis and treatment remains 'highly biased toward the Euro-American constructs' (Kirmayer 2006: 136). Consequently, psychiatric discourses and persons who embody these are more globalized than ever. Diagnoses like depression as well as other psycho-pathologies such as attention deficit hyperactivity disorder (ADHD) and post-traumatic stress disorder (PTSD) have grown in popularity over the past three decades worldwide, including in India (Lang and Jansen 2013). Nevertheless, medical anthropologists and transcultural psychiatrists also have shown the bi-directionality of the diffusion of explanatory models and lay and professional vocabularies (Weiss et al. 1988; Jadhav 1994). However, the global expansion of diagnosis and illnesses in the context of the global mental health movement (see http://www.globalmentalhealth.org/) is pre-eminently a one-way street. While diagnoses like 'hysteria' and 'multiple personality disorder' (Strauss and Kurz 2018) are applied in Indian clinical contexts, a diagnosis like 'possession' remains a 'culture-bound' syndrome and does not travel globally. According to China Mills and Suman Fernando (2014: 190), the framing of 'mental health' or disorder as a global priority and the push for a global norm for mental health and a standard approach for all countries and health sectors not only ignore local realities but also work to discredit and erase and replace local frameworks for responding to distress (Davar 2014).

During my research, I encountered Zaara, a young woman in her early twenties, in the psychiatric ward of the private hospital, who was diagnosed with an eating disorder (bulimia) and borderline personality disorder. Zaara, who hailed from a rich family and an upper middle-class background, held regular phone calls with her aunt, who lived in the United States, to discuss her diagnosis and treatment options with her. One day she shared her belief with me that eating disorders seemed not to be treated with ECT in the United States. She therefore planned to challenge the treatment decisions of her Indian doctors, who had regularly prescribed ECT for her condition. Zaara's case illustrates that the processes of the global expansion of treatment modalities and 'psychiatric narratives' are complex and use manifold channels before they are embodied by individuals and become personified. Disorders of food consumption have long been discussed by medical anthropologists as common 'idioms of distress' with a shifting meaning according to the sociocultural context (Nichter 1981). Eating disorders like anorexia and bulimia are often discussed as typical 'culture-bound syndromes' of Western countries in the social sciences, at once mirroring gender ideals and concepts of beauty and tied to a certain experience of the body-mind and practices of self-control, transformation and discipline (Gremillion 2001; Orsini 2017; Cheney, Sullivan and Grubbs 2018). The emergence of diagnoses like bulimia or multiple personality disorder in Indian psychiatry take place in the context of changing social structures and organization, such as in metropolitan cities like Mumbai, which correlate to a shifting experience of the body and the self (Strauss and Kurz 2018: 163). India's middle and upper classes have become immersed in evolving urban and cosmopolitan cultures that are progressively oriented towards consumption and individualistic values, which certainly also involves a modification of available and suiting idioms of distress within the respective sociocultural contexts (Ulrich 1987).

Psychiatric disease categories as well as bureaucratic classifications have '"extra-logical origins" because they correspond to forms of social organization and the "sentimental distinctions" that enable the systematic arrangement of ideas' (Strand 2011: 274; see Durkheim and Mauss 1963). In clinical everyday life, this becomes palpable in moments when patients' unexpected or disapproved behaviour challenges a mental health professional's knowledge and value system. During my fieldwork, I observed a situation in the OPD where a woman claimed to have a drinking problem. I was surprised as well as a little shocked by the reaction of the psychiatrist and medical officer, who openly and loudly ridiculed her. In this case, the woman had placed herself outside the rules and conventions concerning the sociocultural 'sphere of madness': women do not drink and therefore also do not suffer from alcohol addiction. Laughter was the doctors' way of dealing with a woman who was not 'mad' in the conventional way. At Asha, some mental illnesses are perceived as 'madder' than others, which illustrates how psychiatric diagnosis is enmeshed with sociocultural values and gender stereotypes. Additionally, the meaning and functions of diagnosis are mostly obtained from the bureaucratic and administrative context – for statistical purposes, psychiatrists and administrations have developed an institutionally specific diagnostic approach and, for example, do not provide any rubric for women suffering from alcohol addiction. As I elaborate in Chapter 4, rather than the well-being of patients or their families, bureaucratic structures serve the well-being of the psychiatric institution, to uphold its pre-existing structures.

Diagnostic categories refer to certain sociocultural and institutional 'narrative templates' that are made use of in diagnostic storytelling in order to situate patients in a 'disease story' with an imputed past and future (Davenport 2011). Because female patients at Asha are rarely diagnosed as 'addicted', no sociocultural 'narrative template' that 'female addicts' could occupy as their disease story is available. This illustrates how bureaucratic as well as disease classification systems attain an important communicative, regulative and didactic role in local psychiatric cultures like Asha. Furthermore, modern 'diagnosis as a process' (Godderis 2011) forms certain logics of practices to facilitate the production of 'factual accounts' (Hak 1998). Clinical practices aim to transform the patient's and family's illness narratives into filled in forms and disease categories that are collected in a patient file (Bayetti, Jadhav and Jain 2019: 144). In Chapter 4, I show how these translations are facilitated by interpretation processes that are informed and shaped by professional ideologies and sociocultural values. Consequently, even if the International Statistical Classification of Diseases and Related Health Problems (ICD) and the meanwhile globally exported DSM (Diagnostic Statistical Manual of Mental Disorders) were originally designed to assimilate divergent psychiatric cultures (Nuckolls 1992), each professional psychiatry tends to construct and implement its unique system of diagnosis and classification. This is illustrated by the vernacular interpretation and application of the diagnosis 'gender identity disorder' by a psychiatrist at Asha, which I explore in more detail in Chapter 7.

Paper Narratives

'Paperwork' is of particular importance at Asha. Documents and files play an important and often decisive role, and bureaucratic rites of passage monitor the entry ('admission') and the exit ('discharge') points of the psychiatric institution. I adopt an approach put forward by Matthew Hull (2012b), who suggests treating documents not as mere 'instruments of bureaucratic organizations' (ibid.: 253) or 'representation' (ibid.: 254) but instead as 'graphic artifacts' (ibid. 2012a: 1). Drawing on the theoretical approach of Bruno Latour and acknowledging the agency of things, he stresses the 'generative capacity' of bureaucratic documents and their ability 'to make things come into being' (ibid. 2012b: 259). Accordingly, Hull understands bureaucratic documents as 'constitutive of bureaucratic rules, ideologies, knowledge, practices, subjectivities, objects, outcomes, and even the organizations themselves' (ibid.: 253). Furthermore, they also may be 'sometimes diverted to purposes far from the administrative rationales that produced them' (ibid.: 260). At Asha examples for this are the 'voluntary boarder' (VB) admission and the 'leave of absence' (LOA) discharge (see Rekha's and Varun's cases in Chapter 3). If families were not able to produce all necessary documents for a 'reception order' (RO) admission, patients could often be admitted under the VB label; the superintendent then gave the family a month to hand in missing documents (see Hemant's case in Chapter 5). Most patients are discharged from Asha by LOA discharge, which they have to renew once every month when they come to the OPD to collect medicines. This procedure spares families from having to complete the whole paperwork once again if the patient's readmission might be necessary in the future. At Asha, to comprehend and be in control of official documents equalled being in charge of one's own or a relative's psychiatric treatment. Documentary writing has been recognized as an essential element of modern governance and as a central component of colonial government in South Asia (Hull 2012a: 7). The British colonial government was called *Kāghazī Rāj* (Document Rule) due to the fact that every single act was documented in a 'complete system of records' (ibid.). This system of documentation had developed from the communication practices of the English East India Company, the trading corporation that preceded the government of colonial India. Hull relates the centrality of writing in South Asian governance to fundamental problems the corporation faced in the seventeenth century in regulating day-to-day actions of officers and employees. It even laid out a structure of governance strikingly similar to today's modern corporations. In 1621 it passed the 'Lawes or Standing Orders of the East India Company', which stated that only through a connection with a piece of paper could an action be construed as an action of the Company (ibid.: 8). The 'Lawes' expressed a loss of confidence in people and specified a kind of documentary system in which every document had to be vouched for by another. It was related to making discourse definable through a trustworthy material order, in the context of an empiricist metaphysics that was growing in Britain. The materiality of graphic signs made them useful as 'a palpable sedimentation of the real' (ibid.). In the following century, the

British further expanded their 'graphic regime' (ibid.: 10) of surveillance and control in response to uncertain loyalties of native functionaries: 'Official discourse was anchored to people, places, times, and artifacts through an elaborate use of signatures, dates, and stamps' (ibid.). The mid-nineteenth century British colonial administration was constituted in large measure by various written genres (reports, records and manuals). These 'bureaucratic inscriptional practices' (ibid.: 11) from the colonial period have left their imprint on the contemporary administrative system. As a stereotypic bureaucratic organization, Asha's administrative system produces a bunch of registers that keep track of the number of patients, admission forms, patient diagnoses, the amount of ECT treatments administered, patient deaths occurring in the hospital and patient discharge. From these diverse registers, statistics are compiled that are regularly included in hospital reports. The reports embed the numbers (e.g. admissions for each month of the year), tables (giving an overview of staff, technical equipment, buildings, etc.) and charts (e.g. visualizing the different kinds of discharges, diagnoses etc.) into a narrative describing the facilities and services currently provided by Asha (Ak. Gupta 2012: 155). Reports also draw on the hospital's historical background and on the different activities (e.g. information regarding occupational therapy and different festivals and functions) taking place in the hospital, illustrated by photographs.

Bureaucratic documents play an important role in the production of 'bureaucratic narratives' at Asha. Filled in forms and patients' files, compiled out of diverse documents, constitute the type of narratives that informed my ethnographic narrative. In Chapter 4, I concentrate on one particular narrative routinely produced by a certain bureaucratic practice, namely the filling in of the document 'Patient's Social History' by a social worker. Taken routinely from every patient who is treated at Asha, they are what Jerome Bruner (1991: 18) calls 'narrative accruals'.

The 'Mad' Construction of Reality

A particular kind of illness narrative is one that breaks with common narrative properties and is consequently labelled as 'mad'. In 2012 I participated in an academic workshop during which participants presented excerpts from interviews recorded during fieldwork at psychiatric hospitals. I presented the case of Ramesh, a psychotic patient who was admitted to Asha's so called 'criminal ward'. The chair, a psychiatrist and psychoanalyst, chimed in before anybody else could comment or ask any questions. He announced that he doubted that my material could be used for social anthropological analysis for the fact that the meaning of the words of somebody experiencing a psychotic episode tends to remain obscure and are therefore not accessible for analysis. Ramesh's muttering, he argued, might have just been a string of words that were spoken for the sake of their alliterative sound. After the psychiatrist's comment, we immediately turned to the next workshop participant, whose excerpt he considered more intelligible and sound. This incident left me with several questions and doubts. Was the psychiatrist implying that the narratives of psychotic patients made for useless ethnographic material because their speech did not make sense and therefore could not tell us anything about their sociocultural surroundings? Or was he making the point that social anthropologists have to sort out those narratives that are too 'symptomatic'? When it comes to 'mad' narratives, one major aim of social anthropologists of psychiatry has been to 'depathologize' and 'demedicalize' them in order to show that they have a meaning besides being a medical symptom of a disordered mind and brain (Van Dongen 2002: 25). Counteracting the psychiatrist's advice and implications, by contextualizing and interpreting Ramesh's narrative, I attempt to show in Chapter 6 that the experience of a mental illness, similar to more common experiences, is shaped by cultural meanings and social structures and therefore does not lie 'outside of culture' (Lucas 2004: 146). Nevertheless, stories tend to display certain 'mad' properties when they deviate from, reverse or overemphasize certain narrative principles that are socioculturally agreed upon (Bruner 1991: 21).

To begin with, events incorporated in every narrative occur in a unique sequential pattern over time. According to Laurel Richardson (1995), this is related to the fact that '[t]ime is the quintessential basis for and constraint upon the human experience' (ibid.: 207). Jerome Bruner understands the particular human experience of time and its representation in narratives as a 'mental model' (ibid. 1991: 6). 'Associative flooding' (Kindt and Schecker 1998) that occurs in the context of psychotic experiences can predominantly structure a narrative. It disrupts the ability to organize one's narrative according to the basic principle of diachronicity. Therefore, narratives that are organized associatively and break with this fundamental principle are likely to be unintelligible and labelled as 'mad'. Further, narratives refer to particular happenings. A narrative's particularity 'achieves its emblematic status by its embeddedness in a story that is in some sense generic' (Bruner 1991: 7). An example of this would be the experience of some kind of 'shock' that families of patients often mentioned to me in connection with the onset of a mental illness. The shock could be the death of a parent, conflicts with the in-laws or problems in school. We find shock as a narrative's particularity embedded in explanatory models – that is, in 'notions that patients, families, and practitioners have about a specific illness episode' (Kleinman 1989: 121). Explanatory models include information about the aetiology of illness, and time and mode of onset of symptoms, pathophysiology, the course of sickness and the proper treatment. The contingent components of explanatory models tend to produce generic stories. However, I illustrate in Chapter 6 that Ramesh in his narrative reversed the principle of particularity in that his story does not emphasize a particular event or give an explanation why it happened. Instead, he stresses the social and personal meaning that people's deaths have in the context of his life.

The happenings mentioned in the course of a narrative are relevant to the intentional states of a narrative's protagonists: a narrative account provides 'the basis for *interpreting* why a character acted as he or she did' (Bruner 1991: 7). Happenings in narratives implicitly change the inner qualities of their protagonists. This explains why something could or probably will happen to them. Shocking life events – for example, the mother's decease, quarrels with the in-laws or problems in school – might disrupt a person's inner balance in a way that they become prone to mental health issues. However, a narrative only works if the narrator and their audience share the sociocultural concepts referred to, in order for a character's actions or suffering to be understood. A story somebody tells about a neighbour who urinated behind a bush at a bifurcation on his way to the village and subsequently suffered a possession attack only becomes intelligible if one has the local knowledge that urinating in inauspicious places makes one vulnerable to demons who linger there (H. Basu 2010b: 418). Similarly, misunderstandings or false interpretations might occur because the narrator uses 'mad concepts' or makes apparently idiosyncratic assumptions about a protagonist's inner state. I illustrate this by analysing Ramesh's narrative (which takes up the crime of murder rather surprisingly and abruptly) for the conversational context and his reversal of the principle of inner state entailment. By reversing the narrative principle and negating the intentional state entailment in his narrative, Ramesh purifies the narratively constructed reality of his deeds and guilt.

A narrative's whole and its parts rely on each other for their viability: 'a story can only be "realized" when its parts and whole can, as it were, be made to live together' (Bruner 1991: 8). A listener interprets the narrative that is put together by the speaker. How a narrative is interpreted and if its content is doubted or questioned depends on the way it is narrated and adapted to the narrational context. Bruner mentions two processes: 'narrative seduction' and 'narrative banalization', which commonly suffice for the audience to take a story 'as it is', eluding a conscious interpretation (ibid.: 9). Whether we 'buy a story' depends on the reason a story is apparently narrated – 'the issue of *intention*' (ibid.: 10) – as well as on the background knowledge of both the narrator and the audience and how each interprets the other. Sociocultural as well as psychological variables determine the context sensitivity of a narrative. The experience of psychosis or other challenging inner experiences often constitutes a strong inner narrative force. Accordingly, the narrator becomes less adaptable to the narrational context and at times even ignores or does not consider the existing context knowledge of listeners (see 'Personale Asyndese' in Kindt and Schecker 1998). Stories that lack context sensitivity tend to be odd and unintelligible, and their narrators are likely to be perceived as 'dotty' or 'mad' by others.

Narratives serve communication and social interaction and construct a 'social reality', but furthermore they are important tools to tell 'our story' and to understand ourselves as meaningfully being in the world: 'The self comes to know itself through its own narrational acts. In narrative constructions of past, present and future, of relations of sameness and difference, the self is given content, is delineated and embodied' (Rapport 2004: 75).

The understanding of one's self and several self-related processes, though, is often fundamentally disrupted in the case of mental problems and crises (Jenkins 2004: 35). Therefore, tellers of 'mad' narratives are often obsessed with (re)constructing and rescuing a meaningful self by conveying it to their listeners, who at times feel bombarded with apparently inappropriate personal and repetitive information. Take Rosie, the model and actress, as an example (see Chapter 3), who experienced her stay at Asha as a film crew's test that was supposed to evaluate her abilities as an actress. Every time I encountered her during my research, she spoke at length about her 'aptitude check' and how much she despised having to endure this hospital stay in order to pass it. Stories that are considered to be worth telling are those that show an implicit canonical script that has been breached, violated, or deviated from (Bruner 1991: 11). This narrative property is obviously highly dependent on the sociocultural context, norms and expectations. 'Mad' stories often ignore sociocultural conventions by transgressing or creatively transforming them. They often do not concern particular breaches of a canonical script, but with their narrations and performances 'mad people' constitute a breach themselves (Van Dongen 2002).

Whether a narrative is considered acceptable or not does not depend on its correct reference to reality or its verifiability (Bruner 1991: 13). Rather, narrative 'truth' is judged by its verisimilitude. 'Mad' narratives are labelled as 'nonsense' not because they are 'untrue' but because they ignore certain narrative principles. 'Mad' narratives usually do not follow the aim of constructing a verisimilar account but rather try to control and keep together life worlds and selves that fall apart by juggling symbols and personal associations. In order to (re)gain control over their lives and selves, 'mad' narrators may oversimplify causalities, exploit cultural symbols, ignore conversational contexts and become self-centred. Presumably, tellers and listeners of 'mad' stories evaluate them according to very diverging standards. Bruner (1991: 17) argues that context sensitivity qualifies narrative discourse as a viable instrument supporting cultural negotiability. Undoubtedly, competing versions of a story are much more tolerated than diverging versions of arguments or proofs (ibid.). Nevertheless, which narratives are in the end perceived as 'true' or justified also depends on the social power of their tellers, as I show in the context of bureaucratic narratives in Chapters 4 and 5.

To summarize, a narrative is prone to be labelled as 'mad' if it breaks with one or more of the above outlined narrative principles and therefore displays certain 'mad' properties. By manipulating narrative principles, 'mad' narratives tend to construct different and alternative realities than 'sane' ones do. This cannot simply be framed as the product of a deficient brain or disturbed language. It has to be understood as a phenomenon emerging from different needs and intentions, divergent experiences and perceptions and variational environments. Furthermore, the 'mad' reversion and creative transformation of conventional narrative principles reveal the subtle 'work of culture' (Obeyesekere 1990) and the 'magical power of cultural symbols' (Van Dongen 2002: 42). Every human being who possesses the ability to narrate does magic with his or her words to a certain extent. Humans strive to construct a reality in which they feel comfortable living and where their actions are accountable. But narratives are never consummate. Depending on the tellers' inner state and the sociocultural context, narratives lack coherence, plausibility or verisimilarity. Depending on the tellers' local knowledge and their mental and linguistic proficiency, they are able to adjust their narrative to their audience. Therefore, there is no clear or absolute demarcation between a convincing story and a foolish one, an intelligible or an unintelligible story or a conventional or 'mad' story. Telling stories – like most human phenomena – is 'distributed along qualitatively defined continua rather than as defined by discrete and distinct categories' (Jenkins 2015: 3). Whether a narrative is labelled as 'mad' does not depend on the tellers' mental characteristics alone. Rather, cultural norms and social power structures are decisive as well. Furthermore, as I show in the case of Ramesh, even if 'mad' narratives display different properties than conventional ones, this does not render them unintelligible or nonsense per se.

Queered Stories of Gender and Sexuality

A central theme in Indian psychiatry, taken up by the media, by social scientists and particularly feminists, is the mental health of Indian women. Contemporary authors discuss this predominantly in the context of women's marginal socioeconomic status, gender stereotypes, role expectations in Indian society, domestic and sexual violence and their common abandonment in psychiatric hospitals and shelters (Davar 1995, 1999, 2001; Chandra et al. 2003; Addlakha 2008; Pinto 2014, 2015). In this ethnography, I explore the construction and reinforcement of gender roles – female and male – in the context of a mental illness and psychiatry and how long-term patients either draw on or manipulate and transform gender stereotypes in their (illness) narratives and self-representation. Additionally, I scrutinize a patient's 'queer' narrative that challenges seemingly basic assumptions about gender and sexuality and draws on local queer identity categories in the context of globalized biomedical and psychiatric discourses (see Chapter 7).

According to Ian Hacking (2007: 305), sciences have become central in the self-representation and -understanding of industrialized societies since the nineteenth century. He describes different kinds of 'engines of discovery' among them clinical medicine, biology and bureaucracy that have driven the human sciences in 'making up people' – the creation of kinds of people that in a certain sense did not exist before. He mentions the 'discovery' of 'the homosexual' by psychiatry as an example. What is known as 'homosexuality' today was included in a category of vice, namely 'sodomy', throughout medieval times and the Renaissance (Oosterhuis 2000: 21ff.).[6] The first phase in the rise of an autonomous category of homosexuality was marked by the eviration of sodomites and their identification as 'hermaphrodites' (Hirschauer 1993: 78). Whereas in the past men who had sexual relations with other men were only considered 'hermaphroditic'[7] in some cases, towards the end of the eighteenth century every same sex sexual activity marked both involved parties as psychologically and medically deviant and as belonging to a third gender category (ibid.: 79; see Crozier 2008). Stefan Hirschauer (1993) understands the rise of these medical and psychological theories as happening in a certain sociopolitical context that destabilized opposite sex unions (ibid.: 83). The specific 'knowledge' about so called *Geschlechtscharaktere* (sexual stereotypes) (ibid.: 82) correlated with a discourse that saw the sexes as different from but nevertheless as complementing each other (Hausen 1976). The crisis of heterosexual relationships brought with it the need to clearly define and demarcate people who desire their own sex. The result was that these could neither be 'real' men nor 'real' women and therefore a 'third gender' was incorporated into the theory of the complementarity of the sexes. If the female and male 'naturally' attracted each other, there had to be something female in a man-loving man and something male in a woman-loving female: these individuals were assumed to be 'inverted', belonging to an 'intermediate sex'. The related concepts of 'butch' and 'femme' and the effeminate gay man, the 'fag' or 'queen' emerged in this context (Hirschauer 1993: 83f.).

This categorizing of the deviant sex/gender also had an impact on works and approaches in social anthropology that were concerned with queer expressions of gender and sexuality. Serena Nanda (1999) embedded her work on hijras – India's so called 'third gender' – in a social anthropological discourse concerning the social construction of 'sex' and 'gender'. Her ethnography was read as an example of 'alternative gender roles' to dispel the 'Western belief that there are only two sexes and two genders, each naturally and permanently biologically determined and each exclusive of the meanings and characteristics of the other' (Nanda 1999: xi; see Herdt 1996; Nanda 1996). As Gayatri Reddy (2005a) suggests, the anthropological literature in the 1990s situates hijras 'explicitly within the realm of sexual difference, implicating them in the debate on Western versus non-Western tolerance for sexual ambiguity and binary gender categorization' (ibid.: 31). However, Reddy, in her own ethnography on the hijras in Hyderabad, turns away from what she calls 'third gender analysis' in order to 'defer efforts to read the etiology of the sexed body in terms of the primacy of either cultural system or political economy or to reduce it to biology or psychology' (ibid.: 295). Reddy adopts Laurence Cohen's (1995) approach by locating 'the body within a multiplicity of differences' and examines the embeddedness of sexuality in everyday life and experiences. Accordingly, I approach narratives that tackle gender and sexual experiences as embedded in everyday life and social-cultural contexts and do not understand them as a representation of a stable gendered or sexed self. Rather, I assume that narratives are produced within a multiplicity of contexts of being-in-the-world that open the space to reinforce but also to reframe and transform conventional experiences and notions of gender and sexuality.

An important aspect that concerns narratives regarding gender, sexuality and queerness in this ethnography is the experience or display of 'madness', 'mental instability' and 'deviance'. Arthur Kleinman (1989) was the first to systematically describe how humans organize their experiences of illness and crisis as personal narratives. According to Kleinman, personal illness narratives do not only reflect and share illness experiences but also contribute, shape and even create the experiences and narratives of others. The 'plot lines, core metaphors, and rhetorical devices that structure the illness narratives are drawn from cultural and personal models for arranging experiences in meaningful ways and for effectively communicating those meanings' (ibid.). The function of illness narratives varies according to the different purposes they have, the contexts in which they are told – to the family, the practitioner, the health insurer or the social anthropologist – and the questions they are supposed to address – Why me? How to proceed now? What can be done?

Apart from personal illness narratives, Kleinman discussed two more kinds of narratives concerning 'disease' and 'sickness'. The former is embedded in clinical or 'medical' narratives – in a story that functions to guide treatment and healing decisions and name and explain the biological or psychological mechanisms that apparently cause the patient's symptoms. Furthermore, by employing a medical narrative, the healer 'interprets the health problem within a particular nomenclature and taxonomy, a disease nosology that creates a new diagnostic entity, an "it" – the disease' (Kleinman 1989: 5). Renee Anspach describes 'the conception of specific diseases that existed independently of individual patients' (Anspach 2011: xv) as characteristic of a 'modern' diagnostic practice that emerged at the beginning of the nineteenth century. However, besides the pathologizing effect medical narratives and diagnostic categories have, they also form the foundation for certain 'diagnostic communities' (Smith-Morris 2016: 10). In the Mumbaikar context, 'gays', 'transgenders' and 'kothis', who were identified as 'high risk target groups' in sexual health interventions, constitute such diagnostic communities (see Chapter 7).

Secondly, besides medical narratives that guide treatment, there are certain 'sociocultural' narratives that tackle the question of which social sources and macro-social (economic, political, institutional) forces may cause (mental) health problems and can be held responsible for human misery. Those narratives are concerned with 'sickness' and attach cultural meaning to certain symptoms and diseases, often in connection with moral judgement. Take as an example the case of the stigmatization of venereal diseases like AIDS and the association of the HIV epidemic with male homosexuality in the 1980s (Kleinman 1989: 6f., 21ff.). The translation of scientific insights into public health interventions tends to be interspersed with the moral judgements of the health professionals and politicians who initiate them; for example, the provision of 'knowledge' concerning safer sex education in the context of the HIV epidemic (Irvine 2005: 124ff.).

To summarize, personal illness narratives about the experience of chronic illness form a biographic story, and medical narratives around a disease constitute a body of medical knowledge and sociocultural narratives about sickness that materialize as distinct public health interventions. Motives, themes and plots are what link these different narrative levels. We find similar concerns and explanatory models in personal and medical as well as in sociocultural narratives, adjusted to the respective contexts and a narrative's function. Ajay, whom I encountered during my fieldwork in the admission ward, drew on 'hormonal imbalances' and 'female hormones' as an explanation for his 'homosexual' behaviour and him 'feeling female' (see Chapter 7). In contrast, the medical discourse perceives sex hormones as one factor but certainly not the decisive one in determining a person's sexuality. Nevertheless, the identification of certain biological factors that probably 'cause' homosexuality is part of a highly morally loaded sociocultural discourse. Confronting the disapproving moral judgement of his behaviour, Ajay refers to God, who created his body and desires as it is and who cannot be morally wrong. Homosexuality, even if no longer categorized as a psychiatric 'disease', is still perceived as a social disorder, a 'sickness' in many societies and social contexts. Therefore, tracking down its apparent biological causes, employing biomedical explanatory models and propagating biomedical 'treatment' options is still a prevalent sociocultural intervention, with the aim of eliminating homosexual persons from the social landscape.

Reconciling Alienated Opponents: A Symmetric Approach to the Analysis of Narratives from Psychiatry

Modern psychiatry claims to have an objective, rational and scientific approach to mental health as opposed to a subjective, irrational and backward approach. Indian psychiatric medicine in particular demarcates itself from religious or ritual healing practices, which it denigrates as 'unscientific', 'unmodern' and 'false believes' (H. Basu 2014: 191). According to many psychiatrists, 'mental patients' and their families who frequent ritual healing sites are unaware of what they 'really' suffer from, for example 'schizophrenia' or 'conversion disorder'. Psychiatry's claim to be modern results in psychiatric practices that are imbued with 'purification processes' (Latour 1994) that seek to identify and separate the social from the natural. However, as a consequence, clinical approaches are blind to certain characteristics of illness narratives; 'mad' and 'queer' narratives become unintelligible and inaccessible to psychiatrists, and their systematic analysis and interpretation is left to the social sciences. Let me unravel this argument in more detail in the following.

Before disease classification systems came into being, diagnostic processes in general were rather geared towards the patients' narratives, their wording and observations (Mak 2004: 98). Diagnoses tended to be 'fluid, fluctuating, and focused on the individual patient' (Anspach 2011: xv). With the modern medical approach, it is not the patient but the disease itself that has a narrative or exemplary 'clinical course' that includes a history, its present manifestation, a prognosis and an aetiology. The practice of modern diagnosis positions the patient in a clinical narrative that suits the 'clinical signs of disease' (Rosenberg 2002). While these signs were first detected by the physician alone, later diagnostic technologies like medical tests and laboratories changed the practice of diagnosis. It more and more moved away from the patient's and practitioner's subjective narrative and therefore diminished its role. This gave rise to what Paul Ricoeur (1974) calls the 'Hermeneutics of Suspicion'. He argues that an interpretive wall emerged between the patient's experience of illness and the physician's technologically mediated 'pictures' of disease, leading to a clash of the patient's experience with its medical interpretation. Particularly, psychiatry and the branch of psychosomatics developed concepts depicting the discrepancy between disease and illness experience; for example, 'somatizing disorder', 'functional disorder' or 'hypochondriasis' (Kleinman and Becker 1998; Anspach 2011: xvii).

Therefore, biomedical practices operate at the interface of the 'natural' and the 'social' sphere and are preoccupied with the translation of the individual 'subjective' experience into abstract 'objective' knowledge (Gardner and Williams 2015; Myers and Ziv 2016; Tessier 2016; Hollin 2017; Lawlor and Solomon 2017). This means that any narrative that incorporates ambiguous characteristics from the patient's (subjective and social) as well as the practitioner's (objective and natural) sphere runs the risk of being perceived as suspicious or even dangerous in the modern, dichotomous framework (Douglas 1984; Jackson 2005). This is exemplified by the case of a patient who dared to diagnose and therefore 'objectify' himself at Asha. I was shown the hospital structure and all the wards by one of the senior female social workers, 'Gadge madame', one morning. In front of one of the 'chronic wards', we encountered a male patient. The social worker brusquely directed the man to introduce himself – a very typical, paternalistic mode of interaction employed by many of the social workers when interacting with patients. His name was Sunil and he had been there for two years. He was able to understand and speak basic English and – as far as I can remember, and as it appears from my rather fragmentary fieldnotes of this encounter – we three conversed in a mix of Hindi and English. I asked him what his 'problem' was. He responded that he was troubled by 'psychosis'. Gadge madame briskly interrupted him, adopting a very resolute tone: 'Don't diagnose yourself, Sunil!' and then turned towards me and explained that because 'he is educated he knows some things about the things'. Somehow trying to de-escalate what I felt was a very incriminating situation for Sunil, I hastily continued to ask him if he was given the diagnosis by one of the psychiatrists. '*Nahīn*' – 'No,' he answered in a shy and avoidant manner, while throwing an anxious side glance at Gadge madame. In this scene, the agency and authority to narratively frame his experiences according to the medical discourse was gruffly taken away. In my notes, I additionally mention that I experienced the social worker's behaviour towards Sunil as generally 'very depreciative'. Obviously, the expectation was that Sunil was supposed to speak about his problem like an 'uneducated patient', that means he was supposed to use non-medical and experience near language. He was not supposed to adopt an approach and encroach on terms that from the social worker's perspective belonged to the meta-narrative that clinicians employ in order to be able to scientifically frame behaviour and speech as 'symptoms' and eventually reach a clinical diagnosis. This illustrates how in this local psychiatric context, treatment is not perceived as an intersubjective meaning making process that includes the patient as well as the doctor. Rather ailment is treated as a 'disembodied disease' that is completely detached from the personal experience and subjectivity. However, even if the relevance of experience and subjectivity is denied in clinical contexts and patients' life worlds are not supposed to commingle with those of the clinicians, by engaging in certain 'purifying' interactions a particular kind of reality and lifeworld is nevertheless created by the protagonists.

By perceiving itself as the rational natural, biomedicine in its clinical practice becomes highly vulnerable to 'contamination' by patients' illness narratives and their embodied diseases, which represent the 'irrational' social. Ramesh's narrative epitomizes the amalgamation of the social and the natural. It therefore poses a challenge to practitioners, who have to decide if his narrative should be considered 'mad' and unreasonable because it emerges from a biochemically disturbed brain or if it does hold meaningful information about his past or the institutional surroundings. The modern psychiatric approach seeks to classify Ramesh's speech as either symptomatic or as socially meaningful and avoids acknowledging its 'hybrid' characteristics (Latour 1994) and to eventually recognize that disease is shaped by a 'cultural biology'[8] (Kirmayer 2006). Furthermore, if Ramesh's narrative is eventually considered 'mad', it will become an object of psychiatric scrutiny and tendentiously perceived as inaccessible to social scientific analysis.

Particularly psychiatric diagnosis marks the distinction of what is normal and what is not in a certain society or institution

(Jutel 2011: 3). Homosexuality and its in- and exclusion in the psychiatric diagnostic classification system, its labelling as an abnormal 'paraphilia' and later as a normal 'sexual orientation' is a salient example. Protests against the classification of homosexuality as a disease were staged by gay activists at the American Psychiatric Association (APA) conference in 1970. The Gay Psychiatric Association itself drafted a proposal to delete homosexuality from the DSM, and the board of trustees of the APA finally voted to do so in 1973 (ibid. 2011: 34; Kutchins and Kirk 1997). Decisions on the change of homosexuality's status as a diagnosis were not taken 'on the basis of new empirical or scientific evidence but on the basis of social factors' (Jutel 2011: 34). Nevertheless, as long as diagnostic categories are not challenged by a social movement they tend to be considered and treated as psychological and natural facts. Accordingly, when Ajay in his queer narrative 'mixes up' exclusive psychiatric categories ('homosexuality' and 'gender identity disorder') he is framed as 'uneducated' and 'backward'. 'Mad' narratives such as Ramesh's are understood as 'symptomatic', and therefore understanding their 'nature' can inform the psychiatric body of knowledge. Contrariwise, 'queer' narratives like Ajay's, as long as they are not yet part of a queer discourse or movement, are categorized as uninformed and are therefore excluded from informing the further development of the psychological concepts of 'gender' and 'sexuality' (Okely 1991).

Herewith, I suggest that illness narratives, even if not always as salient as in the cases of Ramesh or Ajay, generally serve as a 'vehicle for hybridization' by imbuing the natural or biological with the social. Accordingly, illness narratives as well as biomedical assessments of sickness become highly targeted by 'purification processes' (Latour 1994). 'Mad' narratives like Ramesh's are perceived to be dominated by disordered 'natural' processes and therefore as idiosyncratic, alienated from the social sphere and not accessible to social scientific analysis. In contrast, 'queer' narratives like Ajay's are framed as predominantly shaped by his (uneducated) social background and subjective experiences and therefore as contrary to a clinical assessment, which is informed by scientifically proven psychological categories. The clear distinction between the disciplinary purviews serves to re-establish the social and the natural as separate spheres and medicine as a 'pure' natural science and part of the rational modern. These purification processes eradicate certain explanatory models, as, for example, when Ajay claims to be gay because his body has too many female hormones. His explanatory model runs the risk of being dismissed with the claim that the 'uneducated patient' misunderstood the medical concept of 'sex hormones'. Generally, bureaucratic logics and practices facilitate the shaping and purifying of 'mad' narratives according to the prevailing psychiatric and institutional categories.

Similarly, the medical sphere has to be purified of 'quack' doctors, who are said to exploit people – often financially – by promising to heal incurable diseases with non-scientifically proven treatment methods or promising to cure moral 'sicknesses' that are no longer perceived as medical diseases, such as 'homosexuality'. The campaign 'Queers Against Quacks' carried out by Humsafar Trust as part of the International Day Against Homophobia and Transphobia (IDAHOT) in 2016 exemplifies such a measure: 'The aim of this campaign was to bring out the homophobic "Quacks" or fake doctors who offer "cures" and "treatments" for homosexuality' (MJ 2016). After the campaign, the Indian website 'gaysi' (The Gay Desi) published a post titled: '9 Indian Doctors Who Claim to Have a Cure for Homosexuality' (ibid.). Among others, it named the sexologist Dr Vinod Raina, who runs a private clinic in New Delhi. According to an article in *India Today*, he stated, similarly to Ajay, that homosexuality is caused by an excess of female hormones that can be treated by a hormone replacement package: 'After taking blood samples, we increase male hormones in them' (Sebastian and Vikram 2015). Dr Raina claims to have treated patients for the past fifteen years and promises a 'one hundred percent cure' for homosexuality, taking six to nine months: 'The complete package costs Rs. 1.1 lakh', the article further cites, '[But] you have to pay the cash in advance. We do not accept cheques' (ibid.).

Biomedical therapeutic interventions foremost disregard the social and personal meanings of illness and sickness and therewith do not engage in any social responsibility beyond the 'rational-technical'. Therefore, they merely remain at the level of 'treating' diseases instead of curing them (Kleinman 1989: 28f.). Modern society's fragmented world view leaves medical anthropology, which scrutinizes biomedical practices, in an ambivalent and precarious state, as it finds itself situated between the social sciences that are supposed to explain the socially constructed and the natural sciences that deal with the naturally determined. Because the social is subordinated to the natural, medical anthropology is merely perceived as a discipline that 'helps' medicine to explain how culture and society 'influence' experiences of disease. Accordingly, John Campbell (2000) points out a methodological tension in medical anthropology that is 'the very different concerns, methods and indeed frames of reference underpinning psychological and anthropological research' (ibid.: 105). The clinical translation of individual experiences into medical diseases and the accompanying purification processes hinder the analysis and encounter of human suffering on a phenomenological and existential level. The division of the social from the natural and/or material world and 'realities' prohibits certain questions from being asked. For example: What leads a self-declared Indian 'gay' person to understand himself as a 'female' while in a biomedical discourse homosexuality and transsexuality exclude each other? Which other causal powers are at work here? Which sociocultural narratives influence and construct his reality and bodily experiences? Which social entities produce the biomedical discourse and which the divergent sociocultural narratives? These questions cannot be asked in the positivist oriented psy-sciences, which results in the social ontology of the respective phenomena and illness narratives not being analysed and contextualized adequately (Elder-Vass 2012). In contrast to psychiatry, medical anthropology has the epistemological tools at hand to recognize that phenomena like the gay patient who feels female are a product of biochemical as well as social forces. A symmetric and integrative analytic approach to illness narratives takes into consideration that the causal effects of social entities and sociocultural constructions equal those of material entities. Vieda Skultans (2003) argues that 'understanding human beings requires us to pay attention to narrative as well as characterization' (ibid.: 164). She suggests a dialogical approach to narratives and 'thinking with' rather than 'thinking about' stories in order to make 'room for a greater degree of empathy with the storyteller which in turn makes demands upon our moral imagination' (ibid.: 159). A dialogical approach and an analysis of narratives guided by empathic listening has the potential to complement clinical and bureaucratic practice. Furthermore, it is capable of reconciling the 'alienated opponents' social anthropology and psychiatry by promoting an interdisciplinary conversation that links anthropology to psychology, literary theory, philosophy and linguistics (ibid.: 156). A symmetric approach to the analysis of narratives that I pursue in this work enables a symmetric approach to research and knowledge production in general and attempts to include more voices or narratives than just the 'sound' ones. It furthermore does not ignore the corporeality and embodiment of narratives that renders them so powerful (Van Dongen 2003; Bahri 2017).

Notes

1. The name of the hospital and persons mentioned in this work are anonymized.
2. I was carrying out the research for my Master's thesis at that time. It was about a nongovernmental organization in one of the suburbs of Mumbai that takes care of roadside destitutes with mental health issues (Strauss 2011).
3. Own data collection from the hospital registers.
4. Ganesha statues are predominantly manufactured in the context of the ten-day Ganpati festival. On the festival's last day, the statues are brought to a body of water, often the sea, and submerged in it. Recently, the demand for eco-friendly statues has risen.
5. Outside the Indian higher middle-class, it is not common to know or celebrate one's exact birthday. Many Indians are confronted with having to estimate their birth date or rather decide on one when applying for official documents like a passport or birth certificate.
6. Sodomy as a category is highly informed by Christian sexual morality and comprises all sexual acts that are not geared towards procreation (Oosterhuis 2000: 21ff.).
7. Men could, for example, have sexual relations with younger lovers without losing their status as male. Only if they preferred a passive part in intercourse were they sometimes considered hermaphrodites (Hirschauer 1993: 79).
8. Kirmayer introduced the concept of 'cultural biology' in transcultural psychiatry in order to counterpose the assumption of an 'universal biology' opposed to 'local culture'. He prompts researchers to combine insights from the social as well as the natural sciences in order 'to understand the sense in which culture is a biological category as we unravel the details of the culture-biology interaction' (Kirmayer 2006: 129).

CHAPTER 1

ETHNOGRAPHIC RESEARCH IN PSYCHIATRY

ETHICAL CONTEMPLATIONS AND SENSORIAL ENGAGEMENTS

Lying on my bed, staring at the ceiling of the small, rather dark chamber that I am renting from a Tamil family, I notice mould has covered parts of it. Every year it is transformed during the rainy season, then it finally receives some fresh paint in October. Still almost half an hour is left until my mobile phone will set off the acoustic alarm. I listen to the heavy monsoon rain at my window. Its constant swoosh almost drowns out the cawing crows. I don't want to get up. I don't want to go to Asha. Actually, I recognize in this moment that I have never wanted to go there. I have just been regularly going because I somehow feel that I have to and because I don't want my research to fail. Everything in me seems to dislike this hospital and its staff. I turn to lie on my side and wrap the thin blanket a little tighter around me.

Pictures start to surface in my mind – a scene that my co-researcher Rini and I witnessed a few days ago. We were sitting in the female unit when a new patient – a woman in her sixties – was dragged in by five attendants. They pulled her hair and twisted her arms. The woman was screaming and protesting. 'She doesn't want to be here,' stated a startled Rini, pointing out the obvious. Through the gate that separates the female from the male unit, we saw three men. At first Rini didn't feel comfortable approaching them, but finally we both agreed to go and talk to them. One was in his mid-twenties, and it turned out he was the son of the patient that had just been brought in. He looked shy, and he seemed overwhelmed by the events. He was accompanied by his uncle and somebody who called himself a 'social worker'. Apparently, he was there to help the family with the paperwork regarding the admission, which involved giving permission to the attendants to cut off the hair of the patient; her hair was too matted, and lice are a common problem inside the wards. Rini asked the son how he felt about sending his mother to Asha. He answered diffidently that he didn't feel good about it but felt there was not any alternative. His father is deceased, and his mother had not been taking care of herself, refusing to take her medicines. A helper patient came out of the gate, holding a folded sari[1] in her hands. 'It is hers', Rini whispered to me. The helper patient handed over the cloth in a respectful and caring manner. Observing this scene, my mind tried to grasp what it meant to lose one's status as a full moral person when changing into the patient uniform. The son took the bundle and tucked it into a plastic bag. I experienced it all as strangely calm, maybe because it stood in such stark contrast to the violence and the woman's screams just a few minutes ago. The next morning, Rini and I went back to inquire about the new patient. The attendants sent us into a ward accompanied by a helper patient. We found the woman lying on a bed naked without a blanket and seemingly unconscious, her arms tied to the bedstead. She had a black eye; somebody must have beaten her. Rini and I were shocked to see her in this condition. When we ask the helper about what had happened, she explained to us that the new arrival had been a 'very bad patient' so far. After she was brought to the female unit yesterday, she had started to beat and choke the attendants, so she was given an injection and then tied to the bed.

The ringing of my mobile phone rips me out of my thoughts. It is not the alarm, though. One of the social

> workers from the hospital is calling me. 'It rained all night, and the railway tracks are flooded. The trains won't go today. Better you stay at your place,' he advises me. A joyful voice in my head immediately pipes up: I don't have to go today. I thank him for his call, say that we will surely meet tomorrow and hang up. I breathe a huge sigh of relief that I don't have to go to Asha today.

My ethnographic fieldwork affected me in a way that at times hampered me from getting up in the morning. Furthermore, my encounters with patients, their families and mental health professionals provoked deep ethical contemplations concerning my informants' and my own actions in the field. My fieldwork was an intense, sensory and transformative experience. Being in the field and 'doing ethnography' (Madden 2011) meant immersing my whole person and self.

Social anthropological methods ascribe a fundamental epistemological value to the experiencing ethnographer. Participant observation evolved as a legitimized method in the 1920s, but the reactions and emotions that the method evoked in the researcher were not supposed to be mentioned or reflected on in ethnographic accounts (ibid.: 5f.). As a consequence, what 'really' happened during fieldwork remained in a black box, and researchers were expected to keep their scientific observations and their personal, emotional experiences separate (Linska and Strauss 2015: 15). In the 1970s, Georges Devereux (1998) unveiled a new perspective on empirical methods in the social sciences that evolved out of a psychoanalytic approach. According to him, methods are not simply tools to gather knowledge but rather help to control the researcher's anxieties. Therefore, as part of the 1970s' critical self-reflection of the discipline, a postmodern, interpretative, critical and reflexive anthropology embraced the approach of 'observation of participation' (Tedlock 1991). This opened up alternative ways of validating ethnographic research apart from the natural sciences' criteria that imply the causality of 'objectivity-validity-reliability'.

In the context of the 'self-reflexive turn', besides patients and practitioners, researchers turned up as a third protagonist in ethnographies of psychiatry. Sarah Pinto (2014) offers very personal insights throughout her book *Women and Madness in Contemporary India*, such as her own failed marriage – an experience that she shared with the women in the psychiatric hospitals and that determined certain research insights. George E. Marcus (1994) describes this approach as 'self-critique, the personal quest, playing on the subjective, the experiential, and the idea of empathy' (ibid.: 395). This rather self-centred reflectivity can lead to a critical discussion of the epistemological and ethical grounds of anthropological knowledge and supplemented the reflexive-textual turn (Geertz 2006; Clifford and Marcus 2010). In the context of an evolving reflexive anthropology, it also became more common for medical anthropologists to admit in their writings that they identify as 'halfie anthropologists' (Abu-Lughod 1991) – that is, 'someone who grew up half in the world she writes about professionally' (Luhrmann 2000: 3). Tanya Luhrmann, the daughter of a psychiatrist, thought about becoming one herself before she turned to the social anthropology of psychiatry. That authors like Luhrmann feel the urge 'to admit' their halfie status to the reader in the first place is rooted in an epistemological premise that social anthropologists are only able to successfully objectify those social and cultural structures that they did not grow up in or identify with themselves (see also Nakamura 2013: 16). While the ethnographic method is certainly founded on the assumption that the insights of a researcher are at least partly generated by an alienation they experience towards the subjects of their study, social anthropologists no longer have to label their research participants as fundamentally different from themselves in order to validate the insights they gained. Rather, the validity and plausibility of ethnographic writing are based on a reasonable contextualization and interpretation of fieldwork material (Madden 2011: 23). Nevertheless, a rather decontextualized self-exploration and presentation of the researcher's emotions and personal anecdotes that do not follow a systematic approach would not 'tell us anything about the people who are the subjects of the research' (ibid.: 21). A more methodologized form constitutes 'sociological reflexivity', in Bourdieu's terms, which puts into question the 'knowing subject' and dissolves the determining opposition between the passive, to-be-explored object and the active, investigating subject (Bourdieu and Wacquant 1992: 213). Following Bourdieu and his sociological understanding of reflexivity as a methodological tool that objectifies the analyst's relation to the object, contemporary discussions in the discipline revolve around the enhancement of the researcher's self-reflectivity within the field in order to enrich the research process (Pink 2009; Davies and Spencer 2010; Spencer 2011; Linska 2015; Stodulka 2015).

In the following four sections, I discuss the reflexive-methodological approaches I took in my fieldwork. I begin with scrutinizing my own role as a social anthropologist at Asha, a bureaucratic organization. I reflect on how my own sociocultural background, with similar taxonomies and regulations, determined my approach and how I failed to cut the red tape that tended to subordinate people in this psychiatric culture. Subsequently, I reflect on the negotiation processes concerning my role and ethical position within Asha's institutional hierarchies and discuss how these generated a certain embodied knowledge about the institution's social and organizational structures. Furthermore, I discuss how reflecting on my sensorial and emotional experiences during ethnographic fieldwork not only served to identify sociocultural biases but constituted a fruitful methodological tool that generated insightful ethnographic knowledge about the moral landscapes of Mumbaikar psychiatric cultures. Finally, I discuss the process of co-creation of knowledge during my fieldwork by introducing my co-researchers, who were an immense social and psychological support in what was at times a very unwelcoming environment. All sections address ethical concerns I faced during my fieldwork. I tackle ethics as enmeshed with all stages of doing ethnography – as embedded in the fieldworker's actions, their thinking and their feelings rather than a discrete object that only has to be taken into account before or after fieldwork (Lambek 2010: 61). When I refer to 'ethics', I mainly understand it as a term denoting 'sociable practices and culturally-legible frames for assessing and indexing the "goodness" or "rightness" of human conduct: that is, it refers to the quality of human selves vis-à-vis other persons' (Lederman 2013: 590). I understand ethical questions as always concerning concrete situations and people's actions (Brodwin 2013: 14). This means that I evaluate a person's behaviour (my own as well as that of others) not according to an abstract rule, but I ask what it actually does or did to another person, what it caused them to feel and experience and if harmful or unwanted effects could have been prevented or foreseen.

The Complicit Anthropologist: Failing to Cut Red Tape

Getting access to and carrying out field research in public hospitals in South Asia can be challenging due to their rather opaque and 'slow working bureaucracy' (Pinto 2014: 154). Similar to other social anthropologists, I overcame bureaucratic obstacles by drawing on my cultural capital and using social and professional networks to open doors (Addlakha 2008: 23; H. Basu 2009: 33). My affiliation with the Tata Institute of Social Sciences facilitated my entrance into the public institution. My supervisor at TISS, an experienced and well-connected expert in the field of mental health in Mumbai and in India in general, was acquainted with Asha's superintendent, Dr Praveen Shukla. When I discussed my research plans with her shortly after I had arrived from Germany, she made a phone call to Dr Shukla to make sure that he would be happy to take care of 'her student'. The superintendent was willing to consider my social anthropological research at his institution and asked me to come to Asha in order to meet him and submit my research proposal.

Dr Shukla's office was located on the first floor of one of the buildings that comprised the male unit of Asha. Just inside the entrance to this building, to the left, was a small room. All hospital staff had to pass by this room at the beginning and end of their shift to enter their name in a red logbook that had been placed on a desk. Back out into the entrance, a commemorative tablet under the staircase displayed the name of a rich Mumbaikar citizen who had donated a notable amount of money towards the treatment of 'Hindu and high-class patients' several decades before. During colonial times, European and native patients were kept separate, and the spatial and social order in asylums established for the natives was determined by the caste system as an equivalent to the British class system (Ernst 2007: 220). So called 'class wards', which do not exist at Asha any more but still exist in several other psychiatric hospitals in India to this day, accommodate patients from families belonging to higher castes and communities. It is in such wards that food restrictions are taken into account in terms of caste or community status (H. Basu 2009: 33). During my time at Asha, caste and community no longer played a significant role in the spatial organization of the hospital. Social classifications were nevertheless inevitably inscribed into Asha's social structure and everyday practices.

The balcony corridor at the top of the stairs had several benches on either side. These were used by patients and their relatives waiting for their turn to enter the superintendent's office; I came to learn that it was not unusual for families and patients to wait here for an hour or two. While waiting my turn to see the superintendent, I took the time to observe the various interactions that took place. The superintendent's office was where all families who wanted to admit or discharge a family member had to go. Later, when I regularly found myself waiting for the superintendent, an assistant would often beckon me not to talk to particularly 'excited' patients or even family members who became too curious or who from their perspective behaved somehow awkwardly with me.

I waited patiently until an electric bell rang and one of the assistants finally signalled that I was allowed to enter the office room. A huge desk took up the centre of the room. The size of a doctor's writing desk is telling and indicative of his/her rank and status within a medical institution; it later seemed the bigger the desk the more difficult I found it to get in contact with the person who sat behind it. In the Indian context, and in governmental institutions in particular, interactions with persons of high status or rank usually involved talking only when one was spoken to and addressing the person respectfully as 'sir' or 'madam' (Pinto 2014: 53 f., 80, 216). A number of chairs had been placed around the desk of Dr Shukla so that rather than a personal working space it looked much more like an official meeting or conference table. Indeed, the superintendent's office constituted something like a meeting room, permanently frequented by a lot of people, including families who were about to admit or discharge a family member, pharmaceutical agents, who wanted to present their newest psycho-pharmaceutical products, or hospital staff, who needed documents signed. Ironically, the chairs placed around the table were rarely used. Except for myself, I hardly ever observed anybody taking a seat. This was certainly reasoned by the unwritten sociocultural rule that one is not supposed to take a seat in the presence of a person of a higher status than oneself, particularly if this person is standing. Patients constituted an exception here. They were asked to take a seat in front of the superintendent while the accompanying relatives usually gathered around them. A reason for this arrangement is perhaps due to the patients' role as sick persons; patients are expected to rest and are meant to be cared for (Parsons 1951: 428ff.). Therefore, for them to sit is less or not at all offensive in the eyes of someone like the superintendent. However, patients would never take a seat in one of the regular, wooden chairs that surrounded the superintendent's desk but in a cheaper and simpler plastic chair hastily provided by one of the attendants as soon as a patient and their relatives entered the office.

When I came to meet Dr Shukla to discuss my research, he was primarily concerned with the number and kind of patients I wanted to talk to. Additionally, he wanted to know the selection and seclusion criteria my research design followed. Therefore, I described what kind of case studies I wanted to collect and approximated a rough sample description. These were terms and concepts Dr Shukla was familiar with from his medical education, while terms like 'participant observation', 'narrative interviews' or 'recursive method' were rather not comprehensible to him. Once my research proposal had obtained the approval of Dr Shukla, I was allowed to come to the hospital on a daily basis, access all the wards and speak to the staff and patients. Being familiar with bureaucratic routines, I merged in well with the bureaucratic institution and its paperwork. Furthermore, I was able to 'pass' as a serious researcher, even if I actually applied a qualitative research design that was not comprehensible to most of the people in the field. Only once during my research did an attendant ask for a permission sheet and the signature of the superintendent when I was about to tape record an interview with a patient. Unfortunately, I could only show the attendant a sheet that gave me permission to bring my interpreter inside the hospital, therefore I was sent to the vice superintendent, who added 'tape recording' to the permission sheet and signed it.

At the beginning of my research, I pondered the necessity of an informed consent form and the pitfalls of asking people in the field to sign such a document. I eventually took the deci-

CONSENT FORM FOR ELECTIC SHOCK TREATMENT OF PERSONS BRINGING PATIENTS

I am giving consent for electric shock treatment to my son/daughter/husband/wife/brother/sister/mother/father named ____________________ through Dr. ______________(or through a self-appointed doctor).

I am giving consent that for the purpose of giving shock treatment anaesthesia be given/ medicines for unconsciousness/muscle relaxant medicines be used by the doctor.

I understand the procedure for this treatment or I have been explained the same by the doctor and I have been informed about the side-effects and other effects of the same.

I have been given satisfactory information in the language I understand by ____________ and I have read the information regarding this treatment given with this.

I have been given information regarding treatments other than electric shock. In spite of that I am accepting treatment by this procedure.

I have knowledge/I am aware that the possible side-effects of this procedure are head-ache, unconsciousness and that they occur immediately and can last for sometime after the treatment. For a few weeks, the memory is weak, but from a scientific point of view there is no functional brain damage and no surgical support of any form is required.

Despite taking all the necessary and complete care and other medical care accordingly, I am aware that there is a possibility of the occurrence of death. I am also aware that sometimes there is a possibility of fractures.

I am giving the doctors the consent to give any treatment to the patient if suddenly required in another hospital/with the help of another expert.

I have not been given any guarantee that the treatment or the side-effects will cure the patient 100%.

I have been informed that this consent is not applicable for all times and I have also been informed that if this treatment does not benefit the patient, then I can withdraw it at anytime and accept treatment through an alternative procedure.

I am aware of the side-effects because of not giving or stopping the treatment.

Figure 1.1. Consent form for electric shock treatment to be signed by the patient's relative, page 1.

sion against setting up any form. My decision had manifold reasons, one of them being that I did not want to produce one more signed document that patients or their relatives were not able to read or comprehend. There are numerous forms and documents to be attained and signed during the admission process. Because many of the families that frequent Asha did not speak or write

IMPORTANT INFORMATION

I am aware that before electric shock treatment, the patient must stay without consuming any food or water for six hours. I/ my relatives have been made aware of the fact that fits occur after giving electric shock treatment.

I am aware (after consulting the doctor) that, the patient due to his sickness/ because of the severity of the sickness is not capable of giving consent/permission, therefore I am taking the responsibility of giving consent on his/her behalf.

Signature of the Witness — Patient's/Patient's relatives' signature

Date/Time/Place — Address:____________________

____

Doctor's Statement:

I state with certainty (assurance) that I have informed the patient/patient's relative about the benefit and the side effects of the procedure of the available treatment. Shri/Shrimati________________, who is his close relative, was present.

Date/Time/Place — Doctor's Signature

Relative's Consent Form

I ____________________ (name) ____________________

____________________(available close relative) of ____________________

________________ (patient's name) state with certainty (assurance) that I have been informed about the procedure of the treatment, benefit and side-effects of electric shock treatment by Dr. ________________.

I am giving consenting to the below mentioned treatment procedure for the patient. (Patient's name)________________________________.

Figure 1.2. Consent form for electric shock treatment to be signed by the patient's relative, page 2.

the local languages of Marathi or Hindi or were unfamiliar with institutional structures, they were often overwhelmed by the meaning or purpose of the documents deemed necessary in the clinical context (see Chapter 4). Observing these proceedings reminded me that agreeing to something does not necessarily imply that one's consent is 'informed' (Skultans 2007: 250). The necessity of informed consent originates from an understanding of research as a violation or invasion and the a priori presumption of an unequal relationship between the researcher and the researched: '[I]n presuming this relationship of inequality, the doctrine actively reinscribes it' (Bell 2014: 518). Families had to sign manifold declaration forms and give their consent; for example, for treatment modes like electroconvulsive therapy (see Figure 1.1 and 1.2) or necessary hygienic interventions like shaving a patient's head in case of a lice infestation before a patient could be admitted. After I had observed several of these bureaucratic practices, and having spoken to families and patients about who participated in these, I was convinced that signing the various documents, often in the context of an ongoing family crisis, could not be understood as 'informed' or 'voluntary'. The bureaucratic routines did not contain any elements of open discussion, negotiation or real clarification regarding treatment modes but predominantly served to legally safeguard the hospital and was therefore part of a 'regulatory language' (Lederman 2013). This 'regulatory oversight' is an inevitable part of 'modern' institutions of medicine and interdisciplinary research ethics. Within anthropology, to obtain informed consent of one's 'informants' predominantly serves to legally safeguard the social anthropologist in her academic context to which she intends to return after fieldwork. When social anthropology embraced the informed consent doctrine, it meant that 'the differing environs in which anthropologists were working could now be considered largely irrelevant as long as people provided their "informed consent" to being studied' (Bell 2014: 514). The notion of 'informed consent' as well as 'protection of privacy' in research may be described as 'cultural products deriving from Western values of individualism' (Addlakha 2008: 300). Even if the code of the AAA (2011 [1998]) states that the concepts 'may be affected by requirements of other codes, laws, and ethics of the country or community in which the research is pursued' (ibid.: 327), their application can become tricky when the research is carried out in a non-Western context, where, for example, biomedical institutions do not follow individualistic principles (Skultans 2007: 251) or surrogate consent is more often the norm (Addlakha 2008: 23). Therefore, I had to responsibly navigate what Paul

Brodwin (2014) calls the 'ethics of ambivalence' and reconcile my aspiration to carry out an ethnographic research that suffices to meet disciplinary ethical standards with my own moral values and develop ethical stances adapted to respective field situations and persons.

At Asha, the notion of 'consent' was neither a local nor everyday concept that framed the encounters between patients and researchers. It was very common for patients to take part in medical or psychological studies carried out by Indian students completing their research internship at the institution. Because these encounters took place within hierarchical social structures prevalent in a medical institution, patients often were not necessarily aware they could also refuse to talk to researchers. They might even have had the impression that the psychological tests and interviews were part of their 'treatment' because the results were regularly added to their files. I tried to circumvent a reproduction of institutional and power structures and prevent giving the impression that I was conducting a 'clinical interview' when I spoke to a patient. For this reason, I avoided the examination or nurses' room as places of interaction and instead tried to arrange to sit down somewhere outside the building on one of the swings or benches. Sometimes I consciously broke with the hospital rules in order to distance myself from the institution, by, for example, bringing in small gifts like chocolate or jewellery for patients. Hospital outsiders, like students, were prohibited from giving anything to patients when they went into the wards. I certainly cannot claim that I managed to emancipate myself from the biomedical and bureaucratic institution and its often patronizing structures completely. Although I tried to avoid bureaucratic structures by not engaging in paperwork myself, my Western appearance and educational status inevitably correlated me with the medical institution. When I recorded patients' social histories in the outpatient department (see Chapter 4), I sat beside the social worker, who filled in the respective forms, and I was introduced by him as a research student to the families and patients he spoke to. Certainly, they identified me with the medical institution in this situation, and I, by recording their conversations with the social worker and taking notes, replicated its bureaucratic everyday practices.

The Ignorant Anthropologist: Negotiating Fieldwork within Organizational Hierarchies

When a psychiatrist or medical officer entered an examination room, it was not unusual to observe a social worker quit their task immediately and jump up in order to offer their wooden chair and take a seat on a plastic chair or leave the room altogether if no other seat was available. This exemplifies how the wants and needs of a superior within a social hierarchy are prioritized over those of their inferiors. Additionally, those down the hierarchical ladder usually engage in much more 'interpretative labour' and imagination work, continuously anticipating the wishes and intentions of those above them (Graeber 2015: 71). However, hierarchical orders did not remain uncontested. At Asha there was underlying tension between social workers, occupational therapists and the medical staff that regularly used to surface during the monthly staff meetings. The people at the top would often use bureaucratic measures in an attempt to fix pressing problems emerging from a lack of resources at the hospital. During one of those meetings, the medical staff discussed the necessity of reducing the high number of patients who could not be rehabilitated because their families abandoned them in the hospital. From the perspective of the superintendent and doctors, a rise in the number of confirmed addresses would result in an increased number of patients that could be escorted home by hospital staff if their families were not willing to discharge them. Therefore, the social workers were to be held responsible for a reliable and more regular confirmation of patients' addresses. But the social workers raised their voices in protest, claiming that this measure would mean an increased workload for them and that the decision did not take into consideration their needs and resources. In general, social workers did not feel acknowledged and respected by superiors and the medical staff at the hospital with regard to their work and efforts. Their university degrees, formally equal to those of the medical doctors and psychiatrists, did not grant them the rank in the social hierarchy that they thought they deserved (see Chapter 2).

Carrying out ethnographic fieldwork at Asha meant that I had to carve out my own position within its hierarchical and social order. Certainly, it was also my initially not-being-aware of the hierarchical stratifications at Asha that led me to ingenuously join the social workers in chatting and sitting in their allotted cubicle on the hospital premises. Only after some time did I recognize that students of social work, with whose field internship my research coincided, never spent much time chatting with the social workers. Instead, they approached them in a very respectful and rather distanced manner. However, at the beginning of my research I was an often-seen guest in the social workers' office. They shared and exchanged their food with me, and particularly the female social workers were curious about my background and liked to chat with me and share anecdotes from their family lives. After some time though, I sensed that they had adopted a somewhat weary attitude towards me. It took me some time to figure out the reason for this change in relationship. From the beginning of my research, I was very eager to move around the hospital, to interact with patients and speak to all the staff. In contrast, the social workers kept a distance from the wards, gave preference to spending little time with patients and most of them preferred light chit-chat over detailed discussion of their work. They continuously struggled to shed a positive light on their role and social status in the hospital. Nevertheless, they, quite obviously, faced limited resources, time constraints and suffered from a low hierarchical status that withheld from them any influential power within the institutional structures. They were well aware of the critical voices regularly aimed at them in staff meetings by TISS students or the medical superintendent, who accused them of avoiding work, responsibility and exploiting their civil servant status. The increasing mistrust towards me and suspicion about my role in the hospital soon led to my separation from the group of social workers and an end to our common lunch sessions.

Though I tried to spend some time in all the wards and every department, I did not manage to develop any long-lasting or trusting relationships that survived the duration of my fieldwork. Once I was invited to the home of one of the female social workers who lived in the hospital staff quarters nearby. I attended the house warming party of one of the occupational therapists and the marriage celebrations of one of the medical doctors that all the hospital staff were invited to and that took place in a hall nearby. But beyond these rare occasions of social inclusion, I remained a loner on the hospital premises. I often felt isolated and alone while navigating the different wards, occupational departments and administrative offices. I was adhering to a strict schedule and detailed research questions that I had written down accurately at home before I entered the field. I never experienced what I was doing in the hospital as an 'immersion'. Rather, it felt like I was continuously busy hunting down the people I wanted to talk to and chasing after bureaucratic papers, files of patients and hospital registers. Gitte Wind frames the constant uncertainty of her role as a researcher in hospitals in The Netherlands and Denmark as a feature created by the field and conceptualizes the process she was engaged in as 'Negotiated Interactive Observation' (2008: 79). Similar to her, I felt uncomfortable not being able to 'really participate' in the activities of my 'informants' and had the impression of failing in becoming 'one of "them"' (ibid.: 87).

During my encounters with medical doctors and psychiatrists, social hierarchies and status differences surfaced and became palpable in very concrete ways. In particular, my interactions with senior psychiatrists brought remarkable challenges with them. The higher their rank and status, the less accessible, approachable and on time they were and the more flexibility and patience was expected from my side when I wanted to meet them. Once I called the head of a psychiatric department in another government hospital in order to get an appointment. Surprisingly, she said that she would have time right now and invited me to see her as soon as possible. Afraid that I would not get another appointment in the near future, I immediately stopped what I was doing and rushed to the hospital. Sarah Pinto aptly describes the particular 'aura' that seems to encompass Indian doctors of high status; they are '. . . a near-mystical being, all but absent, present as though on a whim, but with absolute authority' (Pinto 2014: 81). However, the behaviour of some of the junior medical doctors I experienced as patronizing and dismissive at times. When I entered the doctors' room in order to meet one of the psychiatrists for an interview one day, I was welcomed with pejorative comments regarding my research, and my questions were met with giggling and what appeared to me to be childish behaviour. During the interview, which I was eventually able to carry out, the psychiatrist appreciably resisted being guided by my questions. Instead, he reversed our roles and asked me questions about Germany and how psychiatry works there. This kind of behaviour is perhaps more comprehensible if one considers that psychiatrists and people working in a mental hospital in general have a marginal and stigmatized position in Indian society (Nunley 1992). The doctors' behaviour may be interpreted as a 'kicking down' gesture to put me in my place within the institutional hierarchy, which, as a student and as a social scientist, was definitely below theirs. I often literally had to run after them in order to be able to speak to and interview them. I completed some of my questionnaires[2] while they were seeing patients, which means that I could not record any of the interviews and was only able to scribble down notes.

Similar to interactions with those at the top of the hierarchical ladder, the interactions with those at its bottom had their pitfalls. It was a particular challenge to find a quiet corner to speak to patients. The wards were crowded and staff rooms busy. Therefore, I carried out interviews while sitting under staircases and in the middle of corridors. At times we were interrupted by people rushing in and reclaiming their space such as in the attendants' room. It was not comprehensible for most of the staff anyway why the foreign woman wanted to speak with such people. My concern stemmed from the context that patients occupied at the lowest position within the institutional hierarchy; they were expected to obey the staff's instructions, and usually nobody asked them about their needs, wishes or opinions. I was worried that patients would just agree to speak to me because they thought that they had to or because a staff member had instructed them to do so. As marginal and often resource-lacking settings that are supposed to 'control the out of control', psychiatric institutions are often spaces of violence and negligence (Nagaraja and Murthy 2008; Heckert 2016). This became apparent in various situations during my research. An interview I carried out with a female patient in the occupational therapy department (OTD) together with one of my co-researchers was soon brought to a close when the patient realized that time was running out for her to be able to go and eat lunch on the ward and that if she got to the ward late the attendants would likely beat her. From then on, in order not to put any of the patients at risk, I made sure interviews were commenced long before lunch was served.

In research contexts that concern vulnerable and marginal groups, ethical questions become crucial. Acting ethically in a social system whose rules and morals one is about to study poses a methodological contradiction because 'the anthropologist is frequently forced to make a choice or select a plan of action in an environment of conflict between different customs, principles, and values that normally shape action' (Appell 1978: 3). Additionally, decisions might have to be taken on the basis of limited information and under time pressure. Only after I understood the hierarchical and social structures prevalent at Asha was it possible for me to circumvent situations in which attendants were about to 'pick' a patient in order to be interviewed by me. Methodology chapters of ethnographies of psychiatric settings commonly include the ethical standards and guidelines the authors have set for themselves during their research (Estroff 1985: xvii; Van Dongen 2004: 9f.; Addlakha 2008: 23f.; Pinto 2014: 120). In contrast, occasions on which anthropologists fail to fulfil their ethical demands are rarely reflected on in ethnographic analysis. However, the complex realities that fieldwork takes place in tend to put the anthropologist in a state of what Sylvie Fainzang (2014) denotes as 'ethical dissonance' – where meeting one ethical principle means failing to meet another, which forces 'anthropologists to make choices that are necessarily arbitrary, since they depend on their own ideological, philosophical, or political options' (ibid.: 18). The following anecdote from my fieldwork in the psychiatric department in the private hospital illustrates how ethical practices balance 'deliberately at the point of conjuncture between inevitably-multiple and potentially-dissonant reference frames' (Lederman 2013: 592).

> Shanaya, a young woman in her late twenties with whom I regularly sit down and talk to about her 'alcohol addiction' and other problems, greets me as I enter the ward. Today she opens our conversation with 'They give ECT to everybody here!' I wince because I am not supposed to speak with patients about their ECT treatment. We are standing in the middle of the ward, surrounded by other patients and maushis.[3] I lower my voice to share with her that one of the maushis just showed me a list of four patients who re-

ceived ECT today. Shanaya, who seems not to recognize or at least not to care that the topic makes me feel uncomfortable, turns to one of the maushis and asks her how many of the patients in the ward currently receive ECT. When the maushi doesn't reply to her question, she repeats it with a slight variation: 'How many patients here get "injections"?' The maushi turns to me and asks me reproachfully why I would speak about ECT to patients. I defensively answer that it was Shanaya who brought up the topic. Not paying much attention to the maushi, Shanaya goes on to tell me that she has already received four ECTs and that seven more are left. She is aware that ECT treatment is not disclosed to the patients, and they are simply told that they will 'get an injection'. However, Shanaya knows very well that the injection is part of the ECT treatment – that it puts her to sleep for a short time for the ECT to be carried out – and that if she is asked to go without food in the morning the maushis will be taking her to a room for such treatment. She also shares with me that the Dr has threatened to double the number of ECTs if she doesn't behave well. Shanaya does not like that 'everybody receives ECT'. I feel slightly uncomfortable under the maushi's critical gaze throughout our conversation. I do not know what to reply to Shanaya or which position to take concerning ECT treatment and the obvious 'lying' to patients.

Later that day I meet one of the psychiatrists, Dr Sharma, and ask him why ECT treatment is not discussed openly with patients. He explains to me that ECT is stigmatized and that telling patients would only 'excite' them. However, at the time of discharge they are told about their ECT treatment. So some of the patients who have been admitted to the hospital before or who come to the day care centre are already aware of ECT treatment.

When Shanaya wanted to discuss the issues concerning ECT treatment with me, I experienced ethical dissonance. I felt torn between sincerely responding to Shanaya's needs and queries on the one hand and abiding by the institutional rules and norms on the other. I navigated the situation by faithfully answering her questions as much as I was able to with the maushi listening, but if nobody had overheard our conversation, I would not have respected the institutional rules. I would have followed my own conviction that every person has the right to be informed about what is being administered to their bodies and that there is no justification for deceiving patients to 'protect' them, and I would have discussed this topic openly with Shanaya. I agree with Dilger et al. (2014), who argue that ethical regimes have to acknowledge that social anthropology has to operate within 'epistemological grey zones' and to provide a certain 'flexibility'. Therefore, social anthropology should stress the relevance of a systematic (self)-reflexivity 'with regard to the various positionalities and value systems we adopt and encounter in our anthropological engagements' (ibid.: 8). Furthermore, I tried not to 'neglect to examine the points of view of the "Other of the Other"' (Fainzang 2014: 19). By listening to more than one side – that is, not just the doctors but the patients, caretakers and families – I could outline a proper ontology of apparent 'malpractices' in the psychiatric setting like the so called 'shock therapy' (see Chapter 2). In the private psychiatric institution, patients and their families enjoyed a comparatively high status within the institutional hierarchy compared to Asha. They were treated as 'customers' that had to be convinced of the effectiveness of the psychiatric treatment they were paying for. However, families often expressed doubt concerning the quality of treatment provided. Some of them asked me if I thought that the hospital's treatment options were good and worth their money. In these situations, I tried to provide them with an orientation rather than with an 'opinion'. I mentioned the official position of the hospital concerning ECT treatment, but as well gave them an insight into the situation in Germany, where ECT is mainly used in cases of severe depression where antidepressants have not worked. Carrying out fieldwork in psychiatric settings required me to cultivate a moral self, informed and constructed in relation to my ethnographic field. As a moral person who exists, acts, feels and thinks '*in relation* to others and their ways of being' (Dilger, Huschke and Mattes 2014: 5), I underwent constant changes and transformative learning experiences that at times were emotionally unsettling. Often I wondered if the best fieldworkers are those who can tolerate, acknowledge and live with a certain degree of 'moral ambiguity' that acting in the field inevitably produces (Appell 1978: 3).

Ethical discussions and decision-making are inseparable from 'immediate life circumstances, social roles, political interests, and cultural beliefs' (Brodwin 2013: 14). Further, the ethical can only enter the everyday life if one assumes that everybody experiences 'contemplative moments of moral reflexivity' (Parkin 1985: 5) – a felt 'mismatch between the inherited ideals and what the immediate situation demands' (Brodwin 2013: 17). Becoming conscious of formal values and ethical rules that permeate a person's local world means they may 'seek out alternative values to rethink that world or reorient their action within it' (ibid.). Shanaya's comments on ECT practices – her critical view of 'ECT given to everybody' and of the doctor's behaviour, who tried to discipline her by threatening to 'give the double amount of shocks' – can be understood as an attempt to question formal values and moral practices in the local world of the ward. Ethical practices, in psychiatry as well as in social anthropology, concern the right and wrong, the obligatory and the forbidden and the legitimate use of (professional) power.

Dilger et al. suggest treating the anthropology of ethics or moral values 'jointly with the ethics of *doing* anthropological research' (2014: 4). Therefore, the ethical and moral values of all persons involved in research, including those of our interlocutors in the field, can be scrutinized and be the subject of a critical analysis. Psychiatric practice traditionally revolves around 'the twin imperatives of care and custody' (Brodwin and Velpry 2014: 524). Those two do not constitute a polarity. Rather, they exist as a continuum. Part of this is building up a 'professional persona' (ibid.: 525) that allows one to push back against people's opposition to forced 'treatment' measures. For many who work at the clinical frontline, to apply certain practices of constraint becomes legitimated by the argument that these measures enable them to take care of patients. In the narrative that opens this chapter, the son reasons that the admission of his mother to Asha is necessary in order to secure her care, which he is only capable of managing if his mother starts to take her medication again. Similarly, the helper patient justified the violence against the newly admitted patient as self-defence, labelling it as a kind of self-care. Attendants' first priority was to remain safe themselves, also to be able to further carry out their care-taking role. Attendants understood themselves as an important, if not the most important, moral force in the wards that carried the responsibility of recivilizing patients.

Ethical concerns in everyday interactions may be expressed by words, silence and body language as well as via emotional outbursts (Brodwin 2013: 11). However, even if, for example, Shanaya uttered valid ethical concerns, her voice was not powerful enough to change the moral world within the organizational structures. In rigidly and hierarchically organized institutions, certain ethical voices are prone to being ignored as irrelevant. They therefore do not contribute to ethical discourses or initiate a reorientation of social actions or ethical rules. I overheard a patient who had just been admitted to Asha loudly shouting from his locked isolation cell: 'What gives you the right to lock us up like animals?' This question of course was not taken up as a valid moral claim but dismissed as 'mad speech' and therefore ignored by the people who heard this exclamation. Interestingly, the critical questions and comments from me, the social anthropologist, were occasionally similarly dismissed as 'mad' since they were coming from an 'ignorant foreigner' (see Chapter 7). Additionally, at times I was perceived as a member of a strange, unintelligible and occasionally barbaric moral system. One of the ward nurses, who assumed that I was American, asked me: 'You just shoot incurable patients in America, don't you?'

The Patientized Anthropologist: Using Emotional Reflexivity as Methodological Tool

Emotions[4] and other sensorial experiences 'form part of the anthropological method' (Spencer 2010: 10; see also Pink 2009; Lorimer 2010). By reflecting on their embodied emotions, researchers can 'develop an understanding, a sense of the people and the field and learn through them' (Spencer 2010: 16). George Devereux (1998) stated that the researcher and the researched continuously evoke emotional and psychological reactions in each other that are not adequately taken into account by the positivist scientific tradition. Additionally, Devereux problematized positivist social scientific methods and tried to enhance them using psychoanalytic tools. Michael Jackson (2010) took up Devereux's stimulating thoughts in his work and realized that 'insights that turn out to be *personally* useful may also illuminate the *transpersonal* and *interpersonal* life-worlds that one is seeking to understand' (ibid.: 36).

While conducting fieldwork at Asha, I regularly noted down what emotionally touched me or upset me, and my notes were often rather depressing and gloomy. Doing participant observation at Asha exhausted me and was emotionally draining. I had to regularly force myself to get up in the morning and to interact with staff and patients. I cannot remember even one day that I looked forward to going to the hospital. At best I felt indifferent and just strong enough to endure the day. Some days, I just stayed at home. Only after some time did I begin to ask myself why my field so severely drained me. It appeared to me that the institution 'patientized' me – like it did to everybody else who entered its gates. Erving Goffman (1968) was the first to show how a 'total institution's' social structure fundamentally transforms the patient's self, everyday schedule and posture. Psychiatric hospitals 'act' upon people, rendering them 'patients'. I suffered a lack of social contact in my field. I despised the hierarchical structures I was pushed into. I felt upset by the sometimes arrogant behaviour of doctors and psychiatrists towards me. I hated to be made to wait all the time – once the head of the psychiatric department in the private hospital made me wait for three hours. Sometimes, I was not even sure what I was actually waiting for. I felt almost swallowed up by the institutional structures I disdained. I observed patients becoming 'non-persons' the moment they were admitted to the institution, detached from their social surroundings and relationships. Many patients and families seemed to display a lethargy and passiveness similar to mine. The institution and its hierarchical and bureaucratic structures had deprived us of most of our choices and the integrity that makes it possible to perceive oneself as a complete person – it had 'depersonalized' us (Rosenhan 1973: 256f.).

Dimitrina Spencer (2010: 2) argues that emotional reflexivity is an important part of the social anthropologist's methodological palette because it allows a deeper understanding of one's involvement in the field. Social anthropological analysis necessarily implies a process of abstraction and systematic reflection during which experience is detached from its pure subjective meaning and put into a broader scientific context (Okely 1996). Andrew Beatty (2010), calling for a 'verisimilar' representation of emotions in ethnographies, argues that only a narrative approach can capture an emotion's particularity and temporal dimension. A systematic reflection and contextualization enables social anthropologists to identify the social expectations and cultural value systems a subjectively experienced emotion may refer to and in this way to access an emotion's sociocultural meaning. Ethnopsychoanalysis provides such a systematic approach to analyse the social anthropologist's emotional reactions and relationships in the field. It describes the process of accepting, reacting and acting according to an expectation or role assigned to us in the field by the concept 'countertransference'. Originally, the psychoanalytic term designated the analyst's emotional reactions towards their patient. By paying attention to their own emotions and an 'activity of self-interpretation' (Braddock 2010: 221), the analyst tries to grasp the patient's life and experiential world in the therapeutic process. Ethnopsychoanalysis adopted the concept 'countertransference' and the hermeneutic approach to analyse ethnographic encounters between the field researcher and their informants: 'What that emotional understanding equips the field worker with is a principled basis for seeing how things are for the other from their point of view and what it is that they may unconsciously . . . be communicating, through behaviours and actions which elicit emotion' (ibid.). People in the field transfer their fears, wishes and expectations onto the social anthropologist, who at times complies with those in order to build their field identity around them. In other cases the field researcher may also reject them, which may disrupt field relationships or causing them to fade away (Rhodes 1986: 210). Dealing with the emotions that are elicited by interactions in the field and identifying and negotiating people's expectations of me was not always an easy task. Many of the hopes people pinned on me were related to my skin colour, profession, nationality and/or gender. Some psychiatrists and doctors showed interest in me because they hoped having a contact abroad would advance their own or a relative's career. A medical officer invited me over for lunch in order to introduce me to her son, who wanted to study in Germany. From then onwards, he called me regularly in order to practise his German, which he learned via a tuition course. Some of the social workers at Asha sought to gain my sympathy for their marginalized position in the hospital and maybe hoped that I would join their coalition to oppose the medical staff. When I started to spend less and less time with them, a senior social worker asked me reproachfully 'Why do you avoid us?' Patients, when seeing me enter their ward, often addressed me directly ('Madam! Madam!') and asked me all kinds of favours from calling their relatives or getting them 'out of here' to paying for their operations. Such hopes and demands often left me feeling overwhelmed and uncomfortable.

Francine Lorimer understands countertransference as a 'feeling mode of knowing' that enables the social anthropologist to reflect on feelings and visit different self-experiences without adopting them for oneself (Lorimer 2010: 105). Reflecting on the diverging positions and experiences of the people I encountered in Asha helped me to understand relationship modes and categories, to recognize the diverse expectations people had concerning these relationships, to grasp the image people had of me and to negotiate my way through certain situations. To regularly engage in reflection and self-reflexivity while doing ethnographic fieldwork not only assisted me in participating in the psychiatric setting by embodying the diverse roles the field allotted to me, but additionally enabled me to remain mentally healthy, open-minded and receptive (Lorimer 2010: 103; see also Linska 2015; Strauss 2015). The different dimensions that self-reflexivity in the field concerns – the establishment of meaningful relationships, knowledge production and self-care – can be exemplified by my relationship to two middle-aged, married men who apparently developed romantic feelings for me. Both started to behave possessively sometime after we met for the first time. They wanted to spend more time with me, bought me gifts, wanted to go out for drinks or snacks and became jealous when I spent time with others. Both never openly confessed their feelings – I only deduced these from how they behaved with me. In one case, people started to gossip and comment about our relationship, which made me feel particularly uncomfortable and irritated me, because I still perceived the relationship as being formal. Furthermore, in both cases, I was dependent on the men and a good and functional relationship with them was necessary to be able to carry on with my fieldwork hassle-free. I was quite indecisive with regard to how to deal with these situations or how to address my uneasiness. Subtle signals from my side that were supposed to indicate that I was not interested in any kind of romantic involvement were either not recognized or ignored. In both cases, after the men had tried my patience and become more and more intrusive, I followed the advice of two friends and brought the wife of one of the men into the picture. In the other case, my co-researcher helped me to write a text message that was not too harsh but clearly communicated that I was not interested in anything else than doing my work at the hospital. Despite trying to solve the issues without creating major havoc, both men felt severely aggrieved by being rejected and stopped talking to me after this incident which caused me to lose two very helpful field contacts. I realized that my feelings, wishes and needs had not mattered much in these connections. Both men had seen me as an available woman to have a romantic/sexual relationship with. Our encounters were deeply informed by sociocultural and gendered norms and values that determine how and by whom romantic relationships should be initiated and processed. A fundamental mismatch of expectations, imaginations and how the respective other person actually felt was what finally caused the inevitable disruption. Eventually, discussing the issues and subsequently developing counter-strategies to shape the relationships according to my wishes helped me balance my well-being and gain a deeper, empathic insight into gender relationships and roles (Nadig et al. 2009).

At the beginning of my fieldwork, I was the well-adjusted anthropologist who patiently tried to understand everything around her through observation and empathizing – even the things that provoked strong adverse reactions. However, keeping this up became more difficult the longer my fieldwork lasted. It was only when I wrote down my fieldnotes, or during drinking sessions with Akash, who could relate well to my unsettling experiences based on the internship he had completed at Asha as a social work student (see Introduction), that I allowed my emotions to surface uncensored. The following extract from my fieldnotes exemplifies my at times strong emotional reactions towards the hospital environment and its people:

> On my way to the male unit with Dr Kulkarni, a huge car pulls up beside us. The husband of the clerk from the administration office jumps out and starts shouting at Dr Kulkarni. His wife, the clerk, then also gets out of the car. I had brought her sweets from Germany four weeks before; I had wanted to thank her for helping me collect hospital statistics. Her face had brightened up the moment she recognized the gift in my hands. She felt acknowledged and important in her institutional role. Her appearance now could not be more contrastive: tears in her eyes, and she is standing behind her husband. The latter is at pains to defend his wife's honour and reputation: 'How could you say that in front of everybody? That is not fair,' he accuses Dr Kulkarni. 'This is very bad.' I soon understand that he must be referring to a situation during the staff meeting this morning, when Dr Kulkarni was addressing inefficiencies and morally corrupt practices in the hospital administration. 'How can you accuse my wife of taking *bakshīs* (extra tips)?' Dr Kulkarni asks him to calm down and insists that her aim is to 'change the system' and that 'nobody was attacked personally'. The husband screams at the psychiatrist for a few more minutes before finally taking a seat back in his car along with his wife, and they leave the hospital premises. We continue our walk to the male ward, and Dr Kulkarni comments: 'She [the clerk] is not in control of her emotions. In contrast, I managed to keep a cool mind.'

When putting down notes[5] about the situation later that day, I also recapitulated feelings, thoughts and images the scene had evoked:

> The clerk standing in front of us reminds me of a big, sad hippo. I don't feel any compassion for her. And furthermore, I despise her for letting the husband

> settle the matter for her . . . He isn't inquiring about what exactly happened but just raising accusations. It is clearly not about what happened but about defending the reputation of his wife. The husband is as equally big as her, and so is the family car. A fat, sad and discriminated hippo family. Behind this wall, patients die of untreated coughs and bloody diarrhoea,[6] but that doesn't seem to upset them at all. It is not about understanding and good cooperation/togetherness. Everything is only about one's own fat ass.

Only rarely did my thoughts become as contemptuous, judgemental and accusatory as in the case above. Mostly, my feelings could be understood as an expression of helplessness and powerlessness evoked by the dilemma of witnessing (Behar 1997). When we are confronted with pain and misery in the field, we suddenly also realize and are exposed to our own vulnerability. For me, the clerk and her husband's seemingly indifferent attitude towards the suffering that happened in the hospital, as well as the egocentric behaviour of some of the staff members and the unsuccessful efforts of single protagonists to change a faulty system were excruciating. From my point of view, the scene with the clerk was reflective of two types of people I had observed at Asha. On the one hand, Dr Kulkarni represented those who were selfless and genuinely concerned about the patients, thinking beyond personal gain and working hard to improve the conditions in the hospital. On the other hand, the clerk and her husband represented those who were self-serving, perceiving their government job primarily as a safe source of income and concerned only with status, self-enrichment and self-promotion. The behaviour of the latter evoked anger in me. My rage, revulsion and despair may be interpreted as 'ethical emotions' (Brodwin 2013: 83). Emotions may serve as an engine to realize one's own ethical vision and therefore can play a central role in 'ethical decision-making' (Callahan 1988). Activism or engaged anthropology actively makes use of the transformative powers of such ethical emotions: 'The powerful emotions that arise in the processes of acknowledgement and advocacy – often negative and disabling emotions of guilt and powerlessness – can be productively transformed through this move to doing something concrete in the world' (Smith and Kleinman 2010: 185). In my situation though, I was not able to realize any ethical visions and transform my emotions into concrete actions. I had to remain in the witnessing and understanding position to be able to complete my fieldwork at the institution. This meant my rage against the clerk and her husband transformed into abhorrence, resentment and antagonism, as in my imagination they represented those who I held responsible for the suffering taking place behind the hospital walls. That activism can 'serve as a catalyst' (Huschke 2014: 63) is something I only experienced towards the end of my research at Asha, when I dared to challenge institutional structures and speak for one of the patients (see Chapter 7). Going against the informal rules of good conduct and rebelling against the hierarchical structures in the institution raised suspicion and effectively disqualified me as an acceptable and harmless fellow in the eyes of some of the staff members, though.

However, as social anthropologists, we are no ethicists most of the time. Instead, our aim is markedly different from that of an ethicist's – namely, to withhold judgement and to try to understand the social mechanisms prevalent in the field site (Fainzang 2014: 16). In fact, one of a social anthropologist's main tasks is to empathize with those we are not able to emotionally sympathize or connect with and to understand their reasons and actions, even if they are alien to us. Therefore, as Sylvie Fainzang argues, we either engage in 'moral' or in 'methodological empathy' in the field. I may not morally sympathize with but am able to methodologically empathize with being self-centred, like the clerk and her husband. I can therefore understand that focusing exclusively on one's own family can be a valid and reasonable strategy in an environment that vividly illustrates that those who have lost the support of their families are ripped apart: ego- and ethnocentrism appears as a legitimate moral strategy from a pragmatic point of view. Acting within this moral world is driven by emotions such as the fear of impoverishment.

When Dr Kulkarni dared to criticise the moral behaviour of the hospital staff during the morning meeting she threatened the reputation of the clerk, an important pillar in her moral system and personhood, and therefore was confronted with strong emotional reactions. Dr Kulkarni labelled the clerk's and her husband's performance as an 'over'-reaction that lacked 'emotional control' and indicated 'mental illness'. By contrasting their uncontrolled state with her own 'cool mind', she represented their matter as an irrational one instead of empathizing with the clerk's moral life world, which also prohibited an ethical discussion about corruptive practices.

The Biased Anthropologist: Positionalities and the Co-creation of Knowledge

I grew up in a small village in Germany. My parents migrated from a nearby urban area to the countryside in order to start a family after they had finished their education. We were no locals and additionally a family with a higher educational background, which was rather unusual in this region. I was one of the few children in the village who had several bookshelves in their home, which my younger brother and I explored with much curiosity. When I attended school, I was the only child that was nondenominational in a majority protestant region. My parents grew up in a catholic city but later identified as atheists and were rather critical of religious institutions. My family never really immersed themselves in village life; it was and is still a place that is traditional in its social interactions, and communal festive events take place throughout the year. Therefore, we lived rather secluded from other families and the extended social networks that mark village life. From early childhood onwards, my family background and my rather introverted personality type put me – often deliberately – into the position of a 'participant observer' who tried to fit in but often failed to succeed in that. Now, years later, I feel that these early life experiences forged and continue to forge my self-understanding and my identity as a social anthropologist.

Anyway, even if I am somehow used to not fitting in since my childhood, I never experienced myself as an emotionally distanced 'lonely hero' in the field. Participant observation always comprises an 'embodied relational process' mediated by emotions, which at times can be described as 'a relational observation or relational reflection' (Spencer 2010: 2). Further, I did not do the emotional and reflectional work that fieldwork necessarily entails alone. I was accompanied by several people whom I like to call 'co-researchers' because they helped me to move through my field safely and contributed their views and thoughts. Additionally, they at times supported me emotionally. For a long time in the history of social anthropology, these kinds of people have not turned up in ethnographies and have had the role of 'ghost-workers' (Turner 2010). Nevertheless, they have always been part of the knowledge production process, and it is clear that the co-researcher's effect on the field and its people is no different from the anthropologist's effect. Therefore, Sarah Turner suggests that social anthropologists 'need to stop ignoring the positionality and subjectivity of research assistants/ interpreters in social science qualitative fieldwork, as these factors influence numerous relationships, negotiations and differential access to interviewees and resources' (ibid.: 216). In the following, I introduce my main co-researchers who accompanied me on my fieldwork at the hospital. I have included them throughout the ethnography and provided reflections on our role and positionalities in various (interview) situations. Learning during fieldwork means encountering and engaging with different ways of knowing, being and doing. That is why doing fieldwork presents constant challenges to the anthropologist's self and changes it (Spencer 2011). John L. Wengle (1987) interpreted this process as a symbolic 'death' and 'rebirth'. Spencer (2011: 70) refers to it as 'transformative learning', borrowing the term from educational research (Taylor 1998). Transformative learning may include 'Key Emotional Episodes' (KEE), which denotes the high emotional and physical involvement of the researcher, who 'has lost control and is subordinated to the flow of events' (Berger 2010: 120). KEEs can provide valuable social anthropological insights, if the researcher's emotions are as such not taken as providing an explanation of cultural phenomena, and they may help the ethnographer to empathize and sympathize with his research participants. When I spent time together in the field with my co-researchers, it became clear that I was not the only one who was undergoing a transformative learning process. Nevertheless, it has to be acknowledged that their motivations for accompanying me to the hospital and the perceived outcomes of this particular shared experience differed and that they also differed from mine.

Rini Fernandes accompanied me during my fieldwork in the female unit of Asha. She helped me carry out most of the interviews, which were conducted in Marathi or Hindi, and transcribed and translated all of them into English. To this day we share an emotional friendship connection and understanding. The openness and intimacy of our relationship enabled us to exercise together emotional reflexivity concerning our reactions to situations and persons in the field. We usually reflected on our experiences while having lunch in the nearby shopping mall after having spent the whole morning in the hospital. I was introduced to Rini by a common friend on the campus of the Tata Institute of Social Sciences (TISS), where she had recently completed her MA in Habitat Policy and Practice. She lived with her parents and sister in a middle-class neighbourhood in one of Mumbai's rambling suburbs. Once I wondered why Rini apparently 'changed' her denomination depending on the people we encountered in the hospital. Rini explained to me that her parents had had an interreligious marriage, so she identified as either Hindu or Christian depending on the perceived community category she was interacting with in the field. When we met in August 2011, Rini was about to leave for Lund in Sweden, where she planned to pursue another Master's degree in Gender Studies. Similar to most inhabitants of Mumbai, Rini had never seen one of the asylum-like hospitals from the inside. The more Rini and I visited Asha together the more familiar, oriented and self-confident she was in moving around the wards and interacting with staff and patients. Nevertheless, her insecurities and uncomfortableness in the beginning reminded me of how I had felt myself when first confronted with Asha and its daily routines and, at times, its freakishness. When Rini accompanied me to the hospital the first time, she was curious and excited. We undertook a round of the female wards. In the housekeeping chamber, we encountered a woman who was very busy rearranging plates on a shelf. She was mumbling to herself and said that she must have put these plates on the shelf around three hundred times already. She added that whoever was admitted to Asha would never leave the hospital again. Finally, she pointed to her tummy, looked at us and said that there had been a baby inside until it was cut out by the doctors. When she made a move to lift her frock, Rini winced: 'Oh my god, she is going to show it!'

The woman nevertheless went on to lift her patient uniform and a few moments later was in front of us completely naked. This made Rini feel uncomfortable; she did not really know what to look at and mumbled repeatedly 'Oh god!' and then started to move back and forth nervously. Later, while we were having lunch, she admitted: 'This was my first time [among people with mental health issues] and it was a little shocking for me.' Additionally, it was also the first time she had seen anyone naked in public. By reflecting on her emotional response, we were reminded of the twofold otherness of the place: it was alien to me, the German social anthropologist, but also to her, the native Mumbaikar. After fieldwork, Rini engaged in critical discussions of the manuscript that would be this book with me. It is due to her and a critical reviewer that I took up the question once again of how to adequately represent my co-researchers and the emotional and interpretative labour we accomplished together.

Three different co-researchers assisted me over the course of my fieldwork in Asha's male unit. With all I had a good and cordial connection, but we did not engage in collaborative emotional reflexivity as I did regularly with Rini. At the beginning, a student from TISS who was pursing his Master of Social Work and had already completed an academic education to become a medical doctor joined me to speak with male patients. He planned to write his Master's thesis about 'medical malpractices' and hence had a professional interest in accompanying me. But it quite soon became clear that he was too busy with other obligations to accompany me more regularly. Therefore, Dhaval Joshi replaced him. Dhaval was pursing his Ph.D. in Habitat Studies at TISS, but soon after we started working together he was hired for a job and hence was also not able to accompany me any longer. He introduced me to one of his friends: Akshay Bapat. Akshay is a filmmaker who, at that time, was staying with his natal family in a district in north Mumbai, adjacent to the one Asha was located in. To this day we are in regular contact and met up several times after my fieldwork had come to an end. Right from the beginning, he was inspired by the theme of mental illnesses. After we had started to work together at Asha, he regularly told me about the conversations that came up in his family about his new occupation. For a middle-/upper-class family, Asha was definitely one of the last options they would turn to if somebody in the family was affected by mental health problems; Akshay's relatives imagined Asha as a jail, and it was a familiar point of reference in colloquial jokes and phrases: 'You are crazy. Be careful, otherwise we will send you to Asha!' Akshay shared his vision of making a movie about mental illnesses with me. Indeed, in 2014 he finished shooting a documentary about the NGO where I carried out my research as a Master's student (Strauss 2011). Akshay hails from an upper-class Brahmin family, and it was difficult, if not almost impossible for him, to hide his social background during interactions with patients and hospital staff. When Akshay and I conducted interviews, patients used to ask him for his surname and would identify him as a Maharashtrian Brahmin. But his accent was also a giveaway. S.K. Ratnam, an educated Tamil Brahmin and one of the long-term patients staying in Asha (see Chapter 3), commented during an interview: 'I thought that you may belong to the same caste, because of the way you speak.'

There are several insights I would not have gained from the field without discussions and interactions with my co-researchers. Nevertheless, we did not co-author this book, which was written from my perspective on the situations we experienced together. Therefore, their views and stories about Asha and the people we encountered differ from mine - probably considerably.

Notes

1. A typical female dress; it is a long piece of cloth wrapped in a particular way round the body.
2. I prepared separate questionnaires for each kind of staff at the hospital. This kind of approach was more accepted and appreciated as research work, in particular by the medical staff, than, for example, just 'hanging out' and having random conversations.
3. The ward attendants were called *maushī* (maternal aunt) in the private hospital.
4. For a more detailed discussion of the transdisciplinary concept of 'emotion', see Strauss (2019).
5. Fieldnotes that were rather emotional I usually wrote in my native language, German.
6. Here I refer to an incident that occurred on the same day, which I describe and contextualize in more detail in Chapter 6.

CHAPTER 2

EVERYDAY ROUTINES, LIFE AND SOLICITUDES AT ASHA

The day at the hospital starts around 6.00 AM. Tea is served to the patients in the wards. Subsequently, at 8.30 AM, breakfast consisting of bread, milk and pulses is provided. The nurse in charge starts her shift at 7.30 AM and completes a round of her wards, keeping an eye on the cleanliness as well as the food and water supply. From 9.00 AM onwards, the medical officers, psychiatrists and social workers enter the wards. They do not undertake 'ward rounds' in the actual sense but rather gather round a table in the examination room soon after entering the unit. They then take a look at the patients' files, which the nurses have prepared, and listen to reports about the behaviour and symptoms of the patients. The names of patients who have to be examined by the psychiatrists or medical doctors are called out loudly, and they are subsequently presented to the doctor by one of the attendants. Psychiatrists and medical officers usually do not enter the dorm rooms where the patients stay. Their daily ward rounds end at 1.00 PM, shortly before lunch is served. A meal comprises *capātī* (flatbread), rice, *dāl* (a lentil dish) and a vegetable curry. After eating, most of the patients take a nap. At around 4.00 PM, tea is served. Doctors, occupational therapists and social workers have left the hospital already by this time. Before dinner time at around 7.00 PM, ward routines and chores are taken care of. Some of the patients support the attendants and nurses in completing their tasks. Patients would either chat with each other, chat with the attendants or take another nap before dinner is served. The dinner consists of the same dishes as lunch. Non-vegetarian food is served twice a week: eggs[1] on Wednesdays and boneless chicken on Fridays. On holidays, patients additionally are served sweets as a special treat.

The staff quarters are located adjacent to the hospital. But only some of the hospital staff reside here. Most of the employees commute to the hospital on a daily basis, either by foot, autorickshaw, local train or, in the case of doctors and psychiatrists, with their own car and a private driver. The social workers' office of nine psychiatric social workers is located near the main entrance in the male unit. I spent much time in this office room, particularly at the beginning of my research. I accompanied the social workers on their ward rounds and subsequently had lunch with them. Social workers are supposed to prepare patients and their families for rehabilitation. They are supposed to stay in contact with the patients' families after an admission and inform and counsel them regarding the treatment of a family member's illness. However, the latter task bears several challenges and obstacles, as I discuss in Chapter 4 and further elaborate on in Chapter 5.

Six psychiatrists and nineteen medical officers, including one anaesthetist for the ECT treatment and three gynaecologists, are employed at Asha. Each medical officer and psychiatrist respectively is responsible for up to six wards (one section), which can comprise up to three hundred patients. Additionally, doctors have to cover regular shifts in the OP and ECT department. Officially, their duty ends at 4.30 PM, but some of them can be regularly observed leaving the hospital premises earlier in the afternoon. Over half of the psychiatrists and medical officers are female. This portion is remarkable given the fact that female doctors and psychiatrists constitute a minority among medical professionals in general. The work hours at the hospital prove convenient for those who also have to take care of a family and household chores and at the same time do not want to pursue a committed full-time career. The majority of the psychiatrists and medical officers stem from families in which it is very common to hold a doctorate of medicine. They additionally run a private clinic that opens in the late afternoon.

One matron and two assistant matrons supervise fifteen psychiatric nurses. One psychiatric nurse and one sister is in charge of one section (three sections in the male unit and two sections in the female unit, with each section comprising four to six wards). Nurses in charge have to keep a number of records and registers ('medicine book', 'supply book', 'ECT book') and make sure that everything needed in a ward is in stock; for example, medicine, soap and sheets. Nine out of the twenty-four positions for psychiatric nurses were vacant at the time. A nurse stated that many psychiatric nurses are 'on the waiting list', implying that they would not get a position unless they paid the necessary 'fees' (bribe) to the respective people in the government administration. Besides the psychiatric nurses, eighteen general and ninety staff nurses work in the hospital. Out of these, only five are male nurses.

On one occasion, I asked the nurse matron if she could explain the organizational and staff structure of the hospital to me. She drew it on a piece of paper and then further elaborated on the left portion of the sketch (see Figure 2.1). In her drawing, the matron indicated the importance of the organizational structure of the hospital and its division into different departments. Anti-clockwise in the drawing: 'Day Care', 'ECT' (male/female with an anaesthetist, sister in charge, psychiatric nurse), 'laboratory' (male/female with technician and assistant), 'Occupational Therapy Department' (OTD), 'Outpatient Department' (OPD), the offices of 'social workers', 'medical officers', 'attendants' and 'matron' (located in the female unit), 'administration/clerk department', 'kitchen group' (cook (m/f), dietitian (f)), 'pharmacy department', 'linen department' (linen keeper) and 'tailoring department' (m/f). Furthermore, the matron stressed a more or less twofold structure regarding the staff hierarchy, with the 'medical superintendent' (Head of Department (HOD)) at its top who supervises 'medical persons' and 'nursing staff' respectively. Interestingly, she only added 'occupational therapists', 'social workers' and the 'clinical psychologist' to the drawing after I asked for their particular position in the organizational structure (see the somewhat curvy arrows in the middle of the drawing that she added after she had already drawn everything else). The matron's drawing resembles an organigram that was included in the hospital report; it indicates the different staff positions in the hospital (see Figure 2.2).

The diagram displays the medical superintendent at the top of the staff hierarchy. Additionally, four other important staff positions occupy positions of authority: the deputy superintendent, the class I[2] psychiatrist, the matron/assistant matron and the administrative officer. Occupational therapists, social workers,

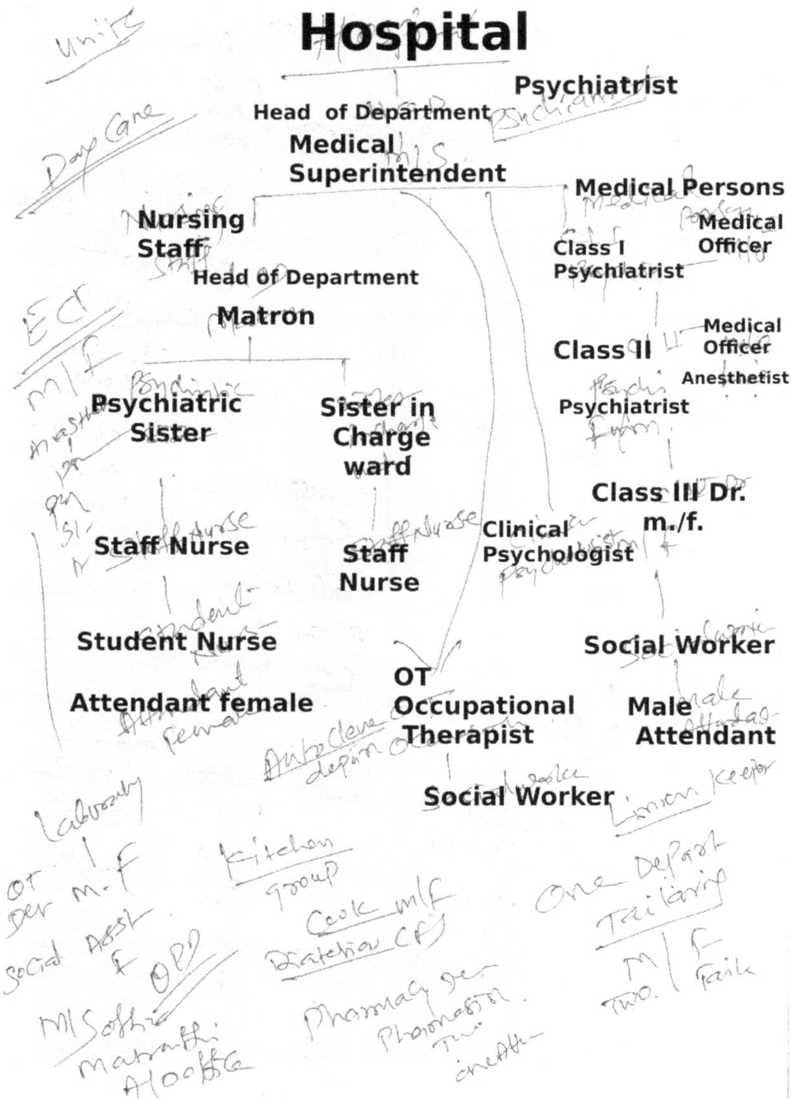

Figure 2.1. The matron's drawing of the hospital's organizational structure.

male attendants and male sweepers are considered subordinates of the deputy superintendent, while nurses, female attendants and female sweepers are subordinates of the matron. According to the organigram, medical officers are supposed to be on the same hierarchical level with social workers and occupational therapists. However, this hierarchy is not reflected in everyday

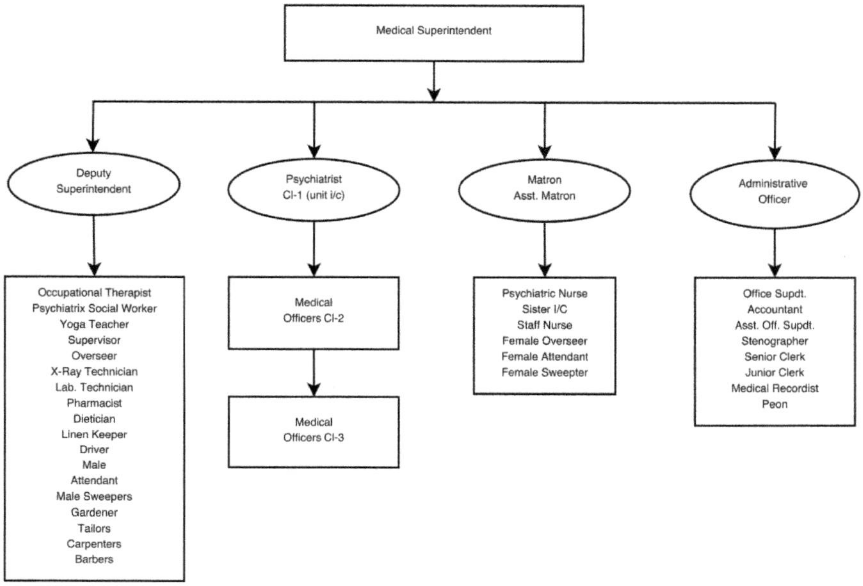

Figure 2.2. Hospital organigram. Generated by the author, based on a diagram included in the hospital report 2011.

interactions, and the matron's drawing depicts this fact more accurately, particularly when we consider the sequence in which she drew it (adding the clinical psychologist, occupational therapists and social workers only after I asked about them). Clearly, the drawing underscores the subordinate position of the staff concerned with rather social and 'soft' aspects of treatment – occupational therapy, psychology or social work – which are perceived as 'inferior' compared to the areas of operation of the medical staff that are associated with the natural sciences and medical facts. Occupational therapists and social workers perceived a contradiction between the official position that they hold and the degradations they experienced in everyday life. This constituted a latent conflict line among the hospital staff. However, even the social workers themselves often perceived allopathic treatment – psychotropic drugs and ECT – as superior to psycho-social interventions in treating mental illnesses. One of the social workers commented on the position for a clinical psychologist that had been vacant for eight years at that time: 'For what patients here need a *psychologist*? These are *psychiatric* patients.'

The staff hierarchy became physically palpable in the seating arrangements and work practices found in the units' examination rooms, in which doctors, social workers and occupational therapists used to write file entries, take case histories or carry out medical examinations. Psychiatrists and medical officers usually sit on sturdy wooden armchairs, while social workers, occupational therapists and students have to put up with one of the less comfortable plastic chairs. In fact, I never witnessed any of the psychiatrists or medical officers sit on one of the plastic chairs. Furthermore, if a social worker or occupational therapist sat on one of the wooden chairs – of which one or two at most were provided for each examination room – and a psychiatrist or medical officer entered, they would immediately give it up to allow them to sit on it. A student of social work reported a situation where a psychiatrist entering the examination room told her – mid consultation with a patient – to get up so she could have her chair. In contrast, patients would sit on stools when doctors or the social worker examined or interviewed them, and they used to sit on blankets spread on the floor while waiting for their turn to be seen. I once inquired about the reason behind patients having to sit on stools and being prohibited from even using the plastic chairs. The attendants and nurses explained to me that many female patients are not able to take care of their hygiene when menstruating, so they were prone to 'spoiling' the chairs when sitting on them. That this practice is also an indicator of social hierarchies is clearly demonstrated when looking at male patients. On one occasion, I invited a male patient to sit on a plastic chair, but upon observing this, a staff member immediately brought a stool for him and directed him to sit on that instead.

The Female Wards

The female wards are only reachable via an additional gate that is guarded by two to three female attendants at the back of the hospital. Families and male hospital staff, excluding medical officers and psychiatrists, are not allowed to enter. Those who enter the female unit have to write down their name in a logbook. When I would enter the female unit, I was sometimes greeted by Rajashree, a woman in her early forties. My appearance once inspired her to start singing a Bollywood song with slightly altered lyrics: 'White girl, white girl, please also visit my ward some time.' Rajashree Milind Adulkar was admitted to the hospital in 2000. Even though her brother visited her regularly and discharged her once for two months in 2008, the hospital had remained her permanent home. She shared this fate with a number of other women. Many of them stayed in one of the 'chronic wards'. The chronic wards accommodate women who either suffer from severe mental illnesses, or whose families cannot or do not want to take them back home. When I entered one of these wards one day together with Rini, a matron was doing her ward inspection round, checking its cleanliness. One nurse, who had been employed in other governmental hospitals before, shared with me that psychiatric hospitals can generally be considered the cleanest: blood and open wounds are rare, and patients clean the wards as occupational therapy. '90 per cent are housewives in the female wards', she explained to me, 'cleaning is in the woman's nature!' Rini had been observing the inspection round of the matron and whispered in my direction: 'Oh my god! It is that hierarchical!', noting how nurses and attendants attentively watched, ready to fulfil any of the matron's demands. During the weeks that Rini and I spent together in the diverse wards of the female unit, we learnt about the social structure and hierarchies that determined the everyday interactions between staff and patients. Even if the attendants were officially organizationally subordinate to the nurses, they obviously had a rather strong position in the everyday life of the ward, and nurses rarely dared to talk back to them: they were in charge of most of the ward chores, provided patients with food and looked after their hygiene and general health condition. There are certain differentiations and hierarchical gradations between the 'attendant' and 'sweeper' category. Sweepers mainly work outside the hospital, where they clean and maintain the premises and take care of the gardening work. While the attendants uniformly wear a white sari with a blue border clearly marking them as civil servants, sweepers usually wear any sari colour. While attendants, as government employees, earn between ten to twenty thousand rupees (depending on their status and length of employment), sweepers, who are hired on contract, earn less than 50 per cent of this salary – between four to five thousand rupees. Additionally, they do not receive any of the allowances government employees are entitled to. An attendant's post comes with certain privileges connected to its civil servant status. For example, if an attendant dies, their spouse can claim the post before somebody else is hired. However, holding a government job also means that one may be transferred to another government hospital at relatively short notice. To be eligible for a government job at Asha, a person has to be a resident of Maharashtra and fluent in Hindi as well as Marathi. The latter criterion disqualifies most of the migrant workers, who come to Mumbai from other states, from applying for an attendant's position, and therefore the posts of sweepers are often occupied by non-Maharashtrians.

Attendants' posts are staffed in compliance with the state's reservation policies. Therefore, a certain percentage of the posts are reserved for people from the so called scheduled or backward casts (SCs or BCs). Rumour has it that attendants from the SCs and BCs tend to be sent to the dirtier wards with a higher work load; for example, to an admission ward, which accommodates patients who have been recently admitted and are more symptomatic and rather difficult to handle. Inside the wards, another status differentiation concerns junior and senior attendants. Senior attendants do not have to work night shifts as often as junior attendants. They prefer to work the convenient shifts at the gate that involve tracking whoever enters and leaves the unit. Senior attendants commonly act as overseers, who, for example, sit on a centrally positioned chair inside a ward to watch over the junior attendants' work. These are often tasks that are perceived as inferior or 'unclean' and include duties such as delousing patients' hair when they are about to be transferred to another ward. A patient who has not undergone an extensive delousing session, which involves having her hair combed with a lice comb, will not be accepted by another ward's attendants. In the female unit, a ward's reputation is based on its state of cleanliness and the quality of housekeeping as well as the hygiene of the patients belonging to it.

Attendants at times had a key influence on the psychiatric treatment of patients. They are present in the wards twenty-four hours a day[3] and report to the psychiatrist during their morning rounds if a certain patient behaved 'excitedly' or 'violently' during the night. Often, a psychiatrist would prescribe ECT treatment without much hesitation for a patient classified as 'very excited' by one of the attendants. Attendants, besides the nurses, interact the most with the patients and were therefore considered the most knowledgeable when it came to the estimation of a patient's behaviour or condition. Accordingly, they also considered themselves as an important, if not sometimes the most important, component in the process of normalizing patients' 'mad' and uncivilized behaviour. As one of the attendants expressed, 'Nurses only give medicine!' Common tools to regulate and control patients' behaviour are reprehension and corporal punishment. Attendants are known for their rather practical and straightforward manner when managing everyday issues in the wards. Often, their demeanour appeared rather rough and dominant, particularly when interacting with patients. A psychiatric nurse told us about a situation when an attendant loudly scolded a patient because she would not remove her bed sheet for the laundry. The nurse interfered and asked the woman what the problem was; she explained it was her fasting day and therefore she could not touch an 'unclean/impure' sheet that had menstrual blood on it. According to the nurse, attendants were rarely interested in the reasons for patients' behaviours and expected them to follow their orders blindly. The nurse reasoned that their ignorant behaviour was due to a lack of education, empathy and insight into the patients' illness. Attendants were also often criticized for holding back patients inside a ward and not sending them to attend occupational therapy for the sake of having their assistance with ward chores. Dr Shukla shared with me how during his morning inspection he found a sweeper making patients work for her. Observing this, he became angry and consequently fired the sweeper.

The matron's drawing above (Figure 2.2) also illustrates the somehow segregated position of the female support staff, who are supervised by the matron. Dr Shukla used to complain about the staff situation in the female unit in particular. According to him, the staff there behave 'like dictators', but to regulate and supervise the attendants, who do not have any 'concept of mental illness' and are 'only here for salary', proves difficult because of their civil servant status and being 'united and organized in unions', which means that it is not advisable to 'fight with them'. In order to sensitize the attendants to patients' needs, the superintendent attempted to enter a dialogue with them by regularly setting up meetings. Already in the early 2000s, the report 'Status of Women in Mental Hospitals in Maharashtra' published by Shubhada Maitra (2003) had recommended holding training sessions and facilitating development programmes concerning patients' needs. While some measures had been initiated by Dr Shukla, he faced bureaucratic obstacles. Particularly the issue of physical violence against patients had still not been addressed sufficiently, as stressed by Shubhada Maitra, with whom I discussed the conditions in the female wards personally in January 2012. Maitra agreed that some issues such as this one were particularly difficult to solve due to the tightly organized hierarchical structures in the wards and the attendants' organization in unions.

In the above-mentioned report, Maitra additionally documented a bunch of other unmet needs of female patients, which included the provision of undergarments, sanitary pads, clean, colourful and culturally appropriate clothes, storing facilities for the women's belongings and the placing of a mirror in each ward (ibid.: 71). These recommendations were partially implemented during the following decade. Nevertheless, there were still shortcomings concerning the provision of basic standards of care. Not all women had beds to sleep on and had scarce resources; for example, underwear was regularly the target of theft. Furthermore, access to resources was dependent on a patient's position in the ward's social and hierarchical structure. Another still prevalent problem was that women who complained about health problems were often not taken seriously or were labelled as 'attention seeking'. Women told me about gynaecological problems, that they did not menstruate any more (a common side effect of psychotropic drugs) or that they had 'problems with their tummy'. Another often-mentioned problem was skin irritations or rashes.

During my research, I repeatedly came across the characterization of female patients as 'more violent' or 'out of control' than male patients. The reasons given for this phenomenon were manifold. Particularly, psychiatrists stressed that women are brought in for treatment relatively late after the onset of their illness. Accordingly, their symptoms (including violent and 'mad', uncontrollable behaviour) are often worse than those of male patients. Another explanation given by some staff was that women who suffer from a mental illness are more likely to be abandoned by their families and therefore would develop an angry, noncompliant and indignant attitude. This explanatory model did not relate their behaviour to the mental illness itself but rather to their subordinated and weak position in the family hierarchy. It was mentioned further, particularly by attendants and nurses, that the female unit lacks male attendants who might be able to control female patients effectively. Vieda Skultans states that female 'out of control' and 'dangerous' behaviour is more readily condemned than the same behaviour from men (Skultans 1991: 325). Women are supposed to be modest and gentle and therefore if women indulge in tearing off their clothes and violent behaviour, it is perceived as more deviant than in the case of men.

Asifa: Doing 'Dirty Work' in Mumbai

I met Asifa Nawaz Ali for the first time in early May 2011, when I accompanied a social worker on a round of her section in the female unit. Asifa was picked up on the street by the police and admitted to Asha by detention order (DO) in November 2010. Her file mentioned as diagnoses 'mental retardation' and 'behaviour problems'. I met Asifa again two months later together with Rini. Asifa agreed to speak with us, and we sat down on one of the swings outside the front of her ward. She shared with us that she was sixteen years old, from a Muslim family and that she had grown up in a village in Uttar Pradesh. Shortly after Asifa's birth, her mother left the family. According to Asifa, her mother had been tortured by her father-in-law. Asifa's father's family had not allowed her mother to take Asifa with her. Therefore, Asifa's paternal grandmother raised her together with her five elder stepsisters. After her grandmother died, her father married a second time, but his second wife died giving birth to a baby girl. Asifa shared with us that she suspected that her grandmother had poisoned her. After his second wife's death, Asifa's father got married yet again, and Asifa was married off to a boy from another village. Soon after her marriage, Asifa gave birth to a baby boy. Unfortunately, her son died soon after she had delivered him. Subsequently, Asifa's husband divorced her, and she went back to her natal family. Thereafter, her father handed her over to a woman who brought her to Bombay.[4] According to Asifa, her father received one lakh rupees for her. The woman made her do *gandā kām* (dirty work). Asifa used to work from early in the morning until 9.00 PM. She was accommodated in the house of her pimp, to whom she had to hand over all the money she earned. In return, she received clothes and food, which regularly included mutton and chicken. After some time, her '*pāgalpan*' (madness) started. After coming back from work one evening, she suddenly started to feel dizzy and her 'head started roaming'. Asifa remembered her colleague bringing her out of the brothel. Subsequently, she was picked up by the police and brought to Asha.

Asifa shared with us that she did not like to wear the patient uniform, a knee-length frock. Instead she would prefer to wear a *salvār kamīz*[5] or T-shirt. At the beginning of her stay, she received underwear. However, it was stolen whilst hanging up to dry. In order to be able to wear sanitary pads when she menstruated, she used to borrow underpants from fellow patients. Asifa did not possess any shoes and wandered around barefoot. Asifa did not like living in the hospital; she got bored very easily. She told us about her previous day when she had slept all day and an attendant scolded her and announced that she would be keeping an eye on her during the coming days. Usually, however, the attendants behaved well with her. Asifa wore bangles[6] and a ring. She explained to us that the bangles were given to her by her friend Parmeen, who stayed in Ward 8 and received the jewellery from her husband. She received the ring from Neela, who stayed in Ward 1 and would always carry a small purse with her. Besides these items, Asifa did not have any personal belongings. Asifa told us about her daily routine in the ward. She used the general comb belonging to the ward and received soap from the attendants as well as oil to wash her hair on a daily basis when all patients used to take a bath together. The attendants helped her oil her hair and she used to help them to bath the patients who could not take a bath themselves. They were only soaped once a week. On the other days, only water was poured over them with a mug.

Asifa's narrative lacked coherence and contained some contradictions. The time frame she presented seemed paradoxical. She also seemed uncertain about her age. When Rini asked her how old she was when she got married, when her father had sent her to Bombay and about her current age, Asifa's answer was always 'sixteen'. It is possible, indeed, that the bureaucratic category of 'age' did not have much meaning for Asifa. Age as an important category to structure one's biographic narrative is rather familiar to urban and middle-class Indians. In contrast, instead of age, getting married or having children are important biographical markers for the poor and in rural regions. During the interview, Asifa wondered why Rini, who was twenty-three at the time when the interview was conducted, was not yet married: 'You are already so old.' Rini explained to her that girls in Mumbai would marry between the ages of twenty-five and thirty, and that, here she pointed at me, the same was true for Germany. Asifa did not miss her husband, nor did she have any desire to get remarried. If she did ever get married again, it would be to a 'decent man'. She described her husband as a drunkard who used to beat her up, exactly like her father. A social worker at Asha had recently sent a letter to her *Māmū*, her mother's brother. When asked about her future, Asifa stated that because of a lack of alternatives, she would return home to stay with her father again. She said that once she was discharged, she would like to study Urdu.

In contrast to the male unit, there was no designated 'old age ward' for senior citizens in the female unit. Nevertheless, Ward 17 was known for predominantly accommodating elderly patients. The few young patients admitted there, approximately ten out of sixty, were helper patients who supported the attendants in running the ward. During the evenings, attendants and helper patients used to gather in the small attendants' room, where they prepared food on a small stove and sat together to eat and chat. At the beginning of October 2011, Rini had already left to pursue her further studies in Sweden, and Kaveri Dadhich, who also studied at the Tata Institute of Sciences, was now accompanying me when I visited the unit. After we had explained that we were interested in the experience of an elderly patient, one of the attendants went to wake up one of the women in Ward 18.

The majority of the patients in this ward seemed to sleep most of the time during the day. We felt bad when we observed the attendant almost throwing the woman out of her bed in order to send her to sit and speak with us, but it was too late to intervene.

Kamalabai and Suman: The Old Age Ward

We sat down with Kamalabai Ganpat Joshi in the nurses' room. She was from a Buddhist community, and her family lived in a suburb of Mumbai. According to Kamalabai's file, she was sixty-five years old and suffered from 'chronic schizophrenia'. She had been admitted to Asha for the first time in 1989. When we asked her about her family, the first people she mentioned were her three daughter-in-laws Geeta, Devika and Sonu. Kamalabai had a daughter, too, who was the eldest of her children. She was married and lived in the railway quarters. Kamalabai only disclosed the names of her sons after we directly asked for them: Gautam, Narendra and Sandesh. Narendra kept discharging and subsequently bringing her back to the hospital, sometimes after only fifteen days. At the time we spoke to her, she had already been at Asha for two months. Although her son had promised to take her home, he had not yet turned up to discharge her. Kamalabai was widowed and hoped that she would be able to go home and stay again with her second son, soon. Although she regularly took medications, she felt that her health was deteriorating. Recently, she fell down and consequently injured her hand and lost two teeth. Her teeth were loose in general. Kamalabai used to apply oil to her scalp in order to soothe her headaches. Oil was regularly provided by the attendants, but she preferred to use the one from her home. Her whole body used to ache when she took a bath in the morning and only cold water was available. Nevertheless, Kamalabai was aware that in such a big hospital like Asha it was not easy to provide warm water to everybody. She remembered earlier times, when her health had been better and she had helped the attendants to fill the water tank and mop the floor.

Kamalabai did not attend occupational therapy because she never went to school. She also considered vocational training in her case to be a waste of time. She grew up in a village near Mumbai, together with four sisters and a brother. Her brother went to school until fourth standard while her sisters remained illiterate like Kamalabai herself. She wished to go home, where her daughter-in-laws took care of everything. She was tired of staying at Asha: 'It's enough!' After twenty minutes of conversing with her, Kamalabai started to feel exhausted. We thanked her for her time and accompanied her back into the ward where she again went to lie down on her bed.

According to her file, Kamalabai had been readmitted to the hospital in May that year because she had not regularly taken her medicine. Furthermore, a fourth son she had not mentioned was noted as suffering from a chronic mental illness as well. A note on the visitor card indicated when her son would be visiting: 'will discharge the patient on 27.9.2011'. When we spoke to Kamalabai, it was already the beginning of October.

Suman Vishwasrao Dere was the second woman from the old age ward we spoke to on this day. Suman was sixty-seven years old and was admitted to the hospital in 1983. When we asked her if she had some spare time, she agreed to talk to us until the afternoon tea was served. We searched for a spot in the ward to sit down but finally settled on one of the swings outside the ward. Suman had no teeth left and spoke quietly; at times it was difficult to understand her. Suman had not gone home even once since her admission. Her illness started when she was young, and her father had regularly brought her to Asha for 'shock treatment' whenever she suffered from a 'heavy head' (*dōkṁ jaḍ*). Because her condition demanded frequent visits to the doctor, her father eventually decided to admit her. Suman hailed from a Hindu family and had two brothers and three sisters, all older than her apart from one sister who was younger. Being the fifth of six children, she studied until the fourth grade. When her mental troubles started, her parents made her quit school, and she used to stay at home and help out with the household chores. Her mother died when she was still a child. Later, she married a tailor with whom she had two daughters. Suman's husband used to beat her up, and sometimes he would even beat the two daughters. 'He never loved any one of us,' Suman told us. Finally, she ran away from his place and went back to her father's house in order to live there. Her husband blamed the family for hiding Suman's mental health issues and therefore for ruining his life. Suman's father sent her to stay in an ashram for some time, but she ran away from there. When she was finally found, her father made all the necessary arrangements to admit her to Asha permanently. At the time we spoke with Suman, neither of her children or anybody else had come to visit her. Her father had died some time ago, her elder brothers were busy with their jobs and her sisters stayed at their husbands' places. Her sisters' and brothers' children were married, and her husband eventually married another woman. Everybody had moved on with their lives, and nobody was there to take care of Suman: 'Now I will stay here until I die; I won't go back home any more.'

Suman had always chewed tobacco and therefore was unsure if she might end up with cancer in addition to her mental illness. She shared with us that she felt very uncomfortable about her body smelling sweaty and that she was glad that we had decided to sit down outside, where a fresh breeze was blowing. Suman thought of her life as a very unfortunate one. She used to laugh about herself sometimes and wondered whether we would also laugh about her misery after this conversation. Eventually, the tea arrived at the unit gate, and Suman said goodbye to us. We had a look at Suman's file and found out that she had been diagnosed with 'schizoaffective disorder'. The psychiatric social worker had sent a number of letters to her family, but apparently there were not many responses. A home visit to the house of Suman's nephew was mentioned in a psychiatric social worker's note in 2009. During the visit, the nephew told the social worker that his father, one of Suman's brothers, died recently. He promised to speak with other family members about Suman's case but also stressed that the other siblings, too, had grown old and feeble. The psychiatric social worker had continued to send letters to the family after her visit, but apparently nobody had replied to these.

The Male Wards

While the female unit is rather secluded and located at the back of Asha, the male unit is much more accessible, located at the main road leading through the hospital together with the outpatient department and many of the administrative departments.

Patients who are allowed to leave their wards often walk this road to the main gate or roam the smaller paths within the unit. Therefore, in contrast to female patients, male patients regularly encounter people from outside the hospital.

James: In Search of the High Life

I met James Peter Rodriguez for the first time in early September 2011, when I was about to leave the hospital after I had spent the whole morning and the early afternoon in the female unit. He was wandering about on the main road and addressed me in English. He told me that his family was Christian, hailed from Goa and introduced himself as an 'old patient' who had been coming to Asha for a long time. On this occasion, he had been at Asha for eighteen days. Being admitted once meant that one could be brought back easily at any point: his father would immediately readmit him after any quarrel between them. James's parents died some time ago and since then his younger brother had been caring for him and bringing him to Asha. Patients like James come to the hospital for short intervals and then go back home for a number of weeks or months before being admitted yet again. This had been the case for James for decades now. When I asked him why he was at Asha so often, he replied that he had an addiction problem – he used to smoke Marijuana. After our conversation had gone on for some time, James told me not to stand in the bright sun and directed me into the shadow of one of the big trees on the hospital premises. He smirked that he knew that foreigners like me adored the bright sun – he had observed this on numerous occasions on the Goan beaches, where many foreigners spend their vacation. James had to take three different kinds of tablets, including one for his sleeping problems. He proudly demonstrated to me that he could name them all correctly. At this point in our encounter, I was feeling very tired, having already spent many hours at the hospital. I said goodbye to James and told him that we would continue our conversation soon.

Two weeks later, Akshay and I visited the old age ward to record James' interview. He was sixty years old at that point in time. We conversed in English, and James's speech was a little blurred as usual. He tended to speak very fast, so we found it difficult to follow him at times. There were two rooms and one common room for forty-eight patients. Each of the dorm rooms contained ten beds. Those patients who did not sleep on a bed slept on mattresses on the floor. According to James, patients did not use to fight concerning who would get the better sleeping places: 'All patients are senior citizens, no?', implying that old men are more peaceable than younger ones, who may more readily engage in arguments and physical confrontations.

When James was admitted this time, he was allowed to keep his rosary, unlike before. At the time of admission, his brother gave thirty rupees to one of the attendants and told him: 'Look after him!' James had worked as a helper patient since the first time he was admitted to Asha: 'If you don't do anything you only go to sleep, you become lethargic, particularly during winter.' Although James came to Asha in order to quit his addictions, smoking remained one of his bad habits. 'I am good in drinking, smoking, hash. What about you? I know you are good at drinking,' he mocked, perpetuating the stereotype that Westerners enjoy drinking alcohol regularly. James suspected that he might have become 'addicted' to his medications as he was unable to sleep if he did not take them.

When James' parents admitted him to Asha for the first time in 1974/5, he remembered his mother paying five thousand rupees to a 'helper' who then took care of the paperwork regarding the court admission (RO). James proved very knowledgeable regarding the legal regulations and rules concerning admission and readmission processes at the hospital. He was discharged from Asha on a LOA (leave of absence). Therefore, there was no need for another lengthy and bureaucratic admission procedure in case of a readmission. Because the LOA expires after sixty days, James used to come to the OPD two or three days before in order to collect his medications and pay the required fifty rupees for its extension. He realized that one day in the hospital would cost him twenty-two rupees and that the fee included food, snacks and medicine, whereas not staying in hospital and just collecting his medicine from the OPD cost him eighty rupees per 5-day blister pack. That meant paying more than a thousand rupees monthly just for the three medications he needed. Therefore, staying in the hospital was the logical option. And every two to three months, James would ask the barber who visited the ward once a week to cut his hair very short, for only forty rupees.

James previously lived in Bandra[7] together with his younger brother and worked as an optician at his brother's shop. James remembered how he had lost his girlfriend when he fell sick for the first time. They wanted to celebrate his friend's sister's birthday, but issues occurred and eventually he went out alone on that night to hang out in a disco. When his girlfriend told James' father the next day that he was 'mentally affected' and was 'doing drugs', his father admitted him to Asha. James was very angry at his girlfriend for telling his father about him doing drugs and was violent towards her after the incident. This caused his girlfriend's mother to tell his mother that if James did not stay away from her daughter he might never get well. Following these events, his girlfriend 'became friendly' with somebody else, immigrated to Canada and left James. When James recollected and told us about his break up he became sad – he still mourned the fact that he never got married.

During our conversation, a helper patient entered the room and started distributing eggs. James took one of the eggs and explained the non-veg policies to us: 'On Wednesdays we get egg curry, on Fridays we get chicken.' He remembered that in the earlier days, mutton and fish were also served. However, due to a surge in prices, it had become too expensive. Many of his friends who also suffered from drug addiction and migraines and led a 'hippie life' used to come to the hospital for treatment. Now these friends had moved – some abroad. James remembered that several years ago there was a building close to the old age ward that stored musical instruments. He used to go there nearly every day with some of the other patients in order to play some music, but the facility was eventually closed down. He said the hospital staff did not follow his suggestion to establish a library. 'They are running the hospital on a raw base', he added, regretfully. Nevertheless, there were events that took place on a regular basis; for example, the sports day in February, where James had won second prize the previous year.

Towards the end of our conversation, James showed us a mark on his head that was the reason he had to undergo a medical examination the following day. He explained to us that the mark dated back to an incident that happened when he was admitted to the sick ward. A ward boy kicked him in the head during his night shift. According to James, the sick ward was one of Asha's worst and dirtiest wards.

After the interview, Akshay and I regularly encountered James. The last time we met him was at the end of September 2011, shortly before my research at the hospital came to an end. He asked us if we knew anything about 'bipolar disorder'. 'A little', Akshay responded. James shared with us that he had just come from the OP department, where he had read about the symptoms on one of the boards. James explained that this illness is characterized by phases during which one feels 'calm' followed by phases of 'excitement'. He then disclosed that he himself displayed precisely these symptoms and so he had to take medication. The drugs seemed to be working because when we asked others about him they would tell us that, nowadays, he 'was only 20 per cent not ok'. When we checked James's file, 'schizoaffective disorder' and 'addiction: Tobacco' were mentioned as his diagnoses.

Similar to the female unit, attendants in the male unit are with the patients twenty-four hours a day and have a particularly close relationship with them. In earlier times, senior male attendants wore a white uniform with a *tōpī* – a cap that is particularly worn by Maharashtrian men. In contrast, junior attendants wore khaki uniforms. At the time of my research, male attendants had stopped wearing civil servant uniforms and instead were dressed in simple plain-coloured overalls. Some of the senior attendants continued to wear a *tōpī*. Sweepers do not wear any kind of particular work clothing but predominantly dress in trousers and shirt. Nine attendants work over three shifts in the admission wards, where around seventy newly admitted and often quite 'excited' (symptomatic) patients stay at a time. Some patients in the ward may be tied up or kept in a separate room in order to prevent them from harming themselves or others. One senior attendant shared with us that ECT is perceived as the last option for controlling a patient's violent or uncooperative behaviour. Attendants regularly prepare reports about patients' behaviour and put those who refuse to eat or behave violently on particular lists in order to report them to the medical staff. Patients who do not sleep, become violent or threaten other patients during the night get an entry in the 'night report', and some of them might be calmed down with injections that can be administered by the doctor on the night shift.

In contrast to the female unit, sweepers in the male unit predominantly complete tasks inside the wards, wherein they clean the toilets, showers, plates and cups as well as the floor in the corridors. While these tasks are predominantly taken on by patients in the female unit, patients in the male unit did not use to do as much cleaning work. Additionally, together with helper patients, sweepers assist the attendants in distributing the food.

The Recreation Hall and Visiting Rooms

The only area that is accessible from both the female and male units is the recreation hall. From time to time, collective activities for patients take place here. For example, the public screening of movies or the performance of traditional dance shows during holidays. The recreation hall is also commonly referred to as 'the temple' or *maṇdir* by staff and patients, as it is used to celebrate the annual occasion of Ganesh Chaturthi, a ten-day festival that typically falls late August or early September. During the festival, the elephant god Ganesha (Ganpati), embodied by a huge *mūrti*,[8] is placed in the hall. Menstruating female patients are not allowed to enter 'the temple', and female attendants make sure that this rule is strictly implemented. Many chronically ill and symptomatic patients are not allowed inside as well. I observed how some of these patients prayed outside in front of one of the windows from where they could see the *mūrti*. Other festivals celebrated at Asha are Diwali,[9] Holi,[10] Gokulashtami,[11] Raksha Bandhan[12] and Shivaji Jayanti[13] and Ambedkar Jayanti.[14] Celebration of these holidays is predominantly organized by the ward staff, including nurses and attendants. NGOs and patients' and ex-patients' relatives support the celebrations with donations.

In the male wards, attendants took the initiative to construct a number of small temples that were then placed all over the unit. Male patients, accompanied by attendants, used to visit these temples during their morning walks. The attendants of one of the admission wards told us that the temple in front of the building had a calming effect on the patients and that the atmosphere in the wards had become more peaceful in general since it was put in place. The female unit does not have temples outside because male ward staff who could take care of the necessary *pūjā*[15] do not frequent the unit. Every ward in the female unit has a little 'home shrine', though, as is common for every Hindu household, and these shrines are usually looked after by female family members.

A part of the recreation hall is also the visiting room for relatives of female patients. The families enter the hall through the male unit. Only in rare cases – for example, if a patient is admitted to the sick ward – are family members allowed to enter the female unit directly. Sometimes families come to the hospital and are told by the attendants that 'their patient' is not well today (e.g. because she has just received ECT treatment) and therefore cannot be brought to the hall. In this instance, the family has to leave without seeing their relative. When families visited, they used to bring them snacks to eat in addition to items that are scarcely available in the hospital, such as underwear or a toothbrush. The male unit accommodates its own visiting room. In contrast to the hall, where attendants receive the visitors, a social worker sits here during the official visiting hours – 9.00 AM to 4.00 PM.[16] The visitors' names, their relationship to the patient, their address and phone number and what they brought in for the patient are noted down in a logbook and on the visitor card in the patient's file. Younger patients are often visited by their parents and siblings. In the case of elderly patients, common visitors include their wives, husbands, siblings and children. Patients are rarely visited by friends. Male patients are brought to the visiting room by attendants or helper patients, who in turn receive a small tip for their services from the patients' relatives. In the visiting room, an information board states the rules that have to be obeyed by the visiting relatives: visiting time is limited to twenty to thirty minutes, visitors are supposed to observe silence while they move through the male unit and they are not allowed to bring homemade or takeaway food from outside into the hospital, with only fruits and biscuits allowed. The last rule reflects a concern that family members might try to poison a family member in order to rid themselves of the responsibility for them. The social worker in the visiting room told us about an incident before this rule was implemented, when a female patient was poisoned with home-cooked food by her relatives during one of their visits. Subsequently, her natal family and in-laws started a public dispute over who actually poisoned her, and the case was never solved. A further visiting rule states that visitors are not allowed to take any signature or written statements from patients without the hospital staff's approval. This rule is supposed to prevent families from pressurizing patients to sign any official document that might concern a property/inheritance matter or a divorce case. Male patients were at times allowed to carry out a meeting with their family outdoors, where they used to sit on one of the benches located around the hospital premises. The visiting room in the male unit also served as a location for AA meetings and a family self-help group that met once and twice a month respectively. Both had been initiated by Dr Shukla.

Abdul: A Hidden Addict

When Akshay and I spoke to 31-year-old Abdul Mohammed Khatri in the admission ward one morning at the beginning of September 2011, it was the first day of Ganpati, and Abdul planned to go to the temple to attend the *pūjā* and the celebrations. Eid[17] had been celebrated on the wards the previous day, and *khīr* (a sweet dish) had been provided to all patients. Abdul's parents visited him on the occasion of the holiday and told him that they would take him home two days later. When he was admitted to Asha, he was supposed to stay for one month. Then his family extended his stay and explained to him that he had to stay longer in order to 'get rid of his habit'.

We sat down with Abdul in the cramped nurses' room after he agreed to speak with us. During the conversation, he addressed Akshay as 'sir', and our interaction was generally rather formal. Abdul appeared distant, and his face remained emotionless. He told us that he was admitted because he used to smoke *charas*[18] and eat *bhang*[19] tablets. His parents came to know about his drug consumption and sent him to Asha to 'free him from his addiction (*nashā*)'. Abdul was admitted to Asha rather than any other addiction centre because it was close to where his parents and two sisters lived. His family had only recently moved to this part of Mumbai. In his old neighbourhood, many of his friends also consumed drugs, but during that time their families had not come to know about their addiction. He worked as a tailor in a shop and used to take drugs while working: 'Your mind starts to fly a bit, so you keep doing your work.'

Abdul's day at the hospital used to start at 5.00 AM. He took a bath with everyone else at 6.30 AM. At 9.30 AM, breakfast was served, and at 10.30 AM the medications were distributed. Subsequently, an occupational therapist came to the unit and took those patients who 'felt bored' to the OT department. Abdul was usually one of these patients and there he engaged in tailoring and sewing from 11.00 AM to 1.00 PM. At 2.00 PM lunch was served, and after that Abdul used to sleep until 6.00 PM, which was the time for him to take his evening medicine dose. After that, dinner was served at 7.00 PM.

Abdul shared his plan to get married during the upcoming year. When his parents had visited him the day before, his father told him that he had seen a girl for him and that they planned to arrange his marriage soon after he was discharged from Asha. None of Abdul's sisters was married yet, and his parents planned to hold Abdul's and his elder sister's marriage at the same time. When Akshay asked Abdul if he planned to remain sober after leaving the hospital and getting married, Abdul responded that this was not in his hands and referred to Allah, who was going to decide everything. Abdul did not think that telling the girl's or his sister's prospective husband's family about his problem or his stay at Asha for treatment was necessary or even recommendable. He was aware that people would think of him as a 'mental patient' and therefore that things like this are better not made public. Anybody who knew about his stay in the hospital or of his drug consumption posed a threat to his prestige in the community. Therefore, his family had told everybody that he had gone on a trip for four months.

When Akshay and I had a look at Abdul's file after our talk, we found out about his diagnosis: 'Cannabis abuse + psychosis + ASPD [antisocial personality disorder] traits'. He had been admitted for the first time six years before, when, additionally, he was suffering from 'chronic alcohol abuse'. His file also contained a three-month-old letter from his sister in which she asked for an extension of Abdul's stay in the hospital because a marriage was about to take place in the house. We spoke with one of the nurses about Abdul, and she confirmed that his discharge was scheduled for the next day. A few hours later she updated us on his case: apparently a politician ('somebody from the *mantrālay*' (ministry)) had called the superintendent and asked him to delay Abdul's discharge further in order to spare his family from Abdul's severe and ongoing problems.

Occupational Therapy

Patients who do not have to be seen by the doctors or receive electroconvulsive therapy (ECT) treatment and who are perceived as 'not too excited' get to attend occupational therapy during the mornings. An Occupational Therapy Department (OTD) can be found in both the male and female unit, where three male and three female occupational therapists are supposed to engage patients in diverse activities and vocational training. Until the early 2000s, patients mostly engaged in tailoring, weaving and carpentry. Recently, a diversification of the activities took place, so it now also includes, for example, gardening, drawing, and the making of candles and sanitary pads. A particular category of occupational therapy is 'ward activities', which entails helping the attendants with certain tasks in the wards. Patients who show good skills in completing these tasks and in supervising fellow patients eventually attain the position of so called 'helper patients' within the ward hierarchy. Outside the hospital walls, a little apart from other hospital buildings, a small Day Care Centre is located, which provides similar activities and occupational therapy options to the OTDs inside the hospital. When I visited it in mid-2011, it was frequented by an average of six patients per day. In order to enable more patients to regularly attend the Day Care Centre, hospital officials planned to establish a pick-up service that would collect patients in the morning and drop them back home in the afternoon. When I eventually came back to Asha in early 2012, the pick-up service had not yet been established.

Mahesh: A Quarrel and its Consequences

I met Mahesh Raju Pawar in May 2011 when I spent the day in the OTD in the male unit. Mahesh was in his mid-twenties and appeared to be shy and socially withdrawn. He rarely made eye contact. One of the occupational therapists, Mr Nakeesh Kekde, shared with me that Mahesh killed his father during a brief psychotic episode. He was arrested in May 2009 and admitted to Asha, where he was accommodated in the criminal ward for about a year. When his mother eventually withdrew her accusations, Mahesh was transferred to one of the general wards. Nevertheless, his family did not want to take him back home because they were afraid of his violent and impulsive behaviour. Mr Kekde suspected that Mahesh's psychotic episode might have been drug induced. He had peddled drugs after he quit school. While I was speaking to Mr Kekde, Mahesh approached the occupational therapist in order to tell him that he did not like the tailoring workshop and that he would prefer to weave or print. Mr Kekde convinced him to give it another try; he explained to him that tailoring would provide him with the necessary skills to get a job once he was discharged from Asha. When I subsequently engaged in a short conversation with Mahesh, he told me that he had gone to school until eighth standard and then had to quit because his family was poor; he had to work in order to contribute to the family income. He shared with me that he was bored with tailoring because he did not know how to do it and that he wished to go back home.

Together with Dhaval, I met Mahesh again almost three months later in August. We sat down in the admission ward for a conversation, which Dhaval lead in Marathi. Mahesh told us that he grew up in a village around three hundred kilometres away from Mumbai and that his family did not have much money. They belonged to the Maratha caste (Kunbi) and were farmers, owning three acres of *kōrḍvāhū* (dry land) on which they grew drumsticks during the rainy season. During the rest of the growing season, the land was infertile because it lacked a water supply. Therefore, his parents additionally used to work as day labourers on the lands of other farmers. Besides working in a shop and selling raisins, Mahesh had also worked as a day labourer and harvested cotton or *bājrā*.[20] Mahesh's father had three brothers, him being the second son. The youngest brother owned much more fertile land and was additionally equipped with a well. One day, Mahesh went to this uncle in order to ask for money. When his uncle refused to give him money, he went to his father, but their encounter escalated, and Mahesh eventually attacked him with a stone. Three months after the incident, his father died of the injuries that had been inflicted on him. During our conversation, Mahesh's face remained blank, and he appeared reserved and somehow distant from his own narrative. When I later went through Mahesh's file, I found that the psychiatrist had diagnosed him with an 'antisocial personality' in the Mental Status Examination (MSE).

Mahesh's relationship with his parents had been tense long before the incident. He used to hand over all the money he earned to his family, but when he asked for some money to spend for himself, they refused to give him any. Furthermore, Mahesh had one sister who got married around 2002. After his paternal cousin (uncle's daughter), who went to school with him and was about his age, got married as well, he asked his parents to arrange his marriage. His mother, however, put him off and told him that he was still young and that he should be patient for some more time. Mahesh remembered that during this time his family had started to call him 'mental'. Therefore, Mahesh suspected that his family thinking of him as 'mad' might have been the actual reason that his parents had refused to arrange his marriage and not, as his mother claimed, his age.

Mahesh related his quick temper and his tendency to lose it and become angry to an incident when he was fifteen years old; he had fallen from a neem tree and injured his head. After that, he fell and hit the same spot two more times and since then his 'mind had not worked properly' any more. It did not hurt, but the 'tension' he felt became overwhelming, and he began getting into fights and no longer listened to his parents. Finally, he was admitted to a hospital near his home village for around one month in 2005. Since then he has to take medication three times a day: in the morning, noon and evening. But even if taking the medicines helped his 'mind to be quiet', another incident occurred in 2006. He ran away from the store where he worked and roamed around in a nearby village for three days. He was picked up by a villager, who informed his family. In 2007, after he had picked a fight with some boys, Mahesh was admitted for ten days to a hospital in Surat, where his father's eldest brother's son lived. After he received treatment there, everything seemed to have gone fine for some time. Then he had an affair with a girl and felt the need to increase the dose of one of his medicines and took three pills instead of one. Then his mind 'stopped working' again, and subsequently he caused the death of his father.

After Mahesh had dropped the big stone on his father's head during the fight, he ran away. People from the village came after him and carried him back to the village police station. Immediately after his arrest, the police took him to the jail in the city. Mahesh did not visit his father in the hospital. Mahesh stayed in jail for a year, not knowing what had happened to his father. He eventually came to know about his father's death when his family came to visit him in May 2010. He realized he had been denied the right to perform the last rites and light the fire of the pyre as would have been his obligation as the only son. Mahesh's mother explained to him that he was 'mental' and informed him that he would be sent to a psychiatric hospital in Mumbai. He asked her to take him back home, promising that he would improve his behaviour and not trouble other people any more. But his mother refused; she did not believe him and said that he surely would beat up somebody again.

In April, his mother and his cousin visited him for what would be the last time. They did not come to visit him often, but when they did they brought him some biscuits. Mahesh explained to us that patients mostly only get the chance to eat foods from outside if they get visitors. Sometimes, family members would even get *pāv bhājī*.[21] When his family visited him, the attendants asked his cousin for one hundred rupees. Mahesh was aware that the attendants did not ask everybody but only those who look well off. They used to ask visitors for a donation in order to finance the construction of a new ward temple or hold a festival. They 'eat the money', as Mahesh expressed it, implying that the attendants were corrupt. At the end of the interview, we asked Mahesh if we could have a look at his file. He agreed and even offered to get it for us.

According to Mahesh's file, he had been declared 'fit for discharge'. Therefore, his family might not have come specifically to see Mahesh back in April that year but had probably been invited to justify their reasons for not wanting him to be discharged. Further, it was mentioned that Mahesh had experienced 'auditory and visual hallucinations' since he was five years old, and his file contained a psychological evaluation. The evaluation was conducted at the end of 2010 by one of the clinical psychology students who was completing an internship at the hospital. It stated that Mahesh had started to see and hear two girls, named Yogita and Pooja, in 2006. The medications he had started to take after his stay in the hospital in Surat apparently had not stopped him from hearing their voices 24 hours a day. They used to say bad things and would not stop when he told them to. Mahesh had started to have everyday conversations with the voices, had fallen in love with them and did not want to live without them any more. While the diagnosis by the ward psychiatrist simply read 'old case of brief psychotic disorder', the diagnostic result of the psychology student sounded much more elaborate: 'Bipolar Disorder, Single Manic Episode, Severe with psychotic features [mood congruent psychotic features], in partial remission'.

'Shock Therapy': A Controversial Topic

Similar to psychotropic drugs, electroconvulsive treatment (ECT) has the reputation of being a very 'effective' intervention in the case of mental illnesses. But unlike psychopharmacological interventions, ECT is a far more controversial topic among mental health professionals and activists, particularly when it comes to so called 'unmodified' ECT, which is administered without anaesthesia (Agarwal et al. 1992; Andrade et al. 1993; Andrade et al. 2000; Andrade 2003; Pathare 2003). In anti-psychiatric and psychiatric critical circles, ECT is suspected of being used by psychiatrists and hospital staff as a kind of punishment and to discipline patients' behaviour (Davar 2014: 272). At Asha, the ECT sessions take place between 9.30 AM and 11.30 AM; specifically, every Tuesday, Thursday and Saturday in the male unit and every Monday, Wednesday and Friday in the female unit. Patients who are about to receive ECT treatment do not have breakfast on these days and are brought to the ECT department by an attendant, where they are asked to wait for their turn. Female patients have to exchange their uniform frocks for a *salvār kamīz*, so that certain body parts and what they are wearing under the frock, are not at risk of being 'exposed' during the treatment procedure. For one ECT treatment, 120 rupees are charged, which is much cheaper than in a private setting, where the charge is around one thousand rupees. During my research, ECT was a topic that popped up repeatedly when I spoke to patients and their families. Psychiatrists, patients and families utter diverse and often contrasting opinions about ECT (Chavan 2006; Andrade 2007; Rajagopal et al. 2012). James recalled that he was admitted to a private hospital to receive shock treatment decades ago. One treatment cost one hundred rupees, which was a big amount of money at that time. Many patients were afraid of being brought to a psychiatric hospital because the ECT treatment was not modified and one did not receive any anaesthesia. Some patients who lived at Asha or had been treated there for decades still remembered receiving electroconvulsive treatment without any anaesthesia. Since the early 1990s, however, unmodified or 'direct' ECT is no longer administered in Asha, and patients receive an injection, so they are not aware of what is happening to them. Suman told Kaveri and me that before receiving her first ECT she also had been afraid of lightening and electricity and how undergoing many (unmodified) ECT sessions had relieved her of her fears. Asifa was also administered ECT treatment not long after her admission. She remembered receiving nose drops and an injection and being tied to an examination couch.

I attended and observed the ECT sessions in both the female and male unit and spoke to the respective psychiatrists in charge as well as the anaesthetist. The ECT treatment is administered behind a curtain on a treatment couch, on which patients lie on their backs. Shortly after the anaesthetist injects them with anaesthetics and a muscle relaxant, they receive their treatment: a device that looks like headphones is put on the patient's head, and the voltage strength is set using a control panel. Dr Dabhekar, who was responsible for the ECT session in the male unit on the day that I attended it, explained to me that the strength of electric current is set appropriately if the patient's toes curl. Six helpers hold down the patient. He or she is then carried over to a mattress on the floor. When the patient wakes after some minutes, they are brought back to their ward accompanied by the attendants. According to Dr Dabhekar, patients in the government setting wake faster after having received ECT than those in the private setting, where patients receive stronger anaesthetics. Patients are not explicitly told that they are about to receive ECT but are instead told that they will receive 'an injection supporting their health'. Nevertheless, after some time most of the patients anticipate or come to know through fellow patients about what happens after they receive the injection. Before a patient can be given ECT, a relative has to sign the respective consent form. Dr Dabhekar explained to me that those patients whose families do not consent to ECT nevertheless have to undergo it anyway: 'It is for their well-being.' Dr Dabhekar was convinced of ECT's effectiveness and its capacity to 'calm down the patient'. Dr Kulkarni, one of the most senior psychiatrists, told me that she would prescribe ECT to around 80 per cent of newly admitted patients. She perceived it as an effective medical intervention, with side effects that were few and manageable (e.g. short-term memory loss). Because most families bring in their relatives in an already progressed state to the hospital, ECT was Dr Kulkarni's first choice of treatment. As a senior psychiatrist, Dr Kulkarni noted that she tended to prescribe more ECT treatment than the younger generation, who received a different medical education to the one she did several decades before. This generational difference in attitudes was further exemplified by Madan, a junior occupational therapists in his early twenties, who exclaimed: 'They give ECT for almost everything!'

Among Indian psychiatrists, ECT is perceived as a very effective treatment for a wide range of psychiatric symptoms and conditions. Gangadhar et al. (2010) point out that in many Western countries the application of ECT is now reserved for the treatment of the most severe cases of depression, but in India '[t]he fact that patients as well as their relatives have a favourable attitude towards ECT may also have allowed more patients to receive and benefit from ECT' (ibid.: 364). However, even after over seventy years of clinical application, the underlying benefits of this psychiatric treatment option remain unclear. Several medical and lay theories promoting ECT's effectiveness exist, and this seems to fuel the continued application of ECT (Jadhav 1994; Perrin et al. 2012), including at Asha. Once a social worker observed me collecting statistics regarding ECT treatment from the hospital registers and commented: 'In May it's more [the application of ECT treatment], because it is hot.'

Even if her statement did not prove true, her comment indicated a general association of mental illnesses with an excess of heat, in this case exacerbated by the sometimes unbearably hot temperatures during the months of May and June before the rainy season eventually relieves Mumbaikars in July. ECT – also referred to as 'shock treatment' – is perceived to 'cool down' a 'heated' mind[22] and is itself associated with a certain kind of hotness. 'English' and 'Western' medicine, as biomedicine is also sometimes referred to in the Indian context, is generally classified as 'hot medicine' with one of its side effects being that its 'heat' tends to weaken the body during treatment (Nichter 1980: 228). Accordingly, a woman whom I encountered while she was visiting her son at Asha told me about her son's physical 'weakness' that he experienced due to the numerous ECTs he had received during the last two decades in order to treat his mental illness. She explained to me that while the shocks 'slowed' down his brain and therefore helped him to behave 'normal' again, they had 'weakened' his body, a side effect that she hoped could be successfully treated during his stay at Asha.

Notes

1. Eggs are not included in the category 'vegetarian' but are considered a 'non-veg' food.
2. Employees within the civil service are distributed into Class I, II and III (doctors and psychiatrists) and superior (administrative officer and matron) staff, whilst Class IV consists of support staff (occupational therapists, social workers, nurses, administrative personnel and attendants). Sweepers do not have the status of civil servants and therefore do not belong to any of the civil service classes.
3. Attendants work the following shifts: 7.00 AM to 3.00 PM, 11.00 AM to 7.00 PM and 7.00 PM to 7.00 AM.
4. Asifa referred to Mumbai as 'Bombay', its official (English) name until 1995, when the government changed it to 'Mumbai'. The driving force behind this change was the Marathi nationalist Shiv Sena party. The city is still referred to as Bombay by some of its residents and by Indians from other regions.
5. The *salvār kamīz* is a traditional outfit worn in South Asia. It comprises a head scarf (for Muslims), *kamīz* (long shirt) and *salvār* (baggy trousers).
6. Rigid bracelets, which are usually made of metal, wood, glass or plastic.
7. A wealthy neighbourhood in west Mumbai.

8. A *mūrti* is an image, statue or idol of a deity or person. In Hindu temples, it serves as an symbolic icon. A *mūrti* is not perceived as the god itself in Hinduism but as the shape, embodiment or manifestation of the respective deity.
9. Diwali is one of the most popular Hindu festivals, also known as the 'festival of lights', which is celebrated every autumn. It symbolizes the spiritual victory of light over darkness and good over evil.
10. Holi, commonly known as the 'festival of colours', signifies the arrival of spring and the end of winter and is for many a day to meet with others and 'play' with coloured powder and laugh.
11. Gokulashtami is a festival that celebrates the birth of the god Krishna.
12. Raksha Bandhan (Sanskrit: 'Tying Protection') is an annually performed celebration rooted in Hinduism and centred on sisters tying a *rākhī* (in the form of a bracelet) round the wrist of brothers as a form of ritual protection. Sisters may receive small gifts of money from their brothers on this occasion.
13. Shivaji is a festival and public holiday honoured particularly in the Indian state of Maharashtra. Celebrated on 19 February, it marks the birth anniversary of the Maratha emperor Shivaji.
14. Observed on 14 April, it celebrates the 1891 birth date of Babasaheb Dr B.R. Ambedkar. Ambedkar is mainly known for his campaign against social discrimination towards the Untouchables (Dalits) and inspiring the Buddhist movement.
15. *pūjā* is a prayer of devotional worship to one or more deities, or to host and honour a guest, or to spiritually celebrate an event.
16. There was no apparent reason why this task was taken care of by a social worker in the male unit. Furthermore, this social worker was visually impaired (blind), but this may have been one task that he was able to do more easily.
17. Eid al-Fitr is a Muslim religious holiday that marks the end of Ramadan, the Islamic holy month of fasting.
18. The hashish form of cannabis.
19. An edible preparation of cannabis.
20. A kind of millet.
21. Fried vegetables with a bread roll, a common street food in Mumbai.
22. A similar concept and explanation model Robin Tribhuwan reports from a tribal community in Maharashtra, where 'madness' is treated by administering a hot iron rod to the temples of a patient (Tribhuwan 1998).

CHAPTER 3

RESISTING THE UNIFORM

SOCIAL DISTINCTIONS AND HIERARCHIES IN THE WARDS

A patient's family and kin group play a major role in Indian psychiatric practice and the organization of the mental health care system in general; they constitute key informants for mental health practitioners (Nunley 1998; Addlakha 2008; Strauss 2011: 150; Bayetti, Jadhav and Jain 2016). The organization of inpatient care at Asha poses a noteworthy exception: in contrast to many other governmental institutions, family members are not allowed to accompany or stay with the patient inside the wards, and therefore hospital staff members are the only people that take care of the patients' everyday needs. This particular conjuncture has, in combination with a lack of resources, several consequences and complicates the situation of patients admitted to Asha. An admission to the psychiatric hospital constitutes an institutional 'depersonalization' to a certain extent. The admission process entails a separation from one's family and familiar social environment. It involves handing over all personal belongings, including clothes, jewellery and wristwatches to the hospital staff. Furthermore, being admitted to Asha inevitably means wearing a uniform that strips a person of their social (status) markers and unmistakeably highlights them as 'mental patients'. If a person undergoes inpatient psychiatric treatment, they are expected to go through a remarkable behavioural transformation and 'improvement' before they can be declared 'fit for discharge' and return back to their families (Addlakha 2001). All these institutional practices mean an admitted person becomes a member of the patient 'communitas', and their stay in the psychiatric hospital is framed as a kind of 'liminal phase' (Strauss 2011: 137).

Being a Long-Term Patient at Asha

Several patients did not leave this 'liminal phase' for years, decades or sometimes never at all. For a number of diverse reasons that I elaborate on in more detail in Chapter 5, they could not be rehabilitated and were not able to return to their families. However, the total institution's impact on people's lives and experiences in general can undoubtedly be rated as tremendous. Living in the wards, particularly if it is long-term, comes with its own routines, social distinctions and hierarchies.

Faiza: A Privileged Long-Term Patient

Faiza Ahmed, whom I found to be charismatic and who had a very uncommon yet appealing way of communicating, was one of the long-term patients at Asha and stayed in one of the 'chronic wards'. During our conversations, I felt both drawn towards and put off by her dominant habitus. Faiza had been admitted to Asha in 2006. Her file mentioned a 'brief reactive psychosis' as her diagnosis, and when I met her, she appeared to be symptom free. Indeed, at that time she had not taken any medications for around seven months. Then the psychiatrist decided that it was necessary to put her on psychotropic drugs again. It was a well-known fact that Faiza enjoyed telling a slightly different story about herself to each different person who asked. As far as what she disclosed to me, Faiza hailed from a Muslim family originally from Jaipur, Rajasthan. Her father was from a Rajput community and her mother Iranian. Faiza had grown up in Delhi and studied at the Jamia Milia University. She had been happy in an arranged marriage with two children before her husband had got involved in racketeering and was eventually shot by the police. After her husband died, she left the children with her sister, who worked as a doctor in the popular Apollo hospital, and came to Mumbai to take up a job.

When I met Faiza, she had already obtained a privileged position in the ward. I saw her frock rolled up to her hips while she sedulously moved round the dorm room, making the beds and changing the sheets. She was the most superior helper patient in the ward and maintained a good relationship with the attendants, with whom she used to joke and to discuss other patients' behaviour. Faiza was the one who got to decide if the ward TV was switched on or off. Almost every ward at Asha is equipped with a TV set. The superintendent, Dr Praveen Shukla, explained to me during a personal conversation that he 'made it a point for every ward to have a TV as a connection to the outside world'. He considered it particularly important that the female long-term patients at Asha had access to media content: 'They are totally cut off from the world, they are cut off from the mainstream.'

Sonia, a social work student who visited the hospital during the time I was carrying out my research, agreed with me that Faiza occupied a superior position within the ward's social hierarchy. She had observed that Faiza did not allow any patients to sleep or rest on the beds during the day. She remembered particularly well an incident in which she had entered the ward and found Faiza sitting on the floor completely naked while two of the attendants were oiling her hair. When the attendants saw Sonia's shocked expression, they asked Faiza to get up and put on her frock.

During the tenth day of the Ganpati festival at the beginning of September, I attended a dance performance that took place on stage in 'the temple'. Several long-term patients performed traditional dances and choreographies, and part of the programme included male patients as well. In front of the stage, the audience, male and female patients respectively, were seated separately on blankets and behind that were chairs, which the staff and I were invited to sit down on. Several attendants made sure that everybody found the seat that had been allotted to them. When a patient sat down beside me due to a lack of space on the blankets, an attendant immediately intervened and sent her outside. During the show, Faiza performed two solo dances. She wore a colourful sari and full jewellery attire, including bangles and earrings. Her long hair, which I was used to seeing tamed in a ponytail, was open and fell over her back and shoulders. She looked beautiful, attracted a lot of attention and her charisma flooded the stage. After the performance, I chatted with another patient, Madhushree, an educated middle-class woman from Calcutta. After some time, Faiza joined us. She had changed back into her patient frock and wore her long hair in a bun again – just the colourful bangles, which clattered together on both of her wrists, were left as a reminder of her stage appearance. Some other long-term patients had joined us as well. Faiza smiled at me, and I realized that I had never really seen her smile that brightly until that day. The atmosphere was relaxed, and the women reacted happily and joyfully when I told them that I had liked the performance, their dresses and stage appearance, and I showed them the short videos I had taken with my mobile phone. Madhushree, though preoccupied as usual with the topic of discharge and reuniting with her husband and her twenty-year-old daughter, suddenly asked Faiza if she was 'also a Bcom' (Bachelor of Commerce). 'Yes . . .', Faiza answered hesitantly. 'Ahhhh', Madhushree sighed, 'what a wasted life'. Faiza's response was a rather forced smile. Madhushree continued to bemoan how her own life was about 'to be wasted' at Asha. When Madhushree went on talking, Faiza's smile vanished completely, and she suddenly announced that she really had to go now because she felt very tired after her performance. Hastily she left in the direction of her ward.

Ratnam: The Hospital as a Safe Space

When Akshay and I entered the old age ward one morning at the beginning of September, the breakfast had just been served and mantras[1] were playing from loud speakers. We asked an attendant about the mantras, and he commented that mornings are pleasure time and that the old patients are supposed to pray to God. The mantras were played until the distribution of the medications was over. Some patients sat in front of a carrom board[2] but did not play. The atmosphere was so calm and peaceful compared to other rooms in the hospital, and Akshay said it brought to mind the fourth life ashram (*sanyās āshram*) of a Hindu male, when he is supposed to completely turn to worshipping and praying during his last phase of life.

S.K. Ratnam had been at the hospital for almost forty years and hailed from a wealthy Brahmin family in Tamil Nadu. He was sixty-four years old at the time when we met him. He used to work as a helper patient in his ward but had then got too old for it. When Akshay and I spoke to him, we conversed in a mix of English and Hindi. When we asked at the beginning of our conversation which language was more convenient for him, he replied: 'Both are convenient. Certain things I can't express in Hindi, certain things I can't express in English.' In Ratnam's file, a psychiatrist had noted the diagnosis 'chronic schizophrenia'. Ratnam was born on 7 July 1947, one month before Indian independence. 'You were born and India became free,' he remembered his father joking. Ratnam grew up in a small town in south-west Tamil Nadu and completed his Bachelor of Science in Chemistry. During his third year of studies, when he was nineteen years old, he suffered his first 'mental attack'. Subsequently, he received 'modified' as well as 'unmodified' ECT treatment, and the doctors told him that he was a 'schizophrenic patient'. Ratnam was aware that 'schizophrenia' was a mental illness because his father was a doctor.

Ratnam described masturbation as one of his 'problems'. Ratnam remembered that he used to observe girls and women 'out there' but that he did not understand what exactly was going on with him. His parents did not speak about anything that concerned sex or girls. His father warned him, though, that he would 'get weak' if he masturbated too much. Ratnam thought that his 'sexual disease' could have been cured if he had been told about it in time. But nobody told him, and therefore he had masturbated regularly until only a few months back. When lunch was about to be served, we paused our conversation with Ratnam so that he could eat, and two attendants sat down with us. They shared an anecdote about Ratnam – that for over six months he used to ejaculate into an old pot of wall paint that was used for renovation work in the ward. One attendant discovered the pot and mistook it for remaining paint and thought about selling it. Both attendants laughed out loud while they were telling their story.

It was rather difficult for Ratnam to recollect what had happened during the decade after the onset of his illness. Nevertheless, he excelled in remembering the dates of certain life events. However, when Akshay and I asked him for more details, he often skipped between themes and topics: 'There is a saying in English, an idle mind is a devil's workshop, that's also my reason for illness.' Ratnam repeatedly referred us to his 'papers' (file) in order to check those details that he could not remember. Ratnam blamed ECT treatment for his poor memory: 'I was given ECT so many times, so I don't remember anything now.'

His family had to spend a lot of money on his treatment: 'My brothers and sisters faced a lot of problems because of me, so now they don't come to see me, nor do they send letters.' Both his parents were now dead, and only Ratnam's three brothers and three sisters were left. His eldest sister was twenty years older than him, and the brother who used to look after him after his parents' death was nineteen years older. Ratnam was certain about the time of his first admission to Asha: May 1974 – he was twenty-seven years old. Since then, he had been discharged and sent home four or five times. From February 1977 onwards, he started to work in the hospital office, where he helped attendants, sweepers and nurses and engaged in stapling and photocopying papers as occupational therapy. He did this work for around fifteen years, and he would also teach the daughter of a nurse for four years. Ratnam was glad that he had been allowed to stay at Asha for such a long time. He felt safe in the hospital: 'In the outside world, I don't understand anything, I don't want to go out.' He told us that the attendants took good care of him and that his stay would spare his family more troubles.

Ratnam had tried to commit suicide many times. One time he jumped into the river from a bridge in Ahmedabad. Another time he took an overdose of tablets when still at his native home in Tamil Nadu. He was saved by his father, who repeated a mantra in order to wake him up from unconsciousness. Another time he stabbed himself with a *kōytā*.[3] Many times in his life Ratnam had 'the feeling' that his mind was confused. When I probed further what he was confused about, he replied: 'I thought that I will also be able to get married. How can I get married when I am not having a job? Nowadays ladies are also demanding high . . . highly paid jobs and all that.' However, he had become less troubled by such issues over the years: 'An idle mind is the workshop of a devil; your mind in its own space can make heaven of hell or hell out of heaven.' During our conversation, Ratnam liked to cite Shakespeare, whose dramas he had read during his studies: 'The kingdom of heaven is within you.'

Ratnam had stayed in almost all the wards, except Ward 13, which was the epileptic ward. The worst ward he ever had experienced was Ward 8, the criminal ward. He was sent there when he used to have suicidal thoughts. The quantity of food that patients received there was scarce. He had to stay in a small, locked room together with four other patients, day and night. He did not befriend any other patients from this ward as they were all locked up and secluded in solitary confinement. Ratnam did not know how to handle criminal patients and was afraid of them. Nevertheless, he was aware that he had been brought there in order to be punished for his bad behaviour: 'If you sow a mango, you will receive a mango tree, if you have sowed paddy, you would receive paddy.' Ratnam hoped that if he behaved well, the attendants would also treat him well.

Eventually, Ratnam was admitted to the old age ward. In this ward, the attendants did not beat the patients, and instead of getting angry with them they would talk to them if there was any issue. Before he finally took the decision not to work any more, Ratnam used to help the sweepers. He received beedis[4] to smoke in exchange and some extra food. There were other patients in the ward who were Brahmin and vegetarian like Ratnam. They would not eat the chicken that was served on Fridays. Before the doctor prescribed a diet that included eggs, Ratnam would not eat the eggs that were served on Wednesdays either. He was aware that not many people liked to talk about caste nowadays. If he did, others would probably make fun of him: 'Because when all are having the same blood, red blood, and this science has proven now, all are human beings, no castes.' According to Ratnam, to know somebody's caste was no longer as important as it had been and therefore he did not know the caste of most of the other patients in the ward.

When Akshay and I checked Ratnam's file, we came across a letter from his brother, who came across as an educated and very eloquent person. He expressed regret that he could not care for his younger brother himself. He and his wife were aged and had meanwhile moved back to Tamil Nadu. The letter also contained some reasons why it was so difficult to keep Ratnam with them: he once tried to kill himself with tablets, and every time he had come back from the hospital so far he had soon become restless because everybody was busy with their daily life. Additionally, the file indicated that Ratnam had had 'problems' with the opposite sex. There was also a copy of a letter that was sent to Ratnam's family after a failed attempt at rehabilitation. It suggested that it might be Ratnam's fate to remain at Asha: 'All along he has felt free and at liberty in the hospital.' The last letter was dated September 2009 and written by another of Ratnam's brothers. He stated that his brothers and sisters could neither take care of him nor visit him because they lived in other places and were too old to travel. All costs for Ratnam's treatment and his accommodation, as a matter of course, would be continued to be covered by his family.

Akshay and I, who both enjoyed our encounter with the eloquent and intelligent Ratnam, tried to meet and speak to him again after the interview. But Ratnam did not feel well and therefore declined to converse with us.

'Mental', 'Normal' and 'Helper' Patients

Patients often vehemently stressed that they were not 'mental' patients but instead understood themselves as 'helpers' who use to support the attendants with their work. Abdul, for example, insisted that he was not like other patients and that he was not '*pāgal bigal*' (mad). Abdul described the everyday issues that surfaced in the ward in a rather blunt way. He perceived most of the patients in the admission ward to be 'mental' patients who would 'eat and shit in the same place'. They smelled of urine, and 'normal' patients like Abdul had to endure it while staying with them. As one of the fifteen helper patients in the ward, he had to manage situations where 'mentals' picked a fight or became violent. Helper patients were supposed to interfere and beat up those patients who irritated others. After disciplining them, they would call a nurse, who then came to give the troublemakers an injection that put them to sleep. Completely uncontrollable patients were locked up in an isolation room until they had calmed down. Abdul realized, though, that most of the helper patients had been 'mental' themselves at one point in time. However, ECT treatment and medication had helped them to recover. Once a patient had recovered, he would leave the admission ward. Nobody stayed there longer than six months. Either a patient's relatives turned up to take them home or they were transferred to another ward 'where they would eventually die', as Abdul expressed it.

Attendants and helper patients often developed close relationships and would sit together and chat and joke with each other. Their relationship was framed by the exchange of favours and goods. Attendants would give helper patients items like shoes and underwear in return for their help in the ward. Female helper patients were allowed to wear jewellery, which was otherwise forbidden at the hospital. Around the time of religious festivals, female attendants also sometimes brought in henna cones so that helper patients could do mehndi.[5] At times, helper patients were paid in tobacco or attendants would buy for them certain items from the outside – often snacks like *vaḍāpāv*[6] or wafers.

Nikhat: An Orphan and Helper Patient

Nikhat Ali Khan was one of the helper patients in the admission ward. Rini and I first met her in July 2011, when we entered the ward one lunch time. She was in her early twenties and had an authoritarian habitus and proud posture. In contrast to other patients who were bossed around by attendants, she could move around in the ward more freely. I overheard the attendants calling her 'Nikhi' and observed her joking around with the attendants. In the mornings, Nikhat used to assist the nurses in distributing medicines. From time to time, I observed her giving certain patients something from a purse that she carried under her blouse. Lunch in the admission ward was served in a long corridor outside of a big dorm room that accommodated around sixty patients. During the night, the women slept here on five beds and several mattresses that were spread out on the floor. During lunch, patients sat on two blankets set out by attendants and helper patients on each side of the corridor. The food, in a huge container, was carried down the corridor by two helper patients while a third, Nikhat, scooped it onto the patients' plates with a big ladle. When we spoke to Nikhat later in the afternoon, she told us she used to eat lunch together with the attendants in a small staff chamber next to the entrance gate of the unit after the other patients had finished theirs.

Nikhat was admitted to the hospital in 2006 because she regularly experienced fits. At that time, she was twenty-one years old. In her file it was mentioned that she suffered from 'epilepsy' and a 'behavioural disorder' with a 'suicide tendency', 'purposeful vomiting' and that she at times had to be forced to eat something. In April 2011, she was declared 'unfit for discharge'. Nikhat hailed from a Muslim family in Aurangabad. When she was nine years old, her parents married her off to an eighteen-year-old boy. She was not happy to be married at such an early age, but her parents did not give in to her pleading to be allowed to stay at home a little longer. 'In case we die, there will be no one to take care of you. Therefore, it is better for you to settle down and get married now,' they explained to her. On the day of marriage itself, Nikhat ran away from her husband's home. Before the police finally picked her up and sent her to an orphanage, Nikhat had completed nine years living on the streets. She had a brother and three sisters who were all older than Nikhat when they had married. They knew her whereabouts and had visited her at Asha once. At times, her uncle came to visit her, too. According to Nikhat, her parents did not know that she lived in a psychiatric hospital.

Nikhat did not like wearing her patient uniform and enjoyed it when she got to wear colourful saris that were given to her by the attendants in the context of festivals like Diwali. Nikhat stated that she did not engage in hitting or physically disciplining patients. If they did not obey, they would be locked up in solitary cells. Attendants, too, claimed that this was how they usually handled patients' disobedient behaviour. However, patients from Nikhat's ward stated that they were beaten up by attendants regularly. Nikhat did not perceive herself as a patient. Instead, she behaved like and talked from the position of an attendant. She used to prepare tea and special food for the attendants, particularly on their fasting days.[7] Because Nikhat occupied a rather high position in the ward's hierarchy, she did not have to do the 'dirty' work, like cleaning the toilets and bathrooms or taking care of 'chronic' and 'unstable' patients and giving them sanitary pads when they menstruated. Latter tasks she delegated to helper patients of a subordinate status.

Nikhat told Rini and me that she had not liked staying at Asha in the beginning. But she had got used to her life in the hospital, and she hoped not to be sent back to the orphanage.

Like Nikhat, many other helper patients also closely resembled attendants and were equipped with the right to discipline fellow patients physically. When we asked her about routines in the ward, Nikhat's identification with the attendants was illustrated by the fact that she spoke of them in terms of 'we'. It was distinctive for the female wards that superior helper patients did not have to engage in any 'dirty' (impure) chores and that they enjoyed the privilege of being invited to eat together with the attendants. From time to time, attendants even treated them to home-cooked or non-veg food or sweets. Reciprocally, helper patients used to prepare tea and food for the attendants.

In the male wards, helper patients used to eat together with fellow patients, even if they were privileged and enjoyed a slightly larger meal portion. However, male helper patients were allowed to sleep outside the common dorm room and at times in a separate room near the locked ward room at night. Female helper patients were only allowed to do so during the day. Mahesh told us that as a helper patient in one of the chronic wards he would help the sweepers to distribute food, wash the utensils afterwards, do the laundry and hang clothes up for drying. When family members came to visit, Mahesh was supposed to bring the respective patient from the locked ward room and hand him over to attendants who then accompanied him to the visiting room. As a helper patient, he did not take a bath with the other patients or share the bathroom. All helper patients in his ward were provided with extra soap from the attendants. They used to break it into pieces and distribute it among each other.

Devendra: A Police Constable

Devendra Yadav was a 48-year-old Maharashtrian who worked as a helper patient in one of the male wards. Akshay and I carried out his interview underneath the staircase in the corridor. Devendra agreed that he would speak with us if we gave him ten rupees. He planned to give the money to one of the sweepers, who would then bring him some tobacco. After we had handed him the banknote, Devendra allowed us to start asking our questions. He seemed confident, self-assured and assertive.

In the mornings, he helped to wake up all patients and took care of storing the mattresses that were put on the ground during the night for those patients who did not have a bed. During the distribution of the medications, he made sure that all sixty-four patients sat in line and nobody missed out on their dose. He helped with changing the bed sheets and cleaning the ward floor. Devendra told us that in exchange for helping the attendants with their work they would treat him well. Additionally, he was allowed to keep a personal shaving kit that his sister had brought him. Other patients had to wait for the ward barber. According to Devendra, the barber used to shave eight patients with just one blade, and therefore he was glad that he could use his own razor and shaving cream. The only thing attendants would not allow him to keep was a mobile phone, because the other 'mental' patients would use it to call their relatives and ask them to come and take them home. Devendra did not use to hang out with the other patients; he was rather aloof and would sit reading the newspaper during the day. He slept in a separate room together with seven other helper patients. His room was clean and had a TV; they used to watch a movie before going to sleep. Besides this he was not treated any differently to anyone else in the ward: he got the same food, and his uniform was changed once a week, like the others. If Devendra felt that his uniform was getting dirty in between, he washed it and left it to dry overnight. Devendra also used to wash together with everyone else in the big shower room. One hose pipe was held by one or two sweepers and everybody had to get naked and stand in front of the jet of water. Up to five patients washed at the same time. Soap and towels were provided by the attendants, and in this manner all patients were usually washed within half an hour. After a while, Devendra did not care any more about getting naked in front of the other patients: 'All are gents!' Of course, the new patients would at first often feel reluctant to remove their clothes, but after some time they all got used to it. If a patient was not able to wash himself, helper patients would step in. According to Devendra, discrimination on the basis of caste or religion did not exist in the ward: 'Everybody mixes with everyone. Nobody is interested in knowing anybody's surname.'[8] However, when Devendra asked for Akshay's name some minutes later and Akshay only told him his first name, Devendra asked for his surname as well.

Devendra appeared agitated during our conversation. He repeatedly got up, walked around and seemed to be nervous and unfocused. At one point, Devendra showed us a newspaper article about a friend who worked at a nearby police station and was awarded for good service 102 times. Devendra, a police constable himself and in service for thirty years, hoped that he would clear fifty awards during the next five years. Akshay asked him why he first used to come to the hospital. 'Because of the drinks,' Devendra answered. He was aware that he did not look like a *dāruīyā* (drunkard), he added, but at times, and particularly with friends, he used to consume hard alcohol. And once he had started drinking, he could go on with it for fifteen days straight. He would declare that he did not feel well and take sick leave from work. Devendra suddenly got up and went to get his purse from the top of the staircase, which he used to store some of his personal belongings. He took out a letter from his office and handed it over to Akshay. 'Here it is written that you have schizophrenia,' Akshay said in a tone of wonderment. Devendra stated that he understood what was written in the letter about alcohol, mental illness, his symptoms and why he was *veḍsar* (insane) – he had this knowledge due to his studies of psychology during his BA. Devendra's purse additionally contained a photo, which he proudly presented to us. It showed him in his police uniform. Devendra used to come home from drinking very late at night, at which point he would drink tea and coffee to sober up but he then could not sleep and so stayed up watching TV instead. His wife would always get angry with him. He felt the only solution to his situation was to come to Asha. According to Devendra, a doctor would have just told him to quit drinking and suggest joining an 'alcohol analysis' group.

During our conversation, another patient named Ajay (see Chapter 7) approached me and asked if I had called his uncle. I informed him that I had not but felt slightly bad because I could not remember whether I had promised him I would call or not. Devendra stood up and putting his hands on Ajay's shoulders guided him back to the locked ward room. After the incident, Devendra shared with us that patients who got too 'excited' and continuously said that they wanted to go home were given an 'injection' in the evenings in order to calm them down and put them to sleep. Devendra and the other helper patients would feed them at dinner time and calm them down in case they started to cry. The medicine that Devendra used to take while at Asha had helped him to sleep in the evenings, and the hospital had structured his daily life, which he wanted to continue at home as well: 'Lunch at lunch time, breakfast at breakfast time and duty at duty time!' On the day we spoke to Devendra, his relatives were about to come to take him home: 'They might have already arrived.'

Resisting the Uniform

A patient's uniform is most salient in marking low status in the ward hierarchy. Particularly women were not comfortable with wearing the barely knee-length frocks and often complained about their clothing. The superintendent was aware of the shortcomings of the uniform and of female patients' unhappiness with it. His long-term plan was to add a design to the uniform, which at that time was just green, blue and red. This measure, though, did not address the most important concern the women had, which was with the inappropriate length of the frock. At the time of my research, it was impossible for the superintendent as well the hospital staff in general to imagine a different style of uniform or no uniform at all.

Sarika: A Failed Housewife

When Sarika N. Prakash was admitted to Asha, she had to get rid of everything personal, including her dress and underwear. When she asked for a new set of underwear, she received underpants that were too big and a bra that turned out to be undersized. In contrast to most other patients, Sarika had her own bed, which had been allotted to her by Faiza at the time she was transferred to the ward. Additionally, she enjoyed the luxury of a locker beside her bed, in which she used to store some personal belongings. Among them were her own soap and a pair of sandals that she received in the OTD for being a 'good patient', as she stated. Moreover, she kept her pyjamas in the locker. She used to wear them when she left the female unit in order to have a phone call with her father in the superintendent's office. 'They are very conservative here,' she commented and told me about being required to change the frock whenever she left the female unit. Compared to most other female patients she did not see any issue regarding the frock's length: 'I mean, even if

I did wear the frock, what would people get to see that they are not supposed to?'

Sarika was just hanging out with Faiza when I met her for the first time in June 2011. During the following months, I often encountered the two women together. They shared an educated, middle-class background and both spoke good English. I asked them for their age during our first conversation, and they told me that they were in their early thirties. A little later, I learnt that both were in their early forties after they had allowed me to have a look at their files. Like Faiza, Sarika took care of several tasks in the ward. While Faiza took care of the beds in the mornings, it was Sarika's duty in the evenings.

Sarika was born to a Hindu middle-class family in Calcutta, and her father divorced her mentally ill mother when she was still very young.[9] Around her fifth birthday, her father took her and her brother to Florida, where she lived until the early 1990s. She met her future husband, a Punjabi, when her father had taken them on a business trip to South Africa. Sarika fell in love, and they ran away to Nigeria. When the two got married, Sarika was eighteen years old, and she soon became pregnant. In 1993, shortly after giving birth to their second son, the family decided to move to Mumbai. After moving to India, though, Sarika struggled with her isolated life as a housewife and with having no friends and contacts in the new city. Conflict with her husband emerged. He was rarely at home and used to spank the children. She started to feel she had lost control over her life, began to lock up the children in the apartment and would wander the streets alone. When her husband came to know about her outings, he did not allow her to re-enter the apartment, and Sarika was banished to the streets. Finally, she was picked up by the police, who brought her to Asha in April 2010.

When I met Sarika in the ward more than a year after her admission, she did not understand why she had had to stay in a psychiatric hospital. She took her medications regularly and had also received ECT treatment at the beginning of her stay, even if, according to her, the treatment had been 'useless' and not changed anything. Sarika shared her sorrows and problems with me. She talked about how she missed her two sons, that her husband had filed for divorce and that she had filed a lawsuit because her husband had beaten her and the children. Sarika told me about the moment she discovered that her husband had been having an affair with a woman who regularly visited their home. 'She ate my food!', she exclaimed. However, her husband had claimed that she was 'just a friend', but according to Sarika, even her sons knew that this was a lie.

According to Sarika's file, she suffered from 'schizoaffective excitement', while the social worker of the ward told me that her diagnosis was 'schizophrenia'. Sarika's file noted shortly after her admission her 'unkempt' appearance, her 'aggressiveness' and 'irrelevant talking' and that she was 'uncooperative'. A note had been added recently that she suffered from the 'delusion' that 'people outside are plotting against her, preventing her from going to her father'. Furthermore, her insight was labelled as 'poor' and her judgement as 'impaired'. Additionally, a nurse had noted her 'grandiosity' and quoted her as saying: 'I have a lot of money, so people behave badly with me.' At the time of our encounter, her main preoccupation was to be discharged. All her hopes laid with her father, who worked as a business man in the United States and had financially supported her ever since she ran away with the man she had once been in love with. In order to discharge Sarika, her father would have to come to India and take care of everything personally.

But although Sarika regularly talked to her father on the phone, he did not seem to be planning a trip to India any time soon. Sarika looked sad when she told me about her family. Her two sons had stayed with her sister-in-law for some time after the separation from her husband. Accompanied by two students of social work, a social worker and a psychiatrist, she had visited the place of her sister-in-law several weeks ago. After the delegation had arrived there though, they discovered that she was not living at this place any longer. Neighbours gave them her new address and phone number. Eventually, Sarika's father told her that her husband had left India together with their two sons to move to South Africa. The superintendent, when I discussed Sarika's case with him, called her father a 'nasty person': though he called his daughter regularly, he refused to take over responsibility.

For women admitted to Asha, the uniform limited gendered practices of social distinction, including particular ways of dressing and decorating their bodies that would usually be exercised by them away from Asha. With these restraints in mind, the hospital asked visitors and students not to give any jewellery or clothing to female patients. For women living in Asha, their appearance nevertheless remained an important part of everyday life, and jewellery still found a way into the wards, often as a present from the attendants or visiting relatives. Women who became friends used to gift each other bracelets and rings. Those who used to perform on special occasions and religious festivals enjoyed displaying themselves in a sari and full jewellery attire on the stage, as Faiza did during the Ganpati celebrations.

Fashion and body decoration and modification were themes that female patients often discussed with me and amongst each other, as illustrated by Sarika and Faiza. They shared their plans with me to lose some weight because they wanted to 'look good'. Accordingly, at the beginning of my research, I often encountered Sarika in the OT, where she regularly came to do some exercise on the training bike. During one of our encounters, they commented on my traditional Indian clothes, which I used to wear while doing fieldwork at Asha. They straightened out my *chūḍīdār*[10] as they said that I was wearing it in a very disorganized way. Faiza remembered that even though she had liked to wear particular suits, her husband had always preferred her in Western clothing. Sarika added that she was not interested in wearing traditional Indian clothes but preferred Western dress; for example, jeans and T-shirt and that she liked Western music and to dance in the disco. She had always preferred to wear big, modern earrings, lipstick and high heels when going out. She repeatedly stressed, though, that she had also always been a 'tip-top' housewife and used to wear a nighty and flat shoes at home. Sarika stated that she felt ready for an 'American husband' and that she would happily consent to such a marriage if her father arranged it for her. 'In America they like housewives now,' she stated. When I met Sarika again in January 2012, her close friendship with Faiza had come to an end. I almost did not recognize Faiza when I encountered her on the hospital premises, because she had gained a lot of weight. She was hanging out with another woman, with whom she seemed to be very close and whom she called 'her wife'. I observed how she used to boss her around as she previously did Sarika.

Distinguishing Habitus

Asha is a place that 'patientizes' and 'depersonalizes' persons. As a typical total institution, Asha regulates and uniformizes in manifold ways the everyday routines and practices taking place behind its walls (Goffman 1968). Nevertheless, the social life and sociocultural norms and values outside the hospital walls are never completely forgotten or considered meaningless inside Asha (Zaman 2005; Bandyopadhyay 2010). The uniform did not eradicate one's social status completely. A patient's community or caste background was often still palpable in their habitus and their speech during interactions.

Rekha: A Traditional Hindu Wife

Rini and I encountered Rekha Mohan Kamble on the steps of the OT department. She was busy doing embroidery on a *tōraṇ*[11] – an activity she used to engage in regularly. We found a table to sit at in the department; she had asked the occupational therapist's permission to be interviewed because she was worried that she could be blamed for lazing around and not doing anything.

Rekha felt her stay at Asha was abhorrent with all the 'mentally ill' people. She was not allowed to keep her own clothes when she was admitted, and if she wanted to groom herself, she had no other choice but to use the ward comb, which was infested with lice. 'Even if you are not mad, you have to live like you are,' she commented. Rekha had to report everything she did to the hospital authorities. Other patients used to sleep on her bed, and because Rekha found that the dishes had not been cleaned properly, she had started to fast regularly. She described how difficult it was to keep hold of one's own soap or anything else because 'mentally unstable' patients were prone to stealing everything. Rekha had started to keep her drawing book and a pencil away on the windowsill to prevent others from taking it. 'I was a good housewife from a respected family. I wasn't from a third-class family. Now my position as a housewife has been snatched away from me, too. I won't get that respect any longer. Everybody calls me mad,' she mourned. However, Rekha repeatedly stressed during our conversation that ultimately it was God's wish that she stay at Asha and that she would keep invoking his name (pray). Rekha kept herself busy with knitting and reading the newspaper to keep her mind engaged. She was aware that many of Asha's patients chew tobacco in order to pass time, but she strongly despised this habit and did not like it if anybody approached her and asked for some.

Rekha was admitted to Asha by her brother in June 2011 – roughly one month before we spoke to her. According to her file, she was 'abusive' and 'aggressive', and she had not been sleeping much at the time of her admission. Her appearance was described as well kept, but her affect was 'inappropriate'. She received the diagnoses: 'affective psychosis', 'B. affection disorder', 'schizo-affective disorder' (which was later crossed out) and 'bipolar disorder'. The onset of her mental illness seemed to have taken place gradually over the course of seven to eight years. While she told us that she was forty-three years old, she was fifty-seven according to her file. Rekha told us about her family, who originally lived in Kacch, belonging to the Kacchi community in Gujarat. Rekha grew up with six sisters and one brother. Her father was a goldsmith, and the family was well off, belonging to the middle class. Rekha stressed in front of us that the family led a very religious life and observed days like *pōrṇima* (full moon) and *amāvas* (new moon) and every fast during festivals. They worshipped 'mother-cow' and did a lot of charity work. The family had cows and buffaloes and was never short of milk. They also possessed a piece of land and had the money to hire labourers to help with the work on the fields. Rekha got married in Bombay when she was nineteen years old. It was a traditional Hindu marriage, *kanyādān*. She was ritually handed over to the husband's family by her brother because her father had died ten days before her marriage. Rekha had been married for thirty-one years and had given birth to two daughters before her husband died. After her husband's death, her in-laws threw her out of the house, and she moved in with her brother. Then her brother's wife died, and according to Rekha, this event caused the family a lot of stress. Therefore, she moved out of her brother's house and was finally admitted to Asha by her brother against her will. Rekha was not aware of any medical problem she suffered from and felt that her stay in the hospital was unjustified. She had the impression that her family wanted to get rid of her. Rekha agreed to the admission to the hospital because she did not want to burden their lives.

The eldest daughter had studied commerce and was already married; the youngest one had studied arts and lived with her sister's family in north Mumbai. Rekha was worried that her daughters were upset with her because she had 'gone mad'. They had not yet come to see her at Asha, and Rekha doubted whether her brother had even told them her whereabouts. Rekha wished to be discharged and go back and live with her brother, who regularly came to see her at Asha. He had promised to take her back home soon and rent a second flat for her. Rekha, however, suspected his words were empty promises. Rekha would never consider staying at her elder daughter's place, because it was inappropriate for women of their community to take care of their ageing mother. This was the obligation of the daughter-in-law. Rekha was concerned that her younger daughter would not find a groom if she studied too much. Rekha herself had studied until the seventh grade and her husband until the tenth grade. He was the only one in the family who could speak English and would from time to time try to encourage Rekha to join an English class. Rekha said that she had shared a good relationship with her husband until he had fallen for *pīne kī ādat* (the drinking habit). Before her husband began to drink regularly, he used to stand up for her and fight for her cause, like when her in-laws would not allow her to go and see her daughters. His brother was the one who got him into drinking. Rekha and her husband did not stay with his parents, but when his mother called him, he would go to see her immediately. And when he eventually came back home from her place, he randomly used to blame Rekha. Rekha felt that life would have turned out better for her if she had given birth to a son instead of a second daughter.

Rini started to cry after she had heard Rekha's story, and Rekha, noticing Rini's reaction, commented: 'Your eyes well up listening to my plight!' When Rini and I reflected on her emotional reaction sometime later, we identified it as a countertransference: she felt herself in the position of a caring daughter, shocked about the fact that somebody could abandon their ageing mother in a psychiatric hospital. When we encountered Rekha some days later in the OT department, she remembered our faces but seemed to be unaware that we had had a lengthy conversation. Rekha started to converse with Rini in Gujarati but did not react when she tried to switch to Hindi – the language in which we conducted the interview. We met Rekha again three weeks later on Rini's last day at Asha, before she had to leave to Sweden. Rekha asked Rini her caste. Rini, who felt uncomfortable answering the question,[12] evaded it by saying that she was a 'Hindu'.

'Rosie': A Fallen Model and Actress

In the case of Rosie, her social status as a model and actress and her distinctive, well-off family and community background became even more accentuated in the context of the mental hospital.

Rini and I encountered Roshani 'Rosie' Seth in the admission ward at the end of July 2011. We observed a psychiatrist doing her morning round. Some of the patients inquired about their medicines and why they had to take them. Monotonously and without even looking up from the file in front of her, to which she was adding some notes, the psychiatrist could only explain that it was necessary. One of the patients caught our attention when she asked in English why she was receiving ECT treatment. When the psychiatrist responded that this treatment measure was definitely 'required', the patient started to cry and became very agitated. Surprisingly for us, nobody seemed to pay attention to the flustered young woman. Rini and I invited the sobbing woman to have a talk with us outside in the corridor, where we took three chairs and asked her to sit down with us.

The woman introduced herself to us as 'Rosie'. She told us that the name 'Roshani', which was mentioned in her file, had been noted down in order to confuse her. She did not remember her last name and asked us to give her a surname that we thought suited her. Rosie was brought to Asha by the police after her bank account was blocked and her landlord threw her out from her flat in a well-off neighbourhood. She had come to Mumbai to pursue a modelling career. She shared with us that she thought that 'they' might have done all this to her on purpose. She perceived her stay at Asha to be part of a movie plot that portrayed her life as a beggar and her survival in a psychiatric hospital. She pointed out that there were small cameras installed all over the hospital premises and in the ward. Given the extraordinary work conditions, Rosie expected 'them' to pay her extra after this shoot was finally over.

Rosie told us that she grew up in an orphanage. She was then adopted, but her adoptive parents had not treated her well. She complained that her body and head hurt after she received ECT treatment. During our conversation, she repeatedly picked lice from her hair. 'Oh my god!' she exclaimed in a theatrical voice in these moments and almost started to cry again. 'I have to sleep with these people,' she said, pointing in the direction of the dorm room, and then she apologized for her unkempt appearance. When I suggested to her that she could ask one of the nurses for some anti-lice shampoo, she immediately turned towards a nurse who was sitting nearby and asked her for it. The nurse informed her that the shampoo was out of stock, and we promised Rosie we would bring her some when we next visited her ward.

Rosie had been admitted to Asha ten days before our encounter. We came to know about this when we had a look at Rosie's file. She was in her mid-twenties, and the ward psychiatrist had diagnosed her as 'schizophrenic paranoid'. A nurse had added a note about a particular 'perception' that led her to feel that she was 'with Barack Obama'.

Four days later, Rini and I visited Rosie again. She told us about the ECT treatment that she had again received and that it caused her to feel a little dazed and furthermore impaired her memory. She appeared calmer and less moody than the last time we met her. She told us that she had been living on the streets since 2008. The police picked her up over a month ago and eventually admitted her to Asha. The moment she had spotted the board stating 'mental hospital' at Asha's entrance gate it shocked her. The police officers had not informed her about where they were taking her. Rosie was delighted when we handed over a small bottle of anti-lice solution. We noticed the fact that Rosie's name and ward number had been written on her under arm. Rosie explained to us that this was done before every ECT treatment so that the hospital staff knew which ward a patient belonged to. On Rosie's left arm, several parallel running scars caught our attention. They seemed to have originated from cuts, and without hesitation Rini asked Rosie if she used to cut herself. Rosie nodded bashfully and murmured that there was this pressure inside her which she had tried to get rid of. She then stroked the marks repeatedly during the rest of our conversation.

She asked us to call the police officer who had brought her to the hospital to ask him if he would discharge her. She told us that the ward psychiatrists had put her off with the remark that she would be discharged within a month's time. She suddenly became very disgruntled when we suggested to her that her family might discharge her instead of the police officer. She told us that she had broken ties with them and did not want to contact them ever again. Her 'real' parents died when she was born, and the parents who pretended to be her parents did not behave as such. Therefore, she had been raised by her uncle and aunt. She blamed her family for delaying her film career for five long years, and therefore held them responsible for the fact that she had not yet become a famous actress. She had had all the important contacts in the film industry and had even written a script; only the actors and a music director were missing. When people saw a photograph of her during a casting, they exclaimed: 'Oh my god, we found our actress.' Of course, right now she was in the middle of an important film shooting, although she disliked that the role of beggar and mentally ill person had been enforced on her without her consent. 'They should have let me take my own decisions!' she protested, 'Why they decided things for me?'

At the end of our conversation, Rosie complained about one of the attendants, who had beaten her. She had resisted when she was asked to eat together with the other patients after returning from the ECT treatment. Rosie asked a helper patient, whom she had befriended, to go and report the attendant's behaviour to the ward nurse. Subsequently, the nurse called over the attendant to interview her about the event. The attendant's version of the incident was that Rosie was very picky when it came to her food and had requested chicken and gravy. Furthermore, she had asked the attendant to serve her before the other patients because she was concerned about their bad hygiene. The attendant argued that she had had to discipline Rosie for her impudence and if she had not beaten her first, she might have been the one beaten up by Rosie. After she had listened to the attendant's statement, the nurse simply let the matter rest.

The life and social status that patients occupied outside the hospital were never fully eradicated – even in the case of long-term patients. Similar to Rosie's case, the habitus of Devendra, the police constable, was accentuated by his position inside the ward. Asking us for money before he allowed us to start interviewing him, he reinforced the stereotype of the corrupt Indian police officer (see Chapter 6). Akshay and I met Devendra again on the first day of Ganpati on the hospital premises. He wore streetwear, and I almost did not recognize him. He was in need of a certificate for his work. Unfortunately, though, it was a holiday, so no administrative staff who could issue his document was present. Devendra opened his purse and gave ten rupees to us. At first, Akshay refused to take it, but Devendra did not give in. He explained to us that one should not sin, and one was supposed to correct one's bad deeds during a religious festival. He did not appear as self-confident and assured as he had a month ago inside the ward. Instead, I got the impression of an insecure and fragile man. He was accompanied by one of his relatives when we encountered him yet again sometime later. At this time, he ignored us and avoided any eye contact.

Food: Marker of Intimacy and Belonging

Female patients generally commented on and complained about the quality of the food more often than male patients. Rosie, for example, was concerned about the cleanliness of the plates and asked the attendants for non-veg food – a demand indicating her upper-middle-class background and the fact that she would have been able to afford to eat meat regularly. The centrality of food practices in the female wards can be understood as linked to the role that food plays in a woman's life outside the hospital. Its preparation, consumption and distribution is pivotal to social and family life and practices of social distinction in India in general (Marriot 1968; Roncaglia 2013; Solomon 2015). Women are in charge of the preparation of food in the domestic sphere and of serving it to their husbands, children and the husband's extended family. Who eats the food prepared by them is meaningful and indicates intimacy and belonging. This is expressly illustrated by Sarika's exclamation 'She ate my food!' when she told me about her husband's affair. Sarika perceived the other woman to have invaded her domestic space, consuming the family's food and the man Sarika perceived as belonging to her. She told me that she sometimes used to prepare *capātī* for the attendants. But even though she had liked to cook for her children and her husband, she despised preparing food for anybody else other than her family. Sarika disliked the hospital food in general, which, according to her, was very 'watery'. Moreover, the tea, according to her description, tasted like somebody had 'added tobacco to it'.

Not surprisingly, poisoning by strangers, envious persons or 'new' family members such as daughter-in-laws are widely associated with mental or possession illnesses in the Indian context (Nichter 1981; H. Bennett 1989; Basu 2008).

Jennifer: Delusions of 'Black Magic'

Jennifer could trace her problems back to being fed poisoned chocolate. I encountered Jennifer Michael D'Monte in the admission ward when I wanted to have a look into the files of patients I had spoken with the previous day. When I entered the ward, some of the attendants held sticks, which they were using to direct patients to sit in the corridor. I recognized the fearful expression of some of the patients as they hastily sat down on a blanket that was spread out on the floor. Here they waited until they were called to collect their medicines one after the other. On another blanket in front of the nurses' room, patients waited to be medically examined. A nurse took a blood sample from a girl while an attendant held her hand. She wore glasses and seemed to be in pain. Sometime later, the girl approached me when I was just preparing to leave the ward. I was a little puzzled when she told me that she had seen my photograph in the OTD. She conversed in Hindi, and I was not sure if I had understood her correctly. I apologized for my bad language skills, and I told her that we might get the chance to talk again during the next few days when I planned to return to Asha with Rini.

Indeed, some days later Rini and I encountered the girl with the glasses again. We spotted her in the OTD, and she agreed to talk to us and did not mind us recording the conversation. Jennifer spoke in a rather low voice throughout the interview so that the other patients in the OTD could not overhear. Jennifer was twenty-four years old, belonged to a Christian family and lived in north Mumbai. Immediately after hearing this, Rini disclosed that she was from a Christian family, too. Jennifer was in her second year of college and was upset about missing so much of her studies due to being at Asha. Jennifer had been admitted because of her 'depression', a problem that started when she was fourteen years old. She suffered from headaches, was scared and had been unable to study for her tenth standard board exam. She used to sit on her bed and think a lot about her future and what would happen to her if she could not complete her exam, even though she was first in her class. Jennifer had stopped eating and was unable to get out of bed. Her hair, really long at the time, had started to fall out. Jennifer related her problems to an incident when she was gifted a chocolate bar by a girl. She was sure she had added some *ashuddh shakti* (impure power) to it. After she ate the chocolate, she had started to throw up frequently and began to fear the presence of other people. When Jennifer stayed at home, she was usually fine, but whenever she tried to go to school she started throwing up again. Finally, after not receiving an appropriate diagnosis for two years, she underwent an appendectomy. Additionally, her professor, social workers, two priests from her community and her principal helped her to recover and prayed for her. She was repeatedly admitted to several hospitals, where she used to receive glucose injections. During her last admission to Asha, her health deteriorated severely: she could not eat or drink anything and had become very thin with a tired-looking face. Additionally, when she menstruated, she used to bleed for an entire month instead of her usual four days and it comprised black clots.

According to the psychiatrist's notes in Jennifer's file, her diagnosis was 'schizoaffective disorder'. At the time of her admission, her behaviour was described as 'abusive and uncooperative'. Another note on one of the observation sheets mentioned a 'delusion of black magic' – an expression that probably referred to Jennifer's story about the 'poisoned' chocolate. The sociocultural 'explanatory model' (EM) (Kleinman 1989: 121) that relates (mental) affliction to poisoning or the intake of impure substances apparently became transformed into a psychiatric symptom and an indication of a 'disturbed' (delusional) mind in the context of modern psychiatry.

Jennifer felt that her parents had 'tricked' her into being admitted to the hospital. They told her that they would be attending a retreat but instead brought her to Asha and convinced her to sign the admission form. Jennifer remembered changing into the patient uniform and leaving the green *chūḍīdār* that she had worn on that day. Her mother had accompanied her until the entrance gate of the female unit.

Her mother suffered from a mental illness herself. She had told Jennifer about her own admission to Asha. She used to think that somebody might have mixed something into her tea, but Jennifer suspected that her mother's illness was connected to falling in love with her father and the disapproval of the match by his father. Although her mother was very beautiful, her family was not very wealthy. Furthermore, her father died when she was five years old, and she was taken care of by a priest. The couple was only able to get married after Jennifer's grandfather had died. Jennifer's mother was thirty-two at that time, and Jennifer's father knew about his wife's mental issues. After the marriage, Jennifer's mother seemed happy and fine until she became pregnant with Jennifer. Her husband worked in Dubai as an asphalt plant operator while she stayed at home alone in Mumbai. She had a troubled relationship with some of the neighbours, and one day somebody threw a dead cat in front of the door. From then onwards, Jennifer's mother behaved in a paranoid manner. She became pregnant a second time with Jennifer's sister, and even though her husband was present at this time, problems occurred. According to Jennifer, the pain her mother experienced during giving birth 'hit her brain'. When she started to undress herself in public and to beat people for no apparent reason, her family decided to admit her to Asha, where she received ECT treatment. The family's neighbours started to refer to Jennifer and her sister as 'the children of the mad woman'. According to Jennifer, people just do not understand the difference between 'being mad' (*veḍṃ*) and 'going into depression'.

Jennifer described her father as a drunkard who used to beat her. Because of her and her mother's health problems, her father had to leave his job in Dubai. He had spent a lot of money on alcohol and on Jennifer's treatment, and he even had to sell his wife's gold jewellery. Jennifer felt hungry and thirsty all the time,[13] and she fought a lot with her father about her eating habits and becoming fat. She had attempted suicide once. This occurred at a time when she had felt mistreated by her father, was not doing well in school and did not have any friends. Jennifer remembered that her father had started to beat her when her mother's illness became worse. While he also used to beat her mother and her maternal grandmother, he had never touched her younger sister. She taught at a preschool and had been the only family member earning money. Jennifer had had a conflict-ridden relationship with her; while her parents came to visit her regularly in the hospital, her sister 'didn't like to see her face'. Jennifer suspected that her sister envied her fair complexion.

Jennifer's grandmother was eighty-four years old, and to Jennifer's dismay, she had problems with incontinence. Jennifer was the one who had to take care of her. She used to bathe her and trim her nails and also made sure that everybody in the family took their medication regularly. Because of her family responsibilities, Jennifer did not have much time for herself. After her father came back from Dubai and stopped earning an income, Jennifer's aunt Mary took care of some of the family's expenses. According to Jennifer, her aunt used to pamper her because she was childless herself and felt thankful that Jennifer looked after her mother. However, Mary had to stop her financial support after she discovered that she had breast cancer.

Jennifer had fallen in love with a boy who was a singer and four years younger than her. He had still never touched her, and they were committed to each other. Even though they liked each other very much, the financial situation in Jennifer's home had not allowed them to get married immediately. Jennifer, worrying about her age, wanted to get engaged soon. Jennifer was afraid that it would cause her and her family 'a lot of problems' if she remained single much longer. Jennifer had the impression that everybody looked at her with 'eyes full of lust', particularly boys from the neighbourhood and the male doctors in the hospital. She asked Rini to come a little closer in order to tell her what she had experienced in one of the hospitals: a doctor had indecently touched her breasts while examining her. After the incident, Jennifer ran out of the examination room and told her parents, but they did not take her seriously. Moreover, six boys in her neighbourhood touched her indecently, which she believed made her breasts grow to their huge size.[14] Jennifer felt ashamed about what had happened to her.

Jennifer did not like that her patient uniform was above the knee. In her opinion, a girl's body had to be dressed modestly so that nobody could 'wag one's finger at her'. She used to feel uncomfortable when she had to undress in front of everybody to wash. If she did not obey the attendants' orders, though, they would beat her. Jennifer disliked the attendants letting patients do their work; for example, cleaning the toilets and carrying the heavy water buckets.

Around noon, attendants brought some of the patients back to the ward, but Jennifer preferred to stay and talk with us. A little later, when she started to think about going back to the ward to have lunch, I offered her a chocolate bar in order to convince her to stay with us a little longer. Another patient and Rekha, who were sat in front of the OT department, had seen me giving the chocolate to Jennifer, so she grudgingly shared it with them.

In Indian sociocultural contexts, disrespect for food or inappropriate eating habits are often taken as an indicator of a mental illness by other family members (Skultans 1991: 326). This is illustrated by the complaints of a son whose mother was admitted to Asha and whom Rini and I encountered in the female visiting room. Rini and I observed how he and his mother were loudly pointing out each other's moral flaws in front of other visitors and patients. The son was furious that his mother, whom he described to us as an alcoholic suffering from psychosis, wandered around and was apparently sleeping with other men. Conversely, the mother was angry that he was beating her and that she was not allowed to see her grandchildren, whom, according to her, he did not treat well. We spoke with the son after his mother had been taken back to the ward, and he told us that she would throw food around at home and that she would demand non-veg food all the time, irrespective of the fact that he only earned eight thousand rupees per month. He thought the latter to be utterly disrespectful behaviour. As Vieda Skultans comments, a family member with a mental illness is often seen as 'either undervaluing family resources or overtaxing them' (Skultans 1991: 327). The mother's behaviour, both abnormal and incongruent with gender norms and her age, threatened the nurturing function of the family and her own role as recipient of that nurture. In this case, the son understood his mother's behaviour as a valid reason to admit her to Asha. Furthermore, he strongly appreciated the fact that patients were regularly physically disciplined by the attendants for inappropriate behaviour and hoped that these measures would put his mother on the right track again. In contrast to most other visitors, the son did not bring any snacks for his mother, reflecting their fraught relationship. The ambivalent role of food in social contexts – a source of status, nurture and intimacy on the one hand but potentially poisonous and dangerous on the other – reflects the ambivalent role the family plays for patients (see Chapter 5). This is further epitomized by the ban on families bringing cooked food into the hospital.

Social demarcation and cohesion in the male unit was not as strongly expressed through food practices as it was in the female unit. Among male patients, rather than its quality or with whom one ate, the quantity of food was the most common complaint. Rather than sharing food, male patients and attendants would sit down together in order to chew tobacco or smoke a beedi. Attendants regularly distributed chewing tobacco among patients. Sharing one's tobacco or giving a beedi to a fellow patient marked friendship. A reason Devendra, for example, felt comfortable and well treated in the hospital was that his family came to see him regularly and provided him with underwear, toothpaste and some money – items that could also be traded in for beedis from the attendants.

In general, hierarchy and social demarcation seemed to be of lesser concern in the everyday practices of the male unit. It was repeatedly stressed by attendants as well as patients themselves that they did not have to help with cleaning the ward, and if they did it was voluntary. For those patients who were interested in chewing tobacco or smoking beedis, though, helping the attendants was a good way of acquiring these. One could also get hold of these items by buying them from the attendants for a few rupees. Patients either received money from the relatives who visited them, as in Devendra's case, or from other patients' relatives, who would tip them for their services as helpers (e.g. bringing a patient to the visiting room). Even though beedis and tobacco were regularly consumed by both attendants and patients, it was officially forbidden at Asha and was perceived as a 'bad habit' by those who did not smoke.

Varun: A Retired Postman

Varun Bekaji Bhandari had been at Asha for two weeks when Akshay and I spoke to him in early September 2011. Varun had been helping the attendants to clean the ward, the dishes and the toilets and received beedis for his work rather than chewing tobacco, as he did not like it. He was sixty-one years old and like Ratnam and James stayed in the old age ward. His family lived in a village in Central Maharashtra, five hundred kilometres away from Mumbai. Varun belonged to a Kshatriya caste and grew up with four brothers and six sisters; his parents had since died. During the interview, Varun asked us for five rupees, which he planned to give to one of the sweepers, who would get him some beedis from 'outside'. For five rupees he would get one package containing twelve beedis, which he would finish off within a day. He asked us not to tell anybody about the money we gave to him. Indeed, after the interview, James asked us if we had given any money to Varun. Keeping Varun's request in mind, I responded that we had not. James told us that Varun's wife had admitted him because he no longer engaged in physical relations with her.

Varun was admitted to the hospital for the first time when he was twenty-six years old. Since then, he had come to Asha once every year. He would either stay two or three months or just for a couple of weeks. He had spent the longest time in Ward 12, the TB ward, where his TB infection had to be treated for six or seven months. Varun stated that he originally came to Asha in order to get rid of the habit of smoking beedis and to quit drinking alcohol. He started drinking when he faced sleeping problems as he realized that he could sleep well after the consumption of alcohol. When we encountered Varun, though, he had already been sober for around fifteen years. However, his wife kept admitting him to Asha because he had 'some trouble with his mind' and used to roam around and ask people for money.

Varun was a retired postman and had two sons and a daughter. Both his sons were computer engineers, and all his children were married. Varun seemed to be a little upset that they had not visited him yet. He liked the old age ward because it was clean, and the attendants would not beat the patients like they used to in other wards. The meals were served on time, and everything was taken care of well. The atmosphere was calm, and quarrels between the patients were rare, so Varun could sleep well. Additionally, the medication he received helped him to sleep.

He used to pray at one of the small ward temples in the male unit every morning. At the time we spoke to him, though, he used to go to the recreation hall, which had become a temple for the duration of the Ganpati festival. Varun told us that he was a devotee of Shirdi Sai Baba, whose framed photo he carried with him. He ritually took a bath and prayed in front of him. Thirty years ago, when Varun was admitted to Asha for the first time, patients used to wear white cotton instead of blue and green polyester uniforms. They were served *kaṇde pōhā*[15] for breakfast, and medication was administered with milk. A typical breakfast was also bread and *ūsaḷ*.[16]

During our conversation, Varun was reluctant to answer our questions and was generally not very talkative. After half an hour, Varun eventually asked us to conclude the interview. He wanted to leave to help the sweepers clean the dishes. When Akshay and I checked his file, we found Varun's diagnosis: 'chronic schizophrenia'. Additionally, his file contained a letter in which his wife had asked for a certificate that attested her husband's mental illness in order to get hold of his monthly pension of six thousand rupees. Varun's wife stated in the letter that she had to interfere because after her husband had collected the money from the post office every month, he would spend it all within half an hour, and nothing would be left for the family.

Patients at Asha employed diverse strategies of defiance and survival. Certainly, an admission to Asha strips many patients, particularly women, of their social and family status. But they adjust and accustom themselves to new social structures and hierarchies inside Asha. By building relationships with fellow patients and attendants, patients are able to access important social, emotional and material resources that equip them for life within the total institution.

Multiplied Narratives and Inconsistent Representations

The narratives of and about patients, including staff stories and statements and different paper narratives consolidated in their files, do not constitute coherent accounts but were often rather inconsistent. The different narratives that surrounded one patient seemed at times contradictory, drawing multiple and conflicting images of a person's life story and what had previously been the problem and what was still an issue (Pinto 2012). This is illustrated vividly by Faiza, whose 'case' had often been allocated to social work students. As mentioned, it was a well-known fact that Faiza enjoyed telling a slightly different story about her past to each different person who talked to her; the social work students interviewed her every other year.

Mahi, a social work student, prepared a case study about Faiza that I later found enclosed in her file. Mahi stated that Faiza desperately wanted to go home at the time of their first meeting. She described how Faiza came to Mumbai from Delhi and lived in a shared apartment. At the office, her superior 'took advantage of' (= sexually harassed) her, and she subsequently left her job. Sometime after this incident, Faiza started to roam the streets aimlessly. She did not remember how she was finally brought to Asha. Mahi hailed from Delhi herself and visited the address Faiza had given to the social workers. She found the house deserted; Faiza's family had apparently moved away. Mahi spoke to their neighbours, but nobody seemed to remember Faiza. During a personal conversation in 2011, Mahi revealed to me that towards the end of her internship she came to know more details of Faiza's story. Faiza had apparently taken up a job as a bar dancer when she had first come to Mumbai. Mahi suspected that this might be the reason why her family did not want to get in touch with her.

Another student, Sonia, was told by Faiza that her sister had married a man without her parents' knowledge. When her sister got pregnant, the family came to know about her husband and sent them both away. Faiza told Sonia that she felt that this incident had influenced her life negatively. Faiza's marriage was arranged with a man from a rich family, and her parents were not aware that he was involved in drug peddling. The couple used to travel a lot and did fall in love with each other after the marriage. When Faiza's husband died, her mother-in-law, with whom Faiza was never on very good terms, expected her to marry his younger brother. Faiza refused and went to Mumbai instead to work for Kingfisher Airlines. Her family asked her to send them three lakh rupees for a car, and a conflict arose that resulted in Faiza taking sleeping pills and being brought to Asha by the police.

Yet another narrative about Faiza I came across in a news article in the superintendent's office, where I had to wait for a psychiatrist who had promised to take me on her round through the wards. I was sat gazing idly at all the paperwork strewn on the superintendent's desk when I spotted a local newspaper report about the festival that had taken place at Asha in January that year. The article mentioned the patient 'Faiza Azis', who was described as 'a gifted dancer' that was preparing to be discharged to join her sister in Delhi. The article quoted Faiza, who said that she felt very excited about leaving the hospital. However, in reality Faiza was still at the hospital, and her file did not mention anything about being discharged let alone a return to her sister's place. Was the story made up by Faiza or by the reporter? If it was in fact the latter, Faiza's long-term stay might not have matched the objective of an article wanting to promote an image of modern mental health care and progressive psychiatric treatment.

Looking at the stories and narratives about mental illness in Indian media and popular culture, it becomes apparent that they integrate psychiatric patients' images into local contexts and traditional and popular explanation models of 'madness' and its treatment (H. Basu 2011: 74). In particular, Bollywood movies have served to shape people's image of people with a mental illness since the 1950s (Bhugra 2006; Pinto 2015). This is also apparent on present-day Indian TV programmes. Jennifer could relate her own suicide attempt to an episode of 'Hello Sakhi',[17] in which they discuss if a child's suicide attempt was the parents' fault – something that Jennifer felt was true. In recent years, the mental health movement has made increasing use of documentary films and feature films to educate and inform the public about mental health issues and their appropriate treatment (H. Basu 2018).

The portrayals of patients that comprise this and the last chapter differ concerning age, length of stay at the hospital, status and role within their respective wards, therefore they may indeed cover a broad range of aspects and experiences that concern institutionalized life in the hospital. However, they are not exhaustive and do not represent all experiences that were possible or prevalent in the hospital at the time of my research.

Notes

1. A sound or phrase that is repeated in prayer or meditation.
2. Carrom is a tabletop game that involves flicking a large, weighted wooden disc at smaller wooden discs and is very popular in South Asia.
3. A particular kind of blade that is used for harvesting in agriculture.
4. A thin cigarette or mini-cigar filled with tobacco and commonly wrapped in a leaf tied with string or bound with an adhesive at one end.
5. Mehndi is a form of temporary body art usually drawn on the hands or legs. Decorative designs are created using a paste made out of the powdered dry leaves of the henna plant.
6. Typical Maharashtrian street food that consists of a deep-fried potato dumpling inside a bread bun.
7. Staff who were Hindus often observed a fasting day in the name of a god at least once a week. Particular deities are associated with certain week days, and to fast on that particular day is believed to be beneficial and pleases that deity. The fast is usually broken in the evening after sunset.
8. Asking for somebody's surname is often equated with asking for somebody's caste. Particularly in north India surnames are an indicator of somebody's caste.
9. Sarika's story was included in Natalie Gies-Powroznik's (2016) working paper on the mental health of Indian women; they met after Sarika was discharged from Asha four years later. The summary of Sarika's life before her admission to Asha is based on this source and informal talks I had with Sarika and others.
10. Tight pants similar to leggings, usually combined with a *kurtā*.
11. A door decoration, usually a string that is embellished with marigolds and mango leaves on the occasion of Hindu festivals and weddings.
12. The constitution of India officially prohibits caste discrimination. Accordingly, some particularly middle-class Indians who perceive themselves as educated and 'modern' do not feel comfortable speaking about their caste or caste in general. Often they associate the caste system with 'backwardness'.
13. A common side effect of the medicines she had to take.
14. According to Rini, it is a common belief that a girl's breasts grow larger if a lot of men touch them. Mothers often use this story in order to discourage their daughters from engaging in intimate relationships.
15. Popular Maharashtrian breakfast dish, with rice as one of the main ingredients.
16. Maharashtrian dish made out of different kinds of beans.
17. A Marathi TV programme.

CHAPTER 4

A MACHINE FOR THE PRODUCTION OF INSCRIPTIONS

PRACTICES OF PAPERWORK AT ASHA

The hospital premises are surrounded by a high stone wall. Visitors have to enter through the big main gate that has 'Regional Mental Hospital' written in Marathi on its arch. When entering the hospital, one faces a big notice affixed to the entrance door – one of many that are spread around the hospital. It informs visitors that one is not allowed to enter Asha without permission or a specific purpose and that the visiting time for patients is between 9.00 AM and 4.00 PM. After the admission of patients, their relatives have to wait ten days before they are allowed to visit them for the first time. Furthermore, one should not give any beedis, money or matchboxes to patients. Finally, the board announces that taking photos is prohibited on hospital premises. After the hospital gate is opened in the morning, different kinds of people frequent Asha during the day. The hospital staff come in for work, families come to visit, admit or discharge somebody from the hospital, agents are there offering their services during admission and discharge and representatives of pharmaceutical companies come to promote their products.

Once a family has decided that taking care of a family member at home is no longer possible, they have to undergo a lengthy and sometimes troublesome admission process. Some families come here from distant villages and travel for one or two days by buses and trains to reach Asha. This particularly poses a challenge if the ill family member refuses to be admitted to a hospital. Therefore, some patients are not told by their relatives that they are being taken to a psychiatric hospital. Some of them only realize that they are about to be admitted either when the family enters the hospital gate or at the latest when they are brought into one of the wards and asked by an attendant to undress and change into the patient uniform. It has been known to happen that patients who behave violently or refuse to cooperate are tied up in order to be brought to Asha. Sometimes a family is related to or acquainted with somebody working in the hospital, which helps with the admission of 'their patient' – a common expression for an admitted family member. Families who are illiterate, or migrants who hail from outside Maharashtra and are unable to read Marathi or Hindi – who are equipped with less social and cultural capital – are awaited by agents near the hospital gate. In exchange for a fee, they offer to support the family in navigating the hospital's bureaucracy and paperwork. Several documents and forms need to be filled in during the admission process. Before they are able to go through with the paperwork, they first have to take care of other kinds of formalities, such as fees, which are reduced for families considered to be 'below poverty line'. In order to prove that they have less than a certain amount of income per year, families have to produce their ration card.[1] They have to apply for this document in the assigned state government office, and the name of the patient has to be included on the card. To attain all the necessary documents can take several weeks. Furthermore, if the patient does not want to be admitted voluntarily, the family has to apply to the local magistrate to admit the patient under a 'reception order' (RO). In order to obtain a RO, families have to provide two medical certificates issued by two medical practitioners, of whom one has to be a medical practitioner in the service of the government. Several other documents have to be collected and filled in during the admission process in the hospital itself. In the OPD, a social worker fills in the form 'Patient's Social History'. Subsequently, in the admission office, a medical officer fills in the 'Medical Examination' form. The admission is eventually completed in the superintendent's office. Here, a general admission document has to be signed that gives doctors permission to perform particular treatments on a patient during his/her stay. These include both major and minor surgeries, extracting teeth that are loose or rotten, cutting hair that has matted because of knots or that has lice, and check-ups and examinations by medical specialists.[2] A further permission document they are asked to sign allows doctors to give electroconvulsive therapy (ECT) to the patient. Signing the document means consenting to the administration of anaesthetics and a muscle relaxant to the patient and declaring they understand the procedure for this treatment or have had this explained to them by the doctor in a language they understand. By signing, families further declare they have been informed about the alternatives to ECT and the side effects (mentioned among others are unconsciousness, headaches, memory loss and fits and also fractures and death in rare cases). All declarations are written in Marathi. Some family members with whom I spoke on the hospital premises shared that they had signed the documents without really comprehending their contents or even having read it. All documents later become part of a patient's file. After all the paperwork is completed, patients are separated from their families and are brought to either the male or female unit. They have to change into the patient uniform and leave all their valuables with their family or with the attendants. Female patients are brought to the back of the hospital without their family, while the male unit being at the front of the hospital means families can accompany their patient to the door of the unit.

Akhil Gupta argues against seeing bureaucratic paperwork as a 'by-product of state activity, as that which merely records actions that state officials have taken' (2012: 142). Instead, he argues for a perspective that sees the state and its organisations as constituted through paperwork and bureaucratic writing. Bureaucratic organizations or 'machines for the production of inscriptions' (ibid.: 141) generate paperwork that matters for 'its forms and practices' (ibid.: 142); particularly for clients with scant cultural capital. A lot of frustration aimed at the inefficiency of government facilities 'hinges on the requirements of paperwork imposed by bureaucracies' (ibid.: 143). The majority of concerns articulated by the families I encountered in Asha were not about the medical treatment as such but related to bureaucratic issues and hassles.

Files, Forms and Registers: Understanding Psychiatric Treatment Regimes

Gupta (2012) discusses various forms of bureaucratic writing, among them the generation and recording of statistics and reports, forms and complaints, and finally registers and files that store these different types of writing under one cover:

> In the Indian bureaucracy, the key device for the storing and retrieval of information is the file. The file is the critical unit that organizes bureaucratic life. It is a material object, but it attains a life of its own that often looms larger than that of people who are supposedly acting on it. What is written in a file or what is missing from it can exert a much greater influence on a decision than the ideas of the person making the decision. . . . The wheels of government grind to a halt without a file. (ibid.: 145)

What Gupta describes also proves true regarding many aspects concerning the role of files at Asha. A complete psychiatric patient's file contains firstly the admission form (police or court order or a voluntary boarder declaration signed by the patient) and the medical examination form, along with the psychiatrist's and medical officer's notes and empty pages for further comments about the patient's progress, current symptoms and prescribed treatment changes. The latter can also be used by social workers and occupational therapists to add observations of a patient. Then follows a weight chart, the general permission for any kind of treatment signed by a relative, the permission forms for ECT treatment, LAB reports, the ECT chart, the psychiatric case history and the occupational therapy form stating the patient's professional history and skills. The file finally includes the nurses' notes, which encompass observations about the patient's behaviour or current symptoms. For female patients, the file also includes a menstrual cycle chart. The file closes with visiting and discharge cards. Visiting cards indicate if there are any persons visiting the patient, who these people are and how often they visit. Discharge cards give information regarding a patient's prior admissions and discharges and how long he/she stayed at home in between. Psychiatric and medical consultations do not take place without the patient's file put in front of the psychiatrist or medical officer. Consultations can and often take place without a patient being present; for example, when they behave violently and cannot be brought into the examination room. During a consultation, a medical officer may additionally ask the nurses or attendants present about the patient's behaviour within the last few days. They enter any change in treatment on the respective note sheets. Psychiatrists and medical officers, social workers and occupational therapists usually do not discuss a patient's case among each other. Each group has their respective office where they mingle with each other during lunch breaks. Meetings where patients' cases are systematically discussed among all the staff do not take place. Instead, everybody individually checks the respective note sheets or forms in the patient's file on their ward rounds. Psychiatrists, medical officers and most of the social workers and occupational therapists add their notes and comments in English, while nurses and attendants write in Marathi. The files of patients, at least partially, remain in the hospital after a patient is discharged. Information about a patient's treatment and diagnosis are added to their OPD file, while the part of the file that contains the forms, official documents and declarations are brought to the file department. Old files of long-term patients are brought here when their file has to be renewed. At the time of my research, over 20,000 files were stored there, according to the clerk in charge. I once accompanied a social worker to the file department; they were in search of an old file of a long-term patient who was admitted in 1974. He hoped that the file contained details about the patient's sister, whom he thought could be convinced about discharging the patient and taking care of her brother at home. His undertaking to rehabilitate the patient was put to a sudden end, though, when the clerk explained to him that old files are discarded after a certain number of years. Indeed, the file he had asked for was brought here more than a decade before. Because the patient himself did not remember any contact details or the address of his sister, the social worker had to give up hope of being able to rehabilitate him at that time.

In Asha, the file is not perceived as something that belongs to the patient, even though it is about them and their treatment. Instead, the file is perceived as a bureaucratic device and a source of accumulated case information. During the admission process, it merges with the patient's persona to a certain extent, making bureaucratic documents indispensable for central steps concerning treatment. Patients themselves repeatedly referred to their files during the interviews as a source of knowledge about their past and illnesses that they could not remember themselves. Hadas Yaron describes documents as enabling 'one's future as much as they monitor and control the everyday lives' (2009: 7) and argues that 'power is not located in one document, but in the dialectic relations between persons and their documents' (ibid.: 13). At Asha, the file is primarily understood as appertaining to the medical institution. The file, the patient and the institution, represented by the medical professionals working at Asha, form an interdependent triad. In this the file functions as a kind of catalyst that ultimately facilitates a patient's 'treatment' and care. The following anecdote from the field further illustrates these diverse nexuses.

I met Priya, a young woman in her early twenties, in the OPD. She had come to Asha to get hold of her father's complete file. However, this turned out to be more difficult than she originally anticipated. Priya hailed from a Brahmin Hindu family, and her father had suffered from schizophrenia for as long as she could remember. Her childhood was strained, as her father's illness consistently impacted family life. During his time at Asha, he always did much better, took his medication regularly, and Priya had gained a better understanding of his mental problems. She had not long been married to a Christian from Chennai. She described it as a 'semi-arranged marriage'. They had fallen in love, and luckily their parents had agreed to the match and subsequently arranged their marriage. Her parents had lived alone in Mumbai after her marriage. One and a half years before her father had been readmitted to Asha again for several months. Now, Priya was planning on consulting their 'family psychiatrist' in Chennai concerning her father's case. The psychiatrist had asked her to bring as many details as possible about her father's former treatment. The psychiatrist in the OPD told her that she would have to apply in the superintendent's office for the delivery of his file from the files department. He additionally informed her that files were not normally handed over to patients or their families, particularly if the purpose was to seek treatment from another psychiatrist. Confused by this statement, Priya turned to the social worker in the OPD to ask for his advice concerning the contents of the application letter. It soon became apparent that the social worker did not comprehend Priya's concern and why she was interested in taking her father's file home. Consequently, Priya went to the superintendent's office without concrete advice concerning the procedure and which information to include in the application letter. I sat with her while she was waiting for her turn, and she told me her concern for her family's situation. In the end, I did not come to know whether Priya was successful in getting hold of her father's file or not. Her story nevertheless exemplifies how her attempt to extract a bureaucratic device from the surroundings it was designed for provoked not only confusion and insecurity among the staff but more paperwork. The disarray that Priya experienced was due to a request that was not anticipated or encouraged in the closed and self-sufficient administrative system of Asha.

By far the most influential kind of bureaucratic paperwork that shapes the interactions and encounters between hospital staff, patients and their families are forms. Gupta (2012: 144) calls filling out a form the 'prototype of bureaucratic writing'. Forms are conceptualized to the principles of standardization and replicability. Additionally to the forms mentioned, there is a 'feedback form' that the social worker asks patients and their families to fill out after a patient's discharge that is written in Marathi. It was also translated into Hindi by one of the social workers who wanted to make hospital procedures more accessible for those patients and their families who do not speak Marathi. Language constitutes an important part of cultural capital on the hospital premises. While Hindi may be sufficient to converse with everybody at Asha, Marathi is the real door opener because all the staff is Maharashtrian. Caste and class make a difference as well. Doctors and psychiatrists predominantly hail from a higher middle-class background and would have completed their medical education in English. All medical forms that have to be filled in by medical officers/psychiatrists ('Medical Examination'), social workers ('Patient's Social History') and occupational therapists ('Occupational Therapy') are in English and use medical language. In the case of Priya and the social worker, aside from her request being unusual, the way she communicated with him may have prevented him from being of much help. Priya had discussed her problem in English and had maybe thought that in the context of a medical institution it would lend her more respect and enhance the chance to be heard and taken seriously. Or maybe it came naturally to her being from a higher middle-class background. Either way, she did not seem to recognize the fact that the social worker was not really used to English as a conversational language. Although he filled in the psychiatric case histories of patients in this language on a daily basis, he usually did not communicate in English with patients and their families. It is possible that he did not switch to Hindi or Marathi in this case because he did not want to reveal the difficulties he had with following Priya's English.

The language of forms and also their structure and concepts 'enframe and categorize the world' (ibid.) in a particular way that is not accessible to everyone. Furthermore, forms fundamentally mould the communication between patients, their families and the medical professional. Filling in a medical form is one of the rare occurrences in what is a long and exclusive interaction between patients and medical staff. In the following, I take the interaction of a patient and an occupational therapist by way of example. Two days after an admission, an occupational therapist used to meet with a new patient in order to fill in the 'Occupational Therapy Proforma' (see Figure 4.1). Madan, an occupational therapist in his early twenties, explained to me how he approached filling in the form, which is divided into a medical examination part and a part that concerns the patient's vocational skills. Information about the patient's educational and occupational history, his 'habits' (e.g. drinking or smoking) and his past medical history are supposed to help the occupational therapist assign a suitable occupational task. Sometimes that can be challenging, particularly as the hospital does not have very diverse occupational training facilities (see Chapter 2). Therefore, Madan has to be creative at times. Somebody who used to work as a driver, for example, he would send to the tailor OT section because he assumes that he possesses good hand-eye coordination. Most of the time, an evaluation of a patient's occupational background does not meet with any problems. In contrast, the psychiatric part of the examination is not always hassle free. For example, Madan has to decide if the patient's appearance is 'tidy' or 'untidy' and whether or not he maintains eye contact and to

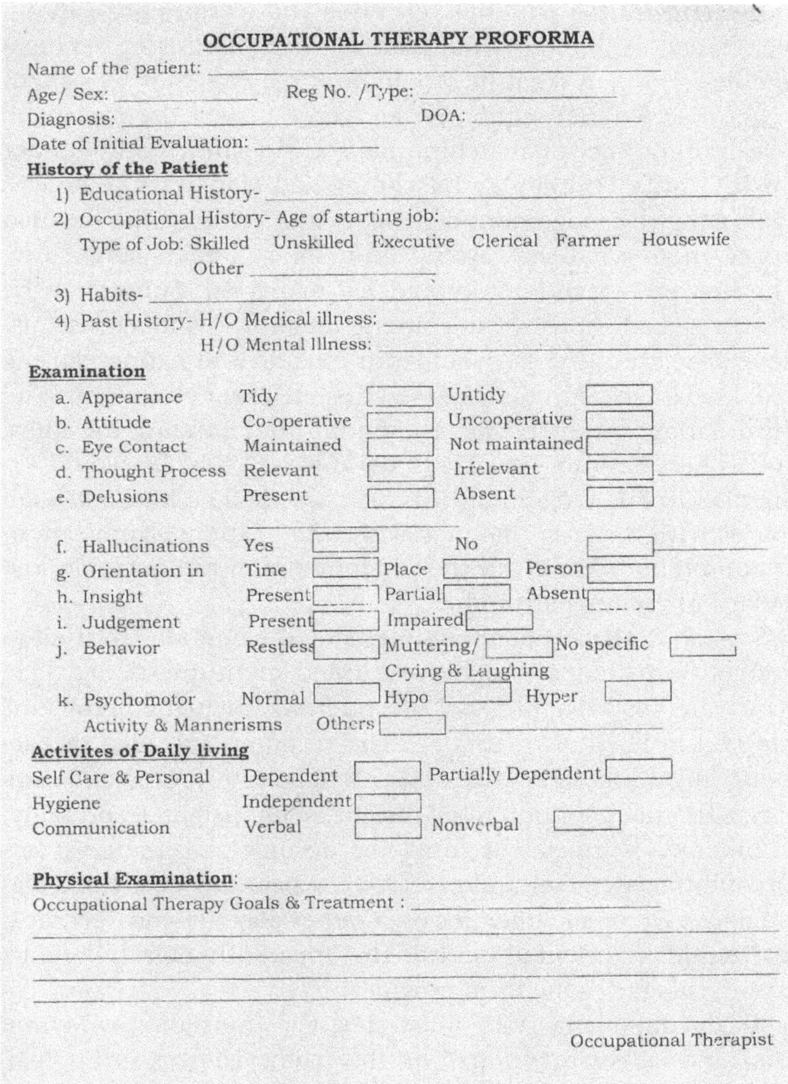

OCCUPATIONAL THERAPY PROFORMA

Name of the patient: __________

Age/ Sex: __________ Reg No. /Type: __________

Diagnosis: __________ DOA: __________

Date of Initial Evaluation: __________

History of the Patient

1) Educational History- __________
2) Occupational History- Age of starting job: __________
   Type of Job: Skilled Unskilled Executive Clerical Farmer Housewife
   Other __________
3) Habits- __________
4) Past History- H/O Medical illness: __________
   H/O Mental Illness: __________

Examination

a. Appearance Tidy ☐ Untidy ☐
b. Attitude Co-operative ☐ Uncooperative ☐
c. Eye Contact Maintained ☐ Not maintained ☐
d. Thought Process Relevant ☐ Irrelevant ☐ __________
e. Delusions Present ☐ Absent ☐
____
f. Hallucinations Yes ☐ No ☐ __________
g. Orientation in Time ☐ Place ☐ Person ☐
h. Insight Present ☐ Partial ☐ Absent ☐
i. Judgement Present ☐ Impaired ☐
j. Behavior Restless ☐ Muttering/ Crying & Laughing ☐ No specific ☐
k. Psychomotor Activity & Mannerisms Normal ☐ Hypo ☐ Hyper ☐ Others ☐ __________

Activites of Daily living

Self Care & Personal Hygiene Dependent ☐ Partially Dependent ☐ Independent ☐
Communication Verbal ☐ Nonverbal ☐

Physical Examination: __________

Occupational Therapy Goals & Treatment : __________

____

Occupational Therapist

Figure 4.1. 'Occupational Therapy Proforma' to be filled in by the occupational therapist.

tick a box accordingly. Questions are also asked about whether the patient has any 'insight' into his condition and whether they behave in a 'cooperative' or 'uncooperative' manner. To fill in these questions demands observational as well as interpretative skills. The occupational therapist has to evaluate a patient's judgement from a patient's reactions and wordings, for example. Madan explained to me that he would do this by asking a middle-aged man what he would do if his daughter was about to get married. Subsequently, he would expect the patient to give him an answer matching his social (parent) and gender (male) status. On the day I accompanied Madan while he was evaluating the judgement of several new patients, he decided to ask them what they would do if their clothes caught fire. The first patient did not know what to answer. Consequently, Madan ticked the box 'judgement impaired'. The second patient answered that he would run outside and extinguish the fire. Madan accordingly assessed his judgement as sound. The third patient stumbled for a moment after hearing the question. Then he burst out laughing and said that he would extinguish it. His judgement was also assessed as intact. Madan shared with me later that he assessed the patient's amusement as comprehensible given the randomness of the question and its lack of contextualization.

Similar confusion commonly emerged when Madan tried to evaluate a patient's 'insight' and asked them questioned like: Why were you brought here? Do you have any mental problem? Are you in need of treatment? The reactions included puzzlement, anger and ignorance and had to be interpreted and categorized as the patient having insight or no insight accordingly. In order to complete the form, the occupational therapist has to continuously label and categorize a patient's behaviour and language. He or she operates on a rather abstract and decontextualized level, oriented towards the apparently objective (diagnostic) categories the form provides.

As the following story illustrates, the translation of symptoms and labels, mentioned on the medical forms in English, into concepts that are comprehensible for patients has its pitfalls. Rini and I observed a psychiatrist conducting a mental status examination during her ward round one morning. She wanted to know if the patient suffered from 'hallucinations' and therefore asked her in Marathi if she had seen any *bhās* (illusions). The woman told her that she would see her children going to school every morning. The psychiatrist said to her that there were no children in the ward. Subsequently, the woman tried to explain to her that she used to see her children going to school in the mornings similar to how she did when she was at home with them. Rini suggested to me that *bhās* might not be a proper translation for 'hallucination' but could have been understood in the sense of 'imagination,' 'idea' or maybe also 'memory' (something somebody sees with one's inner eye) as well.[3]

In the psychiatric setting patients and their language are objects of constant surveillance and categorization. The constant monitoring goes beyond the assessment of a patient's appearance or behaviour as 'tidy'/ 'untidy' or 'cooperative'/ 'uncooperative'.[4] The psychiatric institution in general and the everyday life in the wards is determined by categorizing, indexing and listing patients' diagnoses as well as their eating habits. Lorna Amarasingham Rhodes (2004) shows in her ethnography on maximum security prisons how the ritualistic production of intake documents matches certain categories of persons to certain 'treatment' regimes. Regimes of rehabilitation or punishment take care of 'insane' or 'reasonable' persons. Such 'regimes of control', which work in ways as outlined by Michel Foucault, are also palpable at Asha. Part of these controlling and disciplining regimes is the patient uniform. It has to be worn by every patient, even by those who stay there long-term or for decades. An 'M' or a 'F' plus a number is printed on each patient's uniform. The number refers to the respective ward the patient was admitted to, while the letter indicates if the ward is located in the male or female unit. Male patients who belong to the criminal ward are easy to identify on the hospital premises – their uniform is additionally marked with a green stripe. It was difficult for Dr Shukla, as well as for hospital staff in general, to imagine running a huge psychiatric hospital like Asha without all patients wearing a uniform. When I told a social worker about German psychiatric facilities and that patients would just wear their everyday clothes, she exclaimed: 'But how will you recognize if a patient runs away then?'

Bureaucratic practices, and particularly paperwork, mould and shape everyday interactions and encounters taking place in the hospital. But their ordering, classificatory and controlling functions also comprise pitfalls and ambiguities. Furthermore, such practices are not the only device for framing social reality: it coexists with others (Handelman 1978: 11; Quack 2014). In the

OPD as well as in the admission department, several information boards in Marathi outline particular diagnoses (e.g. 'depression' or 'bipolar disorder') and mental health issues in general (e.g. 'rights of mental patients'). Another series of information boards is concerned with the 'Myths and Facts of Mental Illness' and declares that it is often assumed to be caused by black magic, the evil eye, sins of the past life or the wrath of gods and goddesses. The board contrasts these myths with the 'facts' that a mental illness can be hereditary or genetic, can occur due to physical illness or as a side effect of medicines, can be caused by mental stress and social problems or that someone's personality can make them more liable to becoming mentally ill. The contents of the boards reflect the threat that Indian psychiatrists regularly experience when confronted with religious or other healing approaches. From a modern, psychiatric perspective, practitioners from other healing traditions, often labelled as 'quacks', are prone to 'mislead' or 'maltreat' people who clearly suffer from a mental (and not a spiritual) 'affliction' that is best treated with psychopharmacological medicines (Nunley 1996; Davar and Lohokare 2008; H. Basu 2009, 2014; Quack 2012). The series 'Myths and Facts of Mental Illness' illustrates the psychiatric and 'modern' scientific approach in general, and quite bluntly categorizes the world into black and white: something can either be a 'fact' and therefore true and right or a 'myth', a mere superstition and wrong. The psychiatric approach that claims to build on the scientific pillars of biomedicine tolerates no grey and undefined areas. Indeed, the grey areas that evolve in conversations, practices and encounters, when people and their appearance 'do not comply' with the institutional rules, are constantly erased. In the following, the diagnostic category of 'female addiction' serves as an example. I once sat in the matron's office and copied some of the lists of diagnoses received by patients in the female unit; these had been put into a chart that was updated monthly with much accuracy by the nurses. I recognized that in contrast to the chart in the male unit it did not have any column for 'addiction'. When I asked the matron who was present why this was the case, she answered that women did not 'normally' suffer from addiction disorders. Even if psychiatric categories like 'addiction' or 'depression' are treated as 'objective facts', they obviously do not emerge independently of their social contexts (Corin 1990). The matron further told me that the diagnostic categories for the charts, which besides 'addiction' comprised categories such as 'schizophrenia', 'bipolar affective disorder' and 'personality disorder', were decided on by the former superintendent. They had not been changed or reviewed since then. After the charts have been filled in by the nurses, they are stored in registers and finally used for statistical purposes and included in the hospital report. Even if the diagnosis 'addiction' was never given in the case of women, I encountered women in the wards who were consuming alcohol regularly and told me about their 'drinking problem' (see Tasneem's case in Chapter 5). From time to time, I also found 'alcohol problems' or 'addicted to tobacco' mentioned in some of the female patients' files. But these symptoms never resulted in an official diagnosis and so the chart did not provide a column for 'addiction'. In this way, mental health professionals engaged in 'purifying' activities, as Bruno Latour (1994) would call it (see also Naraindas et al. 2014: 10) – in this case, purifying the institution of ambivalent hybrids ('drinking females') that questioned the social and ontological order.

'What are Your Troubles?': Assembling a Patient's Social History

The OPD constitutes one of the 'bureaucratic hearts' of Asha, where the majority of the institution's paperwork takes place. To the back of the OPD lies the social workers' room, where the 'Patient's Social History' form was filled in by one of the senior psychiatric social workers, Mr Surendra More. Every new out- or inpatient has to have one of these forms, which is added to a patient's file and referred to before they undergo any psychiatric examination or treatment. Mr More's office hours were from 9.00 AM to 3.00 PM. During this time, he usually spoke to between five and fifteen new patients accompanied by one to four relatives or sometimes also friends and neighbours, for around fifteen to twenty minutes. I accompanied Surendra More for a whole week and observed around forty interactions and the process of filling in the form. Nineteen of the conversations I tape recorded, and I asked Mr More to fill in the form on blue print paper. Eleven of the conversations, which were mostly conducted in Marathi, were later transcribed and translated by my co-researcher Akshay.

Psychiatric paperwork is focused on the production of what Tony Hak (1998) calls 'factual accounts'. These are institutionally produced by extracting 'mentionables' from conversations with patients and their families and by reworking them as, for example, 'symptoms' and writing them down in psychiatric reports. Taking patients' social histories was an intersectional process, taking place between families, a social worker and a form, before the patient was brought to the medical officer or psychiatrist. The social workers' room was located to the left of the OPD. One entered it directly from the central waiting area. The entrance did not have a door but a curtain. The room was often not a big enough space for all the relatives accompanying a patient. Mr Surendra More would sit behind a rather simple office table opposite the door. When I was accompanying him, I also sat behind this table on his left side. Two chairs were placed in front of the table. Usually the patient was seated on the right chair in front of Mr More, while a relative considered the main informant and who could provide the most information about the patient was seated on the left. When I wondered about this arrangement Mr. More explained to me that the patient was seated between the wall and one of their relatives to protect others in case of occurring aggressive behaviour. Furthermore, this constellation made it harder for the patient to simply 'jump up and run away'. The patient was not present during every interview, though. In some cases he/she would wait, tied up, in a car or auto rickshaw parked outside of the OPD. In these cases, Surendra More went to have a look at the patient and to check if and how they would respond to his questions. I looked at the following cases in more detail.

Table 4.1. Problems/symptoms of the patients as described by the relatives to the psychiatric social worker (PSW).

	Sex	Age	Accompanied by[5]	Problems/Symptoms (according to relatives)
Case I	Male	20	Father	Three years ago the patient stopped speaking. Takes medicine already, but parents are worried about their son's future.

	Sex	Age	Accompanied by[5]	Problems/Symptoms (according to relatives)
Case II	Male	22	Father and one male relative	Patient is aggressive and has behaved violently, beating and abusing family members. Tried to kill his older brother. Possible reason for patient's illness: unrequited love at college. Patient is tied up in a car outside the OPD during the conversation. Has already been treated but doesn't take his medicine.
Case III	Male	40	Sister- and brother-in-law	Patient mutters, doesn't sleep at night, gets up at unusual times, wanders around, begs at neighbours' doors. His mother, who had been taking care of him and resisted any psychiatric treatment, passed away recently. Now his sister wants to admit him to the hospital.
Case IV	Male	73	His son, cousin (f) and niece	Started muttering, is disoriented, seems not to understand/remember what he does, doesn't recognize distant relatives. Started to have problems after two of his daughters died.
Case V	Female	30	Husband	Patient runs away, hurts herself, doesn't manage to do household work properly or to look after the children. Has fever episodes before attacks, which could not be explained by doctors. Husband wants to admit his wife because he feels overwhelmed by the situation.
Case VI	Female	38	Mother and one more male relative (who speaks Kannada)	Patient runs away, hits family members, throws stones at people, threatens to kill herself, asks for all kinds of intoxicants, eats mud, complains about mother-in-law. Her husband left her and the children because of her illness. Family wants to admit her because her mother, a widow, cannot take care of her.

(continued)

Table 4.1. Continued

	Sex	Age	Accompanied by[5]	Problems/Symptoms (according to relatives)
Case VII	Female	38	Daughter, two men and two women	Patient is violent, urinates/ defecates outside the bathroom, doesn't take bath, throws kitchenware (instead of cooking with it), doesn't take her medicines regularly. Husband divorced her twenty years ago.
Case VIII	Male	37	Father, brother and one man	Patient mutters, runs behind relatives and beats them, faints suddenly. Was in a road accident four months ago, family relates his symptoms to the head injury he suffered.
Case IX	Male	22	Brother, a neighbour and one man	Behaves violently, throws stones at and abuses neighbours, doesn't hear properly, gets nude in public, wanders around the village. Behaved strangely since fifteen years old and was diagnosed as 'mentally retarded'. Old parents cannot take care of him, therefore brother wants to admit him.
Case X	Male	17	Mother	Behaves aggressively with family members, wants to be alone, impaired hearing, speaks only when asked to, doesn't initiate interactions himself, sleeps too much.
Case XI	Male	77	Son and one more man	Patient suffers from 'short-term memory loss'. Bought land and forgot where he has kept the contract, family is afraid that he is cheated out of various things because of his forgetfulness. Family wants medical certificate so that they can apply for custodial care.

Even if the above cases are by no means representative of all patients, they represent some of the typical mental troubles that were prevalent in Mumbai and the surrounding Maharashtrian villages and cities.

Vieda Skultans points out in her study of a Mahanubhav healing temple in western Maharashtra that 'altered behaviour rather than subjective experience is characteristic of madness' (1991: 326). The 'symptoms' described by the families indicate that 'mad' behaviour stereotypically includes a threat or destruction of family ties or of the family's reputation. Accordingly, violent, aggressive or abusive behaviour, particularly against family members was often mentioned during the conversations (Case II, VI, VII, VIII, IX, X). Described as a symptom as well was behaviour that disrupted social and family routines. These included behaviours such as wandering around at unusual hours or taking a bath in the river in the middle of the night (Case III, IX), inappropriate social behaviour; for example, begging at neighbours' doors (Case III), urinating/defecating in inappropriate places and eating inappropriate things; for example, mud (Case VI) and getting naked in public (Case IX). In the case of female patients, relatives complained that they did not take care of the household, the children or preparation of food (Case V, VII) or that they complained about in-laws (Case VI). This illustrates how 'mad' behaviour in the case of women is commonly framed as 'withdrawal of support and services to the family' (ibid.: 327; see also Addlakha 2001). In the case of male patients, this was equated with the patient not working or studying and the fear that he therefore might not be able to provide for his (future) family or himself (Case I, II, IX). Relatives also often critically evaluated behaviour like social withdrawal, the wish to be alone and not mingle with family members or others (Case II, X, IV) and not wanting to communicate (Case I, X). In Cases VIII and XI, the patients were not perceived as suffering from 'madness' by their relatives, even if the patient's manner in Case VIII matched common stereotypes of 'mad' behaviour.

What Surendra More eventually entered on the form often differed from the family's worries or concerns. For example, he omitted the worries of a father about his son's future when he and his wife would no longer be around (Case I). In Case II, he translated the observations and worries of the relatives that their son does not speak much, prefers to be alone and watch TV, does not go out and mingle with friends (described as *ektepaṇā* (loneliness)) into the English psychological term: 'pt [patient] is introvert personality'. Additionally, the social worker anticipated the relative wanting to hospitalize the patient, which was not explicitly articulated by the father. In contrast, other relatives indeed mentioned the admission of the patient as their reason for coming to the hospital (Case III, V, VI, IX). This was usually related to an inability to provide the necessary care for the patient. In two cases, this was related to parents that had taken care of the patient up till then but were not able to any longer due to age or other reasons (Case VI, IX). In one case, the caretaker had already died (Case III), and in another, the husband felt overwhelmed by having to perform well in his job as a headmaster as well as take care of the children and additionally his wife (Case V).

Mr More began filling in the 'Patient's Social History' form (see Figure 4.2) by asking for some basic information about the respective patient, like name, age, address and contact details of the family. He then inquired about the relationship of the patient to the main person accompanying him or her. Even if in most of the cases the patient is accompanied by more than one person, the form only asks for the name of one informant. The form includes the following options: 'Mother', 'Father', 'Husband', 'Wife', 'Brother', 'Son', 'Daughter', 'Uncle', 'Friend' and 'Neighbour'. Before the social worker had to decide whom he perceives to be the main informant in the particular situation and conversation. According to Gupta, we 'can study forms for what is excluded from them as much as for how that which is included is organized' (2012: 145). Interestingly, while 'uncle' is included as a regular informant, its counterpart 'aunt' is missing. Here the form may reflect the 'Ideology of Familial Care-Givers' as outlined by Vieda Skultans (1991: 331). She points out that in Maharashtrian family structures a man's care is perceived as the responsibility of his parents (in a joint family arrangement also including his brothers), his wife's parents and his sons. A woman's care is seen as the responsibility of her husband (even if it is understood that he will unlikely comply with this expectation), her parents and brothers and, later in life, also her sons. In view of this typical care structure, an aunt (mother's or father's sister) is less likely to be the one expected to take over the primary caretaker role; she is perceived as belonging to her husband's family, if married. Therefore, it is much more likely that an uncle would accompany his niece or nephew to the hospital because he either resides in the same household (the father's brother) or he, for example, has accompanied his sister in bringing one of her children to the OPD (the mother's brother).

PATIENT'S SOCIAL HISTORY
Psychiatrics Social Worker Dept.

Date..

Name : ....

Reg. No. .... Date of Adm. :....................................

Age : .... Sex : Male/Female

Address : .... Urban/Rural/Tribal

....

....

Phone No. Office : .... Resi. : ....

Mobile : .... C/o ....

Informant : ....

Relationship with Patient :—

Mother / Father / Husband / Wife / Brother / Son / Daughter / Uncle / Friend / Neighbour /

Other Specify ....

Family History :—

Inter-personal relationship with patient :

Father : ....

Mother : ....

Sibling : ....

Other : ....

Relationship to Patient : ....

History of mental illness in family : Yes / No

If yes : Neurotic / Psychotic / Organic / or if any

Specify : ....

Childhood History :—

Educational Qualification :

Illiterate / Primary / Secondary / upto 10th / 12th / Graduation / Post Graduation / Other

....

Educational Status : Below average / Average / Good / Fair / Excellent / Under Difficult Situation / Regular in Attendance / Irregular Attendance / Dropout /

Specify ....

Occupation : Business / Govt. Service / Pvt.

Service / Retired / Resignation / Dismissed / Other ....

(G.C.P.) O 2805 (10,000–3-2010)

Figure 4.2. 'Patient's Social History' form to be filled in by the social worker, page 1.

The next section in the form concerns the family history of the patient. Here, the information entered by the social worker is usually limited to the whereabouts of the parents, the number of brothers and sisters, if the latter are married or not and if there is any conflict affecting these relationships. This kind of information is particularly important when a patient comes to be discharged. If relatives like spouses or parents are not ready to take them back, social workers often try to contact the patient's siblings to ask them to discharge and take care of the patient. In this section, the social worker also enquires about the 'History of mental illness in family'.

Case I

PSW – Has anybody in the family ever suffered from such a disease?

Father – No.

PSW – Your grandmother . . . grandfather . . .

Father – No.

Case II

PSW – Has anybody in the family ever suffered from such a disease?

Man – Yes.

Father – I was *disturbed*. But I soon became *normal* again.

Case III

PSW – Has anybody in your family ever suffered such troubles?

Sister – No, nobody.

PSW – You mentioned someone.

Brother-in-law – Grandmother.

Sister – My grandmother, my mother's mother.

Case IV

PSW – Had anybody in your family had such troubles?

Son – No. Nobody.

Case V

PSW – Does anybody in the family suffer from this kind of disease?

Patient – No.

Case VI

PSW – Was anybody in your family ill with this type of disease? Until which grade she studied?

PSW – What?

PSW – Let it be.

Mother – [Speaking in Kannada]

Case VII

PSW – Has anybody else ever suffered from such a disease?

Man – Ah?

PSW – Has anybody else in the family ever suffered from such a disease? In their family?

Daughter – No, nobody.

Case VIII

PSW – Has such kind of disease occurred in your family before?

Father – This is not a disease; he went through an *operation*. There was no disease.

Case IX

PSW – Has anybody else suffered from such an illness?

Brother – No.

Case X

Mother – I have another elder son, eighteen years old.

PSW – Do any of the other children have troubles?

Mother – Nothing, nothing to the daughters either.

PSW – Has anybody else in the family ever suffered from such a disease?

> Mother – In the family, in our family occurred a disease, two of my brother's sons – they have been admitted twice.
>
> PSW – No. In your [husband's] family?
>
> Mother – Nobody in my [husband's] family. In my brother's family.
>
> Case XI
>
> PSW – Has anybody in the family suffered from such or a similar disease?
>
> Son – In the sense?
>
> PSW – I mean, has anybody in the family ever suffered from a mental illness etc.?
>
> Son – No, no. He suffers from *short-term memory loss*.

If we pay attention to the wording of Surendra More, in only one case does he use the term *mānsik ājār* (mental illness), which is the literal translation of the English term used in the form, and even in this case only after a relative asks him to specify his question (Case XI). Instead, he tends to be vague, mentioning *asā ājār* (such a disease) eight times, (*asā*) *trās* ((such) trouble/problem) two times or *ashī bimārī* (such an illness) two times. With this kind of wording, instead of labelling the patient's illness as 'mental' right away, he is more likely to evoke memories of similar illness episodes or displays of symptoms within the patient's family, as the question aims at screening the patient's family for any cases of psychiatric or neurological diseases; information the psychiatrist may later build upon when conducting the mental status examination. Further, by avoiding the potential stigma associated with the label 'mental illness', Mr More opens a non-judgmental space for the family members to evaluate if another person has ever behaved is such a disturbing way or has experienced similar troubles – this way he gains more information regarding family health than he may have otherwise. In Case I, he even asks the informant for particular persons, 'Your grandmother . . . grandfather . . . ' in order to trigger memories. Nevertheless, most of the families seem to be aware of what the social worker is implying with his question. This becomes particularly clear in Case II when the father replies with: 'I was *disturbed*. But I soon became *normal* again.', using English terms to describe his mental health. In two cases, the relatives even clarify the social worker's words in stating that their relatives do not suffer from a 'mental illness'. In Case III, the father replies: 'This is not a disease, he went through an *operation*. There was no disease.' The family related the changed behaviour of their son, which started around two weeks before and included behaving violently towards his wife, to a road accident he was involved in around four months before. Therefore, they did not consider their son's illness as 'such a disease', but as being a consequence of the physical injuries he suffered during the accident. Similarly, in Case XI, the patient's son replies: 'No, no. He suffers from *short-term memory loss*'. By doing this he demarcates the illness he perceives his father as actually having with 'such a disease', namely madness. The social worker with his expression 'such a disease' manages to relate the question about mental health issues in the family to a sociocultural classification system that categorizes mental illnesses as different from other diseases, particularly those that are perceived to have physical causes or are not classified as a kind of 'madness'.

Mr. More completes the form by building a conversation and therewith co-constructs a narrative about the patient's illness together with the patient's relatives. This is illustrated in Case X when the patient's mother says, 'I have another elder son, eighteen years old', at this point responding to the question of how many siblings the patient has. Mr. More connects to this information, coming to the next question: 'Does any of the other children have troubles?'. Not every piece of information that is provided during the conversation he considers as pertinent. When the mother in the following reports about the two sons of her brother, who suffer from a mental illness, he doesn't put this information down in the form. Instead he goes on asking if there were any cases in 'her' family, by this referring to her husband's family to which she formally belongs since her marriage. Nevertheless, the social worker does not always succeed in establishing a productive conversation that provides the kind of information he needs to fill in the form: language barriers are a regular challenge he faces completing his task. In Case VI the family discusses the issue amongst themselves in Kannada, a language he does not speak, and eventually, he seems to give up on getting the information he specifically needs to fill in the form: '. . . What? . . . Let it be.' Instead, by asking for the patient's educational status, he tries to get the information to answer the next question, in the section 'Childhood History'. This section also asks about unusual childhood events, like accidents, etc. If no such events occurred, Mr More simply noted down 'normal'. If the patient was an adult, Mr More would also note down his/her occupation and work performance. The next line is specific to the experience of 'Menstruation', giving three options to tick: 'Regular', 'Irregular' and 'Menopause'. In all the conversations I observed, Surendra More did not ask even once about the regularity of a female patient's menstrual cycle and also never ticked any of the categories. Maybe he did not feel comfortable addressing this topic as a male social worker.

Producing Mentionables and Interpretative Work

Yet another section on the second page of the form concerns the patient's marital status and the quality of married life (see Figure 4.3). The conversation below illustrates how Mr More and a patient's family cooperated in producing 'facts' that can be mentioned here.

Case VII

PSW – Is there a father?

Daughter – No.

Patient [the mother] – There is one small boy, Sonu, Sonu.

Daughter – I don't have a father. I mean, there is a father, he didn't die, but there was a *divorce*.

PSW – When the *divorce* took place?

Man – The divorce, I think at the time of your birth . . .

Daughter – I got it. Now I am in my twentieth year.

Sister – About twenty years ago.

PSW – Are you alone [the only child]?

Daughter – Yes, I am alone.

When the social worker asks the daughter 'Is there a father?' (Implying: 'Is your mother married?') and the daughter replies 'No', she immediately recognizes that this response is ambiguous and could lead to the wrong conclusions. She therefore goes on to explain herself: 'I mean, there is a father, he didn't die, but there was a divorce.' When the social worker wants to know

Attendance : Regular / Irregular, if any ....

Quality of Service ....

Menstruation : Regular / Irregular / Menopause

Marital Status : Married / Unmarried / Widow / Separated / Divorce / Remarried

Marital Life : Healthy / Satisfied / Clashes / Stressful / Separated / Any other ....

Personality : Social / Unsocial / Introvert / Extrovert / Mixing / Neurotic / Hot Tempered / Cool Tempered / Religious / Non Religious

Habits : ....

Past History : ....

Duration of the illness : ....

Episode : ....

Treated where and how : ....

....

....

Cause of the present illness : Medicine stopped / Drug compliance / No response to medicine / Any other
If any, specify : ....

View of the relatives towards the illness : Superative / Negative / hatred / over protective / Other

Patient's View towards the illness : Accept the illness / Non acceptance / None of the above due to above illness

Compliance with treatment : Good / Poor

How did you get the information about the illness and the Mental Hospital ?

Remarks :

....

....

....

Psychiatric Social Worker.

Figure 4.3. 'Patient's Social History' form to be filled in by the social worker, page 2.

when exactly the divorce took place, the daughter, sister and another relative actively work on producing the fact 'twenty years ago' to be put down on the form. They are well aware that the relative information 'at the time the patient's daughter was born' does not meet bureaucratic standards. Meanwhile, the reason for the divorce and its impact on the patient, her mental condition and her family life is not discussed at any point. Here, the objective is clearly to produce a 'mentionable' that can be put down in the form by the social worker.

The segments of the form that follow concern the patient's personality, his/her habits (here Mr More asked mostly about 'addictions' like chewing tobacco and drinking) and detailed illness history. The following conversation evolved between the social worker and the family on this point:

> Case VII
>
> PSW – So this problem is present since twelve years?
>
> Man – Yes.
>
> Patient – No since thirty years.
>
> Man – We have admitted her twelve years before.
>
> Patient – It's thirty years, not twelve. Don't take Balaji Tirupati's name.
>
> PSW – Wasn't there any problem before?
>
> Daughter – No, she wasn't ill before.
>
> PSW – It started twelve years back.
>
> Sister – Yes. It's been twelve years now.
>
> Man – The problem is the same since twelve years.
>
> Sister – And she doesn't take medicines.
>
> Patient – Who is Bandya Patil? Don't you know him, he is from Kolhapur.

As it becomes apparent from the excerpt, the patient, a 38-year-old woman, actively takes part in constructing her 'Social History': 'It's thirty years, not twelve.' (See also the excerpt above, when Mr More asks for the father in the family: 'There is one small boy, Sonu, Sonu [son of her daughter].') The social worker reacts to her objection and asks accordingly: 'Wasn't there any problem before?' Nevertheless, even if her voice was not silenced or ignored completely, it was the information her relatives gave to the social worker that was evaluated as the true 'facts' and noted down in the form accordingly: 'Past History: "Mental illness since twelve years"', probably because of her apparent mental instability in mentioning random information and names throughout the conversation. This points to the continuous interpretation work the social worker has to accomplish in order to identify and extract the information from the conversation that is appropriate to the form; these points 'are "found" reflexively and recursively . . . rather than being discovered as "facts"' (Hak 1998: 426).

The following excerpt, too, illustrates the interpretative process that filling in forms necessarily entails:

> Case V
>
> PSW – You are taking medicines right?
>
> Patient – Ask him [referring to her husband].
>
> Husband – She doesn't take them once she has an attack again. S.S. [a relative] came with us to drop us here. And when she got an attack on Friday, he said it's not good . . . don't leave unless she is better. What to do now? It's a big problem.
>
> PSW – Nothing. Take your decision. What he says doesn't matter. Your decision matters. Your decision is important. What I think is that there is no reason to admit her unnecessarily.
>
> Husband – Ok. You give us medicine for a month . . . but if meanwhile her condition worsens, can I admit her then?
>
> PSW – You can bring her at that time. Don't worry. But you have to admit her via court or you have to pay here. But you can do it.
>
> Husband – How does the paying option work?
>
> PSW – There are some government charges, monthly charges.
>
> Husband – How much is it approximately?

> PSW – I cannot tell exactly, but it's around two thousand rupees. Does she do the household work properly? Cooking and all?
>
> Patient – I do. Don't I cook?
>
> Husband – I lost it again in the morning. She gets up . . . Something needs to be done . . .
>
> Patient – Don't I cook?
>
> Husband – See . . . if you would do all these things nicely, then we wouldn't be here.
>
> PSW – How many children do you have?
>
> Husband and patient – Two daughters and one son.
>
> Husband – And I brought her here in a good condition. I am feeling awkward. But no option. I thought, it's holiday, so let's go.

It becomes apparent in the above excerpt that while Surendra More is concerned with producing mentionables by asking the couple the respective questions, the couple, and in particular the husband, is more focused on articulating the tensions at home in relation to his wife's illness. Therefore, the social worker copes with at least two additional tasks in this conversation: responding to the husband's complaints and engaging in a crisis intervention ('Your decision is important. What I think is that there is no reason to admit her unnecessarily'). The social worker's question of whether the patient properly takes care of her household chores or not results in a dispute between the couple. The husband eventually argues: 'If you would do all these things nicely, we wouldn't be here.' Mr More noted down in the form: 'Irregular house work' without commenting or asking more about the disagreements between the couple. Nevertheless, the couple's disagreements were reflected in the form under 'Remarks', the last section of the form: 'relative wants to hospitalize pt [patient]' and 'pt does not want to get admitted, wants to continue medicine'. Under 'View of relatives towards illness', Mr More ticked the option 'superative' [supportive], and under 'Patient's view towards the illness', he ticked 'Accepts the illness' and noted 'pt responding to asking questions'. In order to fill in the last part of the document, the social worker does not ask the patient or their family any questions but relies on his impressions of the family dynamics. 'Mentionables' that are produced in such a way are dependent on what Hak (1998) calls 'nonprofessional' interpretation, which depends on sociocultural knowledge and the experience of the mental health professional and is often influenced by 'ideological commitment' (ibid.: 434). For example, the husband and Mr More seemed to have had a mutual understanding about a housewife's role and the tasks she should be able to perform. Without any further elaboration, the husband's exclamation 'If you would do all these things nicely, we wouldn't be here' was accepted and transformed into a 'mentionable fact' by Surendra More. The social worker reacted in a very understanding way to the position, perspective and needs of his male informant. Maybe this was related to him being a lower middle-class husband and father himself.

Surendra More's attitude, though, was not always accommodating and supportive; this depended on his sympathy with and judgement of the relatives and their situation. This aspect is illustrated in the following excerpt:

> Case IX
>
> PSW – Have you taken him anywhere else?
>
> Brother – No, nowhere.
>
> PSW – You haven't shown him to the doctor yet?
>
> Brother – We don't have that much money.
>
> PSW – You said you showed him in Jalgaon, isn't it?
>
> Neighbour – We are very poor people, sir. He is the only one earning. His parents can't work now.
>
> PSW – I am not interested in this aspect. I am asking, if you have taken him to the doctor in Jalgaon?
>
> Brother – We took him to Jalgaon.
>
> PSW – To which doctor? To which doctor you took him in Jalgaon?
>
> Neighbour – To the government hospital.
>
> Brother – To the government hospital.
>
> PSW – Well, did they prescribe any medicines?
>
> Brother – Yes, they did.

> PSW – So, it made no difference?
>
> Brother and Neighbour – No, no difference at all.
>
> Neighbour – He hears little and . . .
>
> PSW – You have to admit him here via court order. You can't admit him directly. You have to go through the court.
>
> Brother – It's very far to come here . . . We collected money from neighbours to bring him here.

When Surendra More asks the family 'You haven't shown him to the doctor yet?', the brother understands this as an accusation that the family is delaying the treatment of the patient. Particularly rural and 'uneducated' families are blamed for turning to psychiatric treatment too late or not at all by mental health professionals. Therefore, the brother reacts defensively, explaining the delay with 'We don't have that much money'. When the neighbour, too, misunderstands his inquiry ('We are very poor people, sir'), Mr More becomes slightly impatient with the family: 'I am not interested in this aspect.' In contrast to the couple above, where Mr More anticipates and responds to the husband's worries, he does not take up the financial problems and concerns of the family in the conversation but is sternly focused on completing the form. He even further adds to the men's problems by announcing that they have to go through the court to admit the patient, which holds out the prospect of even more paperwork and expenses. At one point, Mr More interrupts a conversation with the brother whom he asked if he 'has parents' (implying if they are still alive): 'Yes, we have but . . .' PSW (interrupting): 'How many brothers are you?' If interruptions take place in an interaction, it represents a breakdown of communicative cooperation: 'An interrupter cuts off the previous speaker, dismisses the old topic, and imposes a new one' (Wilce 1995: 929). Wilce argues that an asymmetrical control of the topic, which can often be observed in conversations taking place within medical institutions, reflects an asymmetry of power. The right to speak, label and interpret in the encounter lies with the social worker, who has the power to let relatives elaborate on their illness experiences (as Mr More does in Case V, with the husband) or cut them off (as in Case IX, with the brother). In the latter case, Surendra More later in the conversation advised the relatives to give medication to the patient, which he promised would have 'a great impact'. When the brother replied: 'He won't take any medications, that is why we have brought him here', Mr More simply handed them over the filled in form and responded: 'Tell this to the doctor and prepare his file.' A similar situation occurred in Case I. The patient's father mentioned at the end of the interview: 'The question is . . . what about his future? . . . after us . . . He will be fine as long as we are there. Our efforts go in this direction.' At this point, Mr More, who had just completed filling in the form, responded: 'Show this [the filled in form] to the doctor in the next cabin. Show it to the doctor and take medicines from here.' The social worker did not leave the relatives' concerns completely unanswered. Nevertheless, his strategy in both cases was to offer a pharmacological solution for the financial, psycho-social and socio-structural problems that were articulated by the relatives (Jain and Jadhav 2009; Bayetti, Jadhav and Jain 2019: 160ff.).

The Social Production of Factual Accounts

The encounters in the social workers' room bring to light two kinds of narratives. One is the contents of the filled in form, which is the bureaucratic narrative. The other one evolves from the conversation between the social worker, the patient and the patient's family. During the encounter, the family does not just passively answer questions and wait for the social worker to fill in the form but brings up their own questions, concerns and worries concerning the ill family member. Whose statements are heard, taken seriously, followed up or written down on the form depends on the social worker's judgement and if he considers them 'mentionables'. This decision is informed by certain 'nonprofessional' interpretation processes that are shaped by sociocultural knowledge and stereotypes – for example, gender and class. Even if the patient is rarely listened to or considered uncapable of reporting his/her own case, they are nevertheless an inevitable part of the constellation. If families turn up without the patient, they will be asked to come back with the ill family member another day. Therefore, the 'Patient's Social

History', treated as a 'factual account' in the psychiatric everyday world, constitutes a co-creation between the social worker, the patient's family, the patient and the form – all bring to the table different forms of agency and sociocultural capital. The form constitutes the inducement of a conversation; it guides and informs the social worker's catalogue of questions. The family eventually articulates their concerns and inquiries within the realm set by the social worker. The latter obviously holds certain 'metacommunicative privileges' (Wilce 1995: 929) that empower him to decide which aspects to take up or just dismiss during the conversation. He also determines the end of an encounter and directs the relatives regarding the next steps they have to take:

> Case V
>
> Man – She searches for scissors, some medicines . . . in this condition . . .
>
> PSW – Is it?
>
> Man – When during such a time everybody is at home, outside . . . kids are there . . . it's havoc . . . I mean she doesn't understand anything at that time. She doesn't do it purposefully.
>
> PSW – Ok. In the neighbouring room there is a psychiatrist, show her to the psychiatrist and report everything. Ok? And prepare a file from that table and show it to the doctor. Tell everything to the psychiatrist and ask her what to do.

The completed form inevitably marked the end of a conversation in all the cases I observed. The relatives were then sent to a neighbouring examination room, shared by a medical officer and a psychiatrist, respectively. The families have to line up in the waiting room opposite the examination room and can enter once it is their turn. First, they encounter the medical officer, who inquires why the family has brought the patient in, if they want to renew their medical description and LOA, if psychiatric re-examination is necessary or if a new patient has to be seen by the psychiatrist in order to receive a diagnosis. Accordingly, the medical officer adds notes to the patient's file and, as may be the case, refers them to the psychiatrist sitting at the neighbouring table. The psychiatrist makes a decision about whether a patient should be admitted or if he/she should be sent home to start or continue treatment based on medications. Medical officers and psychiatrists have an average of two to three minutes for seeing a patient and their families. As I illustrated above, the 'speech economy' (Wilce 1995: 929) that governs health professional-patient-family interactions is inevitably shaped by institutional regimes and power structures. Institutional and biomedical 'treatment ideologies' (Young 1993) determine what 'mentionables' health professionals look out for in conversations with patients and their relatives. They tend to sift out those aspects that seem helpful in pinpointing the patient's illness and are inclined to dismiss others. Therefore, even the 'social' worker is not primarily concerned with the sociocultural and family context of the patient's illness but rather engages in 'cleansing' work that is directed at purifying relatives' narratives from its social baggage.

Notes

1. A ration card is an official document that is issued by the state government to households. With a ration card, a family is eligible to purchase subsidized food grain. The ration card also serves as a common form of identification.
2. Kaveri Dadhich translated diverse documents and forms from Marathi into English. She also accompanied me to the hospital on one occasion after Rini had left for Sweden.
3. A more appropriate translation for 'hallucination' might be the term *ābhās*, which refers to an appearance or phantom of something that is not really there.
4. A patient might be deemed 'cooperative' by the social worker but experienced as 'uncooperative' by the occupational therapist and marked accordingly on the OT form.
5. I only came to know about kin or other relations as far as they were asked for by the social worker or mentioned during the conversation.

CHAPTER 5

NEGOTIATIONS AND IMAGINATIONS IN THE CONTEXT OF DISCHARGE AND REHABILITATION

Asha's admission and discharge procedures are heavily bureaucratic. They constitute the outcome of negotiation and decision-making processes taking place at the intersection of family life and the psychiatric hospital as an institution of care taking. 'Admission' constitutes a transitional marker indicating a switch in social status from family member to that of patient and back again upon discharge. Two important institutions make the decision as to whether a patient is ready to be discharged from Asha or not. One is the family, which decides if a patient's condition has improved to such an extent that he or she can be taken care of at home again. The second institution is the psychiatric hospital. Before a patient is ready to be sent home again, a psychiatrist has to declare them 'fit for discharge'. Additionally, a committee called 'Board of Visitors' (BOV) that meets at Asha on a monthly basis can decide to escort a patient to their family's place in the event that their relatives do not want to discharge them.

The most common kind of discharge at Asha is the 'leave of absence' (LOA), when a patient is discharged on parole (around 75 per cent of discharges between April 2010 and March 2011). This discharge can be granted to patients who were admitted by a 'reception' or a 'detention order' (RO or DO). The LOA can be renewed every sixty days by paying a small fee of fifty rupees and enables the family to come back to readmit the patient without undergoing all the paperwork that would come with a new admission. By reducing the costs of a readmission, an LOA discharge effectively reduces the risks that come with the discharge of a family member. Although the legal purpose of an LOA discharge was initially to enable families to take patients home for a limited time span, it predominantly became an instrument to convince families to discharge relatives by reducing the expected financial and temporal investments in case of an occurring relapse or if taking care of the patient becomes overwhelming once again. At the time of discharge, one of the patient's relatives has to sign a form that formally states that the patient was 'delivered to my care and custody on leave of absence' and that they will have them 'properly taken care of and prevent [him] from doing injury to himself or to others' (The State Mental Health Rules 1990: Form IX). Handing patients over into the family's care and custody is a decisive moment for the institution and its staff and formally releases them from the responsibility to look after them.

However, the hospital booklet states that patients who are admitted voluntarily, the so called 'voluntary boarder' (VB), 'can take discharge any time after they show improvement in their mental status'. Whether their mental health status has improved or not is nevertheless determined by a psychiatrist. This situation constitutes what Paul Brodwin labelled as 'the paradox of consent' (2013: 156). The patient is treated as a 'rational and choice-making moral agent' (ibid.: 158) until they have signed the VB admission form: 'This apparent guarantee of clients' autonomy, however, actually paves the way for involuntary treatment' (ibid.: 159). The document highlights the institution's greater power, and patients implicitly agree to be kept in the hospital involuntarily from their admission onwards. Therefore, the categories voluntary and involuntary start to blur right after the admission form is signed, which constitutes a 'threshold paradox' (ibid.).

From a social anthropological perspective, it is highly questionable if a person who decides to be admitted to a psychiatric hospital would ever be considered an 'autonomous agent' that has made their decision independently. The medico-legal ideal of the 'voluntary admitted patient', having its origin in Western 'bioethics' (ibid.: 12), is particularly problematic in a sociocultural context in which the 'individuum' is rarely experienced as a bounded, singular and individual self (Marriot 1976). Instead, persons tend to be perceived as being enmeshed with other (human) beings and with their environment (H. Basu 2008). Rekha Mohan Kamble, who according to her file was admitted by VB admission, illustrates in Chapter 3 the various social enmeshments that determined her decision to sign the admission form. Her decision cannot be understood as an 'autonomous' one taken by Rekha alone. Rather, it was 'produced' by family dynamics and power structures. Rekha did not 'want' to be admitted to Asha or to live with 'mad people', but on the other hand, she also did not want to stay in the family home, where she was apparently considered a burden. She might have 'consented' to admission as something she saw as inevitable; a prestigious elderly Hindu woman – particularly a widow – would not want to become a family's burden. In the following section, I illustrate in more detail the decisive role that patients' families play in the negotiation processes that may lead to a patient's discharge and, more often, nondischarge.

Going Home or Staying Back: Negotiating Discharge

Part of the evaluation and negotiation process regarding whether a patient's condition has improved to such an extent that he or she can be safely sent or taken home is the examination of a patient's talk by the hospital staff and patients' families. Normative constructions of gender and self play a central role when it comes to the evaluation and judgement of a psychiatric patient's narratives (Addlakha 2001). In the following section, I discuss the stories and experiences of Hemant Dere and Tasneem Fateh Ali, who both fiercely negotiated the issue of discharge with their families.

Hemant: The Pitfalls of Resistance

Akshay and I met Hemant Dere and his family in early September 2011, exactly one month after the family admitted the forty-three-year-old to the hospital. We encountered Hemant's relatives on the ground floor of one of the buildings in the male unit. The superintendent admitted him as a 'voluntary boarder'

(VB), which limits the extension of a patient's stay to thirty days. The family came back to Asha in order to extend Hemant's stay in the hospital. They therefore had to take care of the formalities needed to complete Hemant's RO admission, which meant admitting him through the court. It was common at Asha to grant families a VB admission so that they could meanwhile get hold of all the necessary documents to complete the RO admission. Hemant's wife was accompanied by her sister and nephew, who lived near Asha and had already assisted her during the admission procedure. Hemant and his wife had two children, a son and a daughter, and lived about 400 kilometres away. The wife's nephew, Deepak, who was in his late twenties, took over most of the talking during our first conversation. In contrast, Hemant's wife remained quiet. The family had admitted Hemant to the hospital because he had started to behave violently with others. His file mentioned the diagnosis of 'chronic paranoid schizophrenia'. His nephew told us that he had behaved in a dangerous way long before his admission. The problems started in 2005, shortly after his brother died. The brothers ran a tailor shop together, but they fought frequently. One day, after one of their arguments, Hemant's brother committed suicide by setting fire to himself. The family tried to treat Hemant at their place and did their best to convince him to take his medications. However, their efforts did not work, and Hemant finally ran away from home. Distraught, Hemant's wife called Deepak threatening to poison herself and the children. Deepak started a search for Hemant and eventually was able to track him down around seventy kilometres away from his home wandering around a village. Not long after Deepak had found Hemant and brought him home, the family decided to admit him to the hospital.

After Deepak had told us Hemant's story, he went upstairs to inquire about Hemant. After five minutes, Deepak came back and informed us that his condition had not improved. The family left in the direction of the superintendent's office to discuss further steps to be taken with the psychiatrist. Akshay and I went upstairs to meet Hemant ourselves. He shared with us that nobody from his family had come to see him since they admitted him to Asha. He seemed desperate to go home. When he told us that he used to work as a tailor, it caught the attention of an attendant standing nearby. He came over and asked Hemant to follow him to the nearby tailor room. The tailor section, where some patients were seated on four or five sewing machines, was part of the occupational therapy facility. In this section, patients sewed the very uniforms that they had to wear when admitted to the psychiatric hospital.

Akshay and I continued our round through the male unit. We encountered Hemant's family once again on their way back from the superintendent's office. The meeting was successful, and Dr Shukla had granted them a ten-day extension to take care of all formalities. The family explained to us, as they had to Dr Shukla just minutes before, that it was not possible for his wife to take care of Hemant at home. Extensive treatment at Asha was therefore inevitable, and they wanted to admit Hemant for at least a year. Deepak shared with us that Hemant's daughter no longer wanted to go to school as she was being teased for her '*pāgal*' (mad) father. Akshay reported to the family that we had just met Hemant and observed him starting occupational therapy in the tailor section. Hearing about this, Hemant's wife, rather blank and expressionless until this moment, came to life. She started to interrogate us about her husband's condition. She wanted to hear our opinion on whether we thought that his stay in the hospital would improve his performance at home. Hemant's wife, her sister and Deepak assured us that they did not just want to get rid of Hemant but wanted to see some behavioural change before they could start thinking about bringing him home again. His wife was particularly troubled by Hemant's resistance to take his medication regularly. She even tried to mix the tablets with his food, but he eventually turned to exchanging his plate with that of another family member.

Six days later, we met Hemant together with his family while they were on their way to the superintendent's office. We asked Deepak about Hemant's condition. He told us that Hemant seemed to be quite stable now. Nevertheless, he was still convinced that Hemant should stay at Asha for at least six more months. However, the family still had to attain the second medical certificate, which had to be issued by the superintendent. Deepak did not want to leave the certificate's issuance to chance and tried to increase their prospects of receiving this important piece of paper by contacting a family friend who was on good terms with Dr Shukla. Recently, he had donated a water cooler to the hospital, and Deepak had asked him to call Dr Shukla and put in a good word for the family.

Sometime later, we spotted Hemant's wife, her sister and Hemant coming out of the superintendent's office. They all went to sit down under a shady tree in front of the OPD, where waiting families generally liked to sit in an attempt to escape from the blazing sun and heat. Apparently, they were waiting for Deepak, who was about to finish the paperwork in the superintendent's office. We overheard Hemant arguing with his family and noticed the tense atmosphere between them. He stated that he did not want to be admitted. He claimed that he had a lot of work to do at home and that the amount of food he received in the hospital was insufficient. His sister-in-law explained to him that he did not take his medications and therefore had to be treated in the hospital as an inpatient for some time. Hemant responded that he regularly took his medications in the ward and that he would do so at home as well. When Hemant realized that he would not succeed in convincing the two women to take him back home, he eventually turned his back on them and kept quiet. The family continued to wait for Deepak in silence. When Akshay and I were on our way to the male unit a little later, we encountered Deepak coming out of the superintendent's office. Relief showed on his face, and in his hands he held the second medical certificate.

The case of Hemant and his family illustrates the negotiation processes that determine decisions concerning discharge. A medical indication alone is not decisive concerning the question of a patient's admission and discharge from the hospital. The ability of family members to convince and influence persons in charge is of equal importance. The hospital staff is overtly aware of the powerful position families occupy in these decision-making processes. These interdependencies shape the everyday interactions and conversations between staff, families and patients. For example, I overheard a psychiatrist commenting to a patient during an OPD consultation: 'If you don't take your medicine, you'll have to come here your whole life!' One of the most common reasons for a patient's admission or readmission to Asha is patients' resistance to take their drugs. In Hemant's case, besides his violent behaviour towards family members, his resistance to take his medication was determining the family's wish to admit him to Asha long-term. Assuming a resistance to taking medication could be in part taste-related or to do with ease of use, pharmaceutical companies have extended their product lines accordingly. During my research, sales representatives came into the hospital to introduce pineapple-flavoured 'fluid solutions' for 'uncooperative patients' to the psychiatrists. This comprised a little bottle containing some yellow fluid with an active substance commonly used to treat bipolar disorders. This product line, however, had not been designed for the regular clientele that frequented Asha but the middle and elite-class clientele that attended the psychiatrists' private clinics, where they used to see patients from late afternoon onwards after they were done with their shift in Asha. Only better off families could afford the prices for these fancy medical solutions.

Psychiatrists and doctors were familiar with families who just wanted to 'get rid of' and abandon family members as quick as possible. When Akshay and I once accompanied Dr Gambhire during her consultation hours in the OPD, an elderly woman turned up together with her son, who was around forty years old. The woman told Dr Gambhire that her son would not sit still in one place for long, would often get angry and also beat her at times. Telling this to the psychiatrist, the mother started to cry. Dr Gambhire, however, remained rather unimpressed by this emotional outburst. She calmly requested the mother to stop crying and went straight into asking the remaining questions on her examination sheet. After the old woman and her son had left the consultation room, Dr Gambhire explained to us that the woman was just trying to get her sympathy and trying too hard to convince her to admit her son: 'She is old now and wants to dump him here.' Furthermore, the patient's brother was about to get married. Dr Gambhire suspected that the mother wanted to 'get rid of her son' before her daughter-in-law came to the house.

Actually, there indeed seemed to have been a number of families who saw Asha as a depository to rid themselves of troubling family members when their resources and patience eventually had come to an end. Nevertheless, the majority of families who wanted to admit a family member did not want to abandon them. Some of those had the sincere hope that a stay in the hospital would improve the mental health of their patient. Others, like the parents of a nineteen-year-old boy whom Akshay and I encountered one day in the visiting room, just found taking care of their ill family member on a daily basis to be overwhelming. The father shared with us that their son was hyperactive and unable to communicate. From the age of seven until fourteen, he had not spoken at all. Though the father stated that their life improved remarkably after they admitted their son to Asha, his son's life did not. The hospital did not have the means to take care of his individual and special needs. He wished that somebody could explain to him how his son feels and how to understand him better. Sometime later we spotted the parents while they were spending time with their son on the ward. They sat together in silence. The parents calmly cut their son's toe nails until an attendant asked them to leave and to continue what they were doing outside the ward.

Many of the families I encountered during my research were constantly busy with finding creative solutions to resolve the crises caused by a family member's mental illness. Part of this crisis management was to find a possible spouse and arrange a marriage for one's mentally ill or disabled children. Dhaval and I conversed with two men outside the OPD one day. They had a son and daughter respectively, both being outpatients in the hospital. They came from a rural part of Maharashtra and regularly travelled to the hospital in order to extend their children's LOA and to collect their medications. Additionally, one of the men would accompany other families from the village when they had to bring a mentally troubled family member to the hospital. Both men were concerned with finding a suitable match for their child. One was afraid that if he failed to find a suitable match for his son the consequence might be a bastard child (*hāramī*). He expected the situation to become tense when his other sons finally got married and brought home their wives and started having sexual relations with them. The other man was most apprehensive about there being nobody to take care of his daughter in the future. Both men contemplated possible arrangements to offer to the family-in-law. One thought about renouncing dowry or even transferring property to the son's wife. The other discussed the possibility of letting his son-in-law move into his house and inherit the family's property after his death.

However, when it comes to marriage arrangements for mentally ill children, another common strategy is to hide a mental illness, other invisible disabilities or chronic illnesses or to match children with similar disabilities (Addlakha 2007). Mental illnesses (in contrast to, for example, spirit possession) are perceived to have biological and genetic causes, therefore the whole family would be perceived as being 'afflicted' and would feel threatened by what a psychiatrist in Asha called the 'stigma of inheritance' (see for Das 2001). Admitting a family member with a mental illness to a psychiatric hospital can play a significant role in stigma management, which means families are ambivalently perceived within the hospital environment. They are at once a potential threat to the patient, which is reflected in the precautions taken to prevent a potential act of food poisoning (see Chapter 2), but at the same time depended on to come back and discharge their relatives and take over custody. Therefore, the psychiatrists are often rather cooperative when it comes to the extension of a patient's stay. However, if this becomes a pattern or the family does not respond to a social worker's calls or letters, a patient might be discharged by the 'Board of Visitors' and escorted home even against the family's will. Some families try to avoid being contacted by the hospital or prevent their family member from ever being escorted back by giving a fake address at the time of admission. A social worker has to confirm a patient's address and to check if the family still stays there before they can be brought in front of the BOV.

According to the Mental Health Act 1987, the 'Board of Visitors' (BOV) or 'Visitors' Committee' (VC), as it is referred to at Asha, is required for regular inspection and monitoring of psychiatric hospitals. According to the State Mental Health Rules (SMHR) 1990, it is responsible for 'a. review of admission and discharge of patients; b. inspection of the wards, outdoor patient department and kitchen; c. facilities to be provided; d. suggestion for improvement; and functioning as liaison officer between the Government and hospital' (Mental Health Act 1987: SMHR Chapter VI, 2.). Additionally, during the meetings taking place once every month, cases of patients who are considered as potentially 'fit for discharge' by the medical staff but whose families are reluctant to take them back home are reviewed by the BOV, and every three months medico-legal cases of so called 'criminal patients' are evaluated. The BOV meeting takes place in the recreation hall in the part that provides for the female visiting room. The visitors appointed as supervisors at Asha are the director of Health Services, Mumbai; a commissioner/ representative of the district 'handicapped welfare board'; the Hon. Session Judge of the district where Asha is located; a private psychiatrist, two clinical psychologists, two social workers, the superintendent of the central jail of the district; the civil surgeon of the civil hospital of the district; an executive engineer from the public works department of the district, the deputy director of the health services, Mumbai circle, and the medical superintendent of the hospital. Additionally, two to three of Asha's social workers and occupational therapists took part in the meeting. The patient whose case was to be discussed would be brought in by an attendant who would sit with the patient during the hearing and discipline them if needed. Sometimes the BOV would also summon the family of the patient, but often no relative was traceable or the family was reluctant to show up. The presentation of cases was unstructured, and the BOV members were not given any information about the patient before the meeting started. Sometimes basic information about the patient's case was read out from a file. Other pieces of information were given by psychiatrists, nurses, social workers or attendants. The BOV made the final decision if a patient was fit or unfit for discharge mainly based on the ground of symptoms displayed by the patient, e.g. facial expression and how they responded to the asked questions. To evaluate a patient's condition, the committee only had two or three minutes of time. If patients were declared fit, they were discharged by BOV order.

Tasneem: 'My Parents Don't Love Me!'

When I attended a BOV meeting for the first time, it took one hour and forty minutes. Overall, thirty-one patients were seen, among them twenty criminal patients. One of these patients was Tasneem Fateh Ali. She was forty-nine years old at that time and had been admitted to the hospital two months before. When the social worker contacted her parents and told them that her daughter was ready for discharge, they responded by saying that they were unwilling to take her home because of her 'misbehaviour'. When Tasneem was brought in front of the committee, she was accompanied by her parents. She was a divorcee who had moved back in with her parents together with her son after the separation from her husband. The hearing was short: Tasneem's parents reported on the welfare of Tasneem's son, who was pursuing his Bachelor of Commerce degree and in whom they had observed a change in personality during the last months. They related this to the shame he felt concerning his mother's inappropriate behaviour. The Muslim family was outraged about Tasneem's ignorance of 'their culture'. According to her parents, Tasneem would party with male neighbours, and she drank and smoked. When the committee asked Tasneem for her perspective, she simply stated, 'They are too conservative for me.' The committee then sent Tasneem outside the room in order to discuss her case.

The clinical psychologist with whom I spoke after the meeting stated that Tasneem's behaviour fell short of her family's expectations. This made her rehabilitation rather difficult. One of the senior female social workers described Tasneem as an 'exceptional case'. Instead of taking care of the family unit as was appropriate for a woman, she rebelled against this societal norm. The social worker saw Tasneem's inappropriate behaviour as 'a stigma' that affected the whole family and had led to her son threatening to run away if his grandparents brought his mother back home.

I had a look at Tasneem's file around ten days later. When Tasneem had given me permission to access her file, she also warned me that not everything written in there was necessarily true. Her diagnosis was 'paranoid schizophrenia' and 'alcoholism'. According to her file, she stopped drinking a year ago when she moved back in with her parents. One of the social worker's notes said: 'she is talking well + sensitive in hospital, but gives much trouble to parent at home.' Tasneem's file additionally contained a letter from the housing society based where the family lived, stating that her treatment in Asha had been inevitable. Her inappropriate behaviour such as sitting naked on the balcony disrupted community life. A note in Tasneem's file also mentioned that two days after the BOV meeting took place, the social worker counselled Tasneem. She spoke to her about her problematic behaviour at home in order to prepare her for discharge. The social worker had called Tasneem's parents shortly before, and they had announced that they would come to Asha within five days. When I spoke to Tasneem about her imminent discharge, she insisted that her parents would certainly come because they loved her. Indeed, two weeks later Tasneem's parents came to discharge her.

Around three months later, I bumped into Tasneem's father outside the admissions department. He remembered seeing me in the BOV meeting. Additionally, Tasneem had told him that she used to speak to me. He told me that her condition had deteriorated and that her behaviour was very disturbing for everyone. He described how Tasneem would say that she was 'not mental', would toss her medicine around instead of taking it and threatened to beat up her mother. He held up one of his fingers that was bandaged and described how Tasneem bit him. They had already admitted her to several hospitals, and at each she had stayed for around one month, but her behaviour remained the same. He warned me to be aware of her manipulative behaviour and that she was very intelligent, but also often dissembling. Just a week before, Tasneem had gone to a rave party and consumed drugs. Her father wondered if I could advise him regarding how to deal with his daughter's behaviour. I responded to him that I also, unfortunately, did not know what to do.

Three days later, a Muslim woman wearing an abaya[1] approached me outside the OPD. When she had removed her niqab,[2] I recognized her as Tasneem. She wore red lipstick. She was accompanied by her father, and he told me that they were there because she had problems with her medication. Tasneem's father added slightly mockingly that the medicine at Asha was not good and that Tasneem would therefore be admitted to a 'luxurious, American hospital'. Turning towards me so that Tasneem was not able to overhear what he was about to tell me, he murmured that I should not mention or discuss the topic of 'admission' in front of her. Then father and daughter left in the direction of the OPD.

I met Tasneem one week later. She shared with me that her father had surprisingly readmitted her. Tasneem was aware that a marriage was about to take place in her mother's family, and she suspected that it would trouble her parents if she was around during that time. Additionally, she blamed them for 'poisoning' her son against her. She shared with me that their relationship had been good once. She had even supported them financially when she worked as a teacher in Kuwait. 'My parents don't love me,' she concluded. I shared with her my recollection that when we spoke the last time in the ward she was confident that everybody loved her. Tasneem answered that after her readmission she doubted those words now.

When I encountered Tasneem on that day she was hanging out with her good friend Madhushree who told us that she was supposed to be seen by the BOV during their next meeting that was about to take place within two weeks. She had already been on the list to be seen by the committee members for the last meeting, Madhushree remarked sourly. She was not summoned eventually, because the social worker in her ward had forgotten to check her address. Tasneem interfered at that point and wanted to know more about the formal procedures that are observed when a family is not ready to discharge a patient. The formalities and procedures concerning a hearing by the BOV had not mattered much to Tasneem when she was admitted to Asha previously. Being readmitted, though, seemed to have taken away Tasneem's carelessness and confidence. Now she was interested to know what kind of behaviour was expected from her and if I thought that it would enhance her chances of being discharged if she stopped talking back to her parents. I shared with her that since patients were at the bottom of the hierarchy at Asha, they were expected to behave 'cooperatively' as much on the ward as in front of the BOV. Nisha, one of the helper patients in the ward, additionally gave Tasneem some advice concerning 'good' behaviour in the ward: do not abuse the attendants, take your medications regularly and remain calm in order to become a commendable patient who is ready for discharge.

After this encounter, I did not meet Tasneem again. When I came to the hospital in January 2012, I heard rumours that Tasneem had been discharged the previous October. I do not know if she was finally discharged by the BOV or by her family. However, like Tasneem, many patients gradually started to inquire about how to behave in front of the BOV and with the hospital staff in order to be discharged when they realized that it was unlikely their family will discharge them.

According to the Mental Health Act, the BOV (aka VC) is supposed to have a critical eye on what happens in and around the hospital. During the monthly meetings, social workers, and occupational therapists in particular, were often criticized for their work performance. During one particular meeting, the BOV decided on measures to improve bureaucratic processes in the hospital, but these were soon thrown out by the social workers and occupational therapists, who felt they were being targeted unfairly and resisted to shoulder the blame for things like the low number of confirmed addresses of patients that they were regularly held responsible for. The superintendent, Dr Shukla, was critical of the majority of the BOV members. He found fault with members that regularly turned up for the monthly two-hour meetings but never took any extra time to look round Asha or speak with its patients and staff. 'I think rather than criticizing us, they should work with us. . . . I find only one or two of them are helping us. [The others] are more there for the cap on their head. That they are members of this committee, that is not serving the purpose, isn't it?' One could think of the BOV as an institution of power, execution and decision-making. But the more I attended BOV meetings, the more I had the impression that it was a rather superficial, bureaucratic ritual. The BOV could actually change little about the grim circumstances in the hospital and the at times hopeless situation of patients abandoned by their families. The meetings merely served as a display of power and status. They also inevitably determined the BOV as a morally superior institution, doing much to reinforce the superordinate status of members over the regular hospital staff. This rather prohibited its members from engaging in sustainable problem solving based on reliable information and cooperation with Asha's staff.

The course of the meetings and their spatial arrangement mirrored typical elements of a court hearing. The seats were organized in the shape of a big U, and the chair for the patient was placed centre in front of it. The patient, family and hospital staff were fiercely questioned by the judge and other board members. For the judge, the patient's 'insight' was one of the most important criteria for discharge. The psychiatrists, instead, stressed clinical criteria during the hearing. Additionally, board members sometimes engaged in something like a 'diagnosis competition' and felt proud of their abilities to predict the diagnosis mentioned in the file from the patient's appearance. Other voices or moral and ethical arguments tended to be silenced during the meeting. For example, the families who complained about the patient's behaviour or the social workers' who complained about work load and hierarchical structures. The BOV hearing served as a stage where they could present decision-making, hierarchy and status and the institution and its bureaucracy were celebrated. It therefore functioned primarily as what Handelman terms a 'public event of presentation', where causal effects were more a by-product of the uncertain interaction between the enactment of it 'and the wider social order in which it is embedded, rather than a direct consequence of the internal logic of the event itself' (Handelman 1998: 44).

Between Protection and Control: The Status of Female Inpatients

An information board in the female visiting room announces the agenda Asha generally subscribes to: 'The hospital's purpose is to rehabilitate patients and to rebuild patients' lost prestige in society. This aim is easily achievable with the help of the patient, the patient's relatives, renowned people in society and NGOs.' Nevertheless, in the opinion of various members of the BOV and Indian mental health professionals, the area of social rehabilitation is one of the biggest shortcomings of Asha. This proves particularly true in the case of women, as the following table indicates.

Table 5.1. Length of stay of female patients (compared to male patients) in the years 2002 and 2011.

Length of Stay	**Women (2002)** (see Maitra 2003: 27)	**Women (May 2011)** (own data collection)	**Men (May 2011)** (own data collection)
Up to one year	20.9%	38.1%	64.43%
1–5 years	24.3%	23.51%	15.86%
5–10 years	19.9%	13.56%	06.86%
Over 10 years	34.8%	24.82%	12.86%
Total number of patients	100% (727)	100% (693)	100% (700)

In May 2011, when I started to frequent the hospital, almost every fourth female inpatient had been there for more than ten years. In the case of male patients, it was every eighth. Nevertheless, there had been an improvement concerning the rehabilitation of women compared to the decade before. In 2002, almost 35 per cent of women had been at Asha for more than ten years, according to the report 'Status of Women in Mental Hospitals in Maharashtra' (Maitra 2003). As shown in the table above, only every fifth woman admitted to the hospital left within the first year of her stay. In May 2011 in contrast, 38 per cent of the women admitted to the hospital, almost double the amount in 2002, left the hospital during the first year of their stay. Nevertheless, in 2011 they were still much less likely to be discharged within the first year after their admission to the hospital than men. Almost 65 per cent of male patients were discharged from the hospital within the first year of their stay. Besides the 'gender gap' regarding discharge and rehabilitation, the report also criticized the fact that psychiatric treatment tends to uphold and reinforce normative constructions of femininity (see also Addlakha 2001). During a personal conversation in January 2012, Shubhada Maitra criticized the fact that occupational therapy still focused on monotonous and gender stereotypic work like garlic peeling or embroidery. Maitra stated that the activities, including occupations in the ward taken over by the helper patients, merely kept women busy and supported the hospital staff more than the women, who were not developing lasting skills that might enable them to maintain a life outside Asha. When I spoke to the superintendent, Dr Shukla, about the issue of female long-term patients, he considered it unjustified that most of the blame was regularly put on Asha and its staff. In his opinion, Asha's staff were not the ones who kept female patients in and hindered their rehabilitation. Dr Shukla in our talk wanted society at large to take some responsibility and 'back the women, accept them outside the hospital and bring them in earlier for treatment'. Additionally, he thought the government and NGOs and corporates had to provide adequate services and provide funds: '[I]n India funds are put in front of deities rather than for a noble cause.' According to Dr Shukla, the media should be criticizing these kinds of social attitudes rather than bashing Asha with slogans like 'Governmental hospital holds back patients'.

As guardians of family honour and 'carriers of the burden of morality', a bigger stigma seems to be attached to the mental illnesses of women in Indian society (Addlakha 2008: 35). Vieda Skultans (1991: 325) states the different expectations and evaluations of men's and women's behaviour as the reason for this greater shame. According to Skultans, the three cornerstones of the Maharashtrian stereotype of madness – tearing of clothes, violence towards other family members and lack of attention and irreverence towards the preparation and consumption of food – are more severely condemned in women than in men: 'Women are supposed to be modest and gentle and their most important household task is the provision of meals for the family' (ibid.). Because the woman is in charge of household affairs, family life tends to be disturbed in a more severe way if it is she who suffers from psychiatric problems (Patel 1999; WHO 2004: 25). That women suffering from a mental illness are more likely to be sent back to their natal homes, be abandoned or divorced is reasoned because of their vulnerable position within the kinship structure and the sociocultural institution of marriage itself (Addlakha 2008: 35).

For most women, marriage is biographically very significant, but its sociocultural meanings are highly ambivalent. Marriage and procreation is 'not only central to men's perception of women, but it is also the core component of women's own self-identities' (ibid.). Accordingly, most young women envision marriage as one of the most important milestones in their lives, and many married women find pride and self-assurance in their marital status. At the same time, marriage coincides with leaving one's natal home and moving in with one's in-law family. In her husband's family, the newly wedded bride has to adjust to a foreign social environment, get accommodated with her status and position in the new family and establish new social relationships. These processes often entail high psycho-social stress for young women. Nevertheless, marriage is commonly conceptualized as a cure for mental illness, and to remain unmarried beyond a certain age can be stigmatizing for an individual as well as their families. In this context, it is understandable that young women like Jennifer, portrayed in Chapter 3, are afraid of this kind of stigma and therefore want to get married before they are 'too old' (in Jennifer's case 25). Families are usually distinctly aware that having a mentally ill child who remains unmarried constitutes a twofold stigma. However, from the medical and legal perspective, mental illness poses a threat to marriage alliances. One of the boards in the hospital that is supposed to educate visitors about traditional 'misconceptions' of mental illnesses warns about the consequences of delayed psychiatric treatment. That marriage is a good remedy for a person with a mental illness is listed as a myth, among others. According to the five Indian marriage laws,[3] a marriage can be annulled if one of the married parties was not 'mentally sound' at the time of the marriage ceremony. This provision does not apply if a spouse falls ill after the wedding. Nevertheless, if a newly wedded bride begins showing symptoms of a mental illness, the in-law family will suspect that her natal family was concealing her problems at the time the marriage was arranged (see Suman's case, Chapter 2). It is common for a newly wedded woman to stop regularly taking her medication because she is afraid of raising suspicion within her in-law-home. This behaviour might cause her to relapse, eventually revealing her mental illness. Statistically, psychotic episodes or a psychological crisis are more likely to occur in young adulthood, especially in the context of life-changing circumstances. Consequently, the first onset of a mental illness shortly after a young woman's marriage might not be such a rare case.

A woman and her natal family do not usually occupy a very decisive position in negotiations concerning whether her married status continues or not. When a newly wedded bride starts to show symptoms of a mental illness, her in-law family might just send her back to her family. Further, it was a common scenario for a married woman upon discharge from Asha to discover that her marriage had been annulled during her stay. In contrast, if a man suffers from a sudden onset of a mental illness shortly after marriage it is much more likely that his wife will stay with him and take care of him (Thara and Srinivasan 1997; SCARF 1998). Although the 'Ideology of Familial Care-Givers' as outlined by Vieda Skultans (1991: 331) holds a husband as equally responsible as a wife to remain on the side of their spouse in the case of a chronic mental illness, it is much more common for a woman to take lifelong care of her husband than it is the other way round, as illustrated in the case of Varun Bekaji Bhandari's wife, portrayed in Chapter 3. She had endured thirty-five years of Varun's mental illness despite his behaviour tremendously threatening and disturbing family life. Nevertheless, men's families, including their wives, tend to refuse to take care of them as soon as they become physically threatening, as it is illustrated by the cases of Mahesh (cf. Chapter 2) and Hemant.

Although at Asha families are predominantly recognized for their absence, negligence and by their failure as caregivers, the family and the social network of the patient are nevertheless invaluable for psychiatric diagnosis and treatment. Renu Addlakha (2008) comments that the 'operation of general hospital psychiatry in India is both theoretically and functionally dependent on a strategic alliance between the hospital and the family' (ibid.: 28). In the absence of adequate and acceptable state-sponsored facilities that provide any kind of long-term care for persons suffering chronic mental illnesses, biomedical institutions emerge as a viable option for a periodic reprieve (ibid.: 29). The cases of Kamalabai and Abdul (both Chapter 2) and Devendra, James and Varun (Chapter 3) show how the hospital is seen and used as a regular resource by families but also by patients, who may want to relieve family members of the burden of care taking. Patients may also be caretakers themselves and want to take a break, like Jennifer. In her home, she looks after her ailing grandmother and additionally makes sure that her mother, who suffers from a mental illness as well, takes her medication. Jennifer's stay at Asha therefore relieves her of her daily duties and looking after others in the family household.

Despite the close entanglement of family and psychiatric care in the Indian context, some patients are indeed discharged without the involvement of their families. In this case, the BOV has to be convinced that a patient is fit for a solo discharge. Generally, patients are rarely discharged from Asha completely independently, especially in the case of female patients. Males are more likely to be able to build on cultural capital they have to navigate a solo discharge: a formal education, social networks outside their immediate family circle and possibilities to work and make a living. The superintendent Dr Shukla stated that it was more difficult to discharge female patients on their own because the hospital staff would not know where to send them. Hostels, for example, may take in single men but rarely accept single women. A commonly mentioned concern was that women might start to make a living as sex workers after a solo discharge. Renu Addlakha (2008) comments that 'in the context of mental disorder and its treatment among women, it is the regulation of the female body that emerges as the salient concern of both the psychiatric and familial institutions' (ibid.: 32). According to Addlakha, women's reproductive functions and sexuality are articulated in terms of certain key social categories embedded in caste and religious structures of society: 'purity and pollution, auspiciousness and inauspiciousness, shame and honour, and segregation or purdah (veil)' (ibid.). These social categories become markers of their social as well as their self-identities as is indicated in Rekha's narrative (see Chapter 3). Rekha describes her self-identity before marriage as having been closely connected to her status as a daughter of a well-reputed Hindu family. Later in life, she perceives herself as a devoted wife who is painfully aware of her failure to give birth to a son. The latter diminished her status in the in-law family, and from Rekha's perspective she might not have been thrown out by her in-laws after her husband's death if she had delivered a son instead of her two daughters. Finally, Rekha apparently suffered a lack of support from her natal family, particularly from her brother, after becoming a widow and mentally unstable. Complying with the submissive ideal of a dutiful daughter and devoted wife, though, she never openly criticized her male relatives during our conversation; neither her husband, who was apparently an alcoholic, nor her brother, who admitted her to Asha. In the case of a chronic mental illness or any other disability, Indian women seem to be 'caught between their failure to approximate the culturally constructed feminine self and their actual experiences of the lived impaired self' (Addlakha 2008: 35). Being a female long-term patient at Asha is often experienced as a similarly contraindicative status. As the following case of Maneesha Shirodkar illustrates, female inpatients in general inhabit an ambivalent position between care vs. abandonment, freedom vs. constraint and hope vs. desperation (Pinto 2014: 35).

Maneesha Shirodkar opened the conversation with Rini and me with the statement that everybody was very unhappy in the hospital and would be much happier if they were allowed to go home. Maneesha was fond of jewellery and asked Rini to bring her some earrings, which she planned to wear during the Ganpati festival that was to take place the next month. Around her neck, she wore a *maṅgalsūtra*,[4] which she got from one of the attendants and which she proudly showed us during the course of the interview. Although Maneesha was not on good terms with her husband, she was proud and conscious of her marital status. Maneesha was thirty-seven years old and had lived with her family in one of the suburbs of Mumbai before her admission to Asha almost four years ago. She had suffered from schizophrenia since her mid-twenties and until then had been treated as an outpatient in Asha. Although, she did not know what 'schizophrenia' meant exactly she was aware that she suffered from a mental illness. In the early days of her illness, she used to get angry and beat people. Her father had problems finding a good match for Maneesha, and a number of grooms rejected her. Maneesha explained this as being a *māṅglik*.[5] In her late twenties, her father succeeded in arranging a marriage for her. Her family as well as the family of her future husband belonged to a lower caste (Mahadev Koli[6] and Chambar[7] respectively). Her husband was a divorcee, and Maneesha was about to be his second wife. The first wife of her future husband had left him and taken their two children with her. He was ten years older than Maneesha, and his health was deteriorating. Despite these shortcomings, Maneesha felt that she did not have any choice but to marry him – she was getting older, and it was therefore getting much more difficult to find a suitable match for her. Maneesha's husband used to work as a security guard. After the marriage, he hopped from one job to another, and they did not have any regular income. Therefore Maneesha also started to earn one to two hundred rupees per day by selling Gujarati products like soaps etc. to people on their doorsteps. Even though the couple had a healthy sex life according to Maneesha, she unfortunately did not get pregnant, and they did not have the financial means to undergo any medical examinations or treatment. Furthermore, her husband eventually came to know about her mental illness after the marriage and, additionally, became angry with her when she could not keep up with his expectations concerning household work: 'He always complained that I didn't wash his clothes and didn't cook or clean the floor properly. I mean, although I had been done with all the household chores, he still had complaints.'

Maneesha's family had faced a crisis when her father died of a heart attack some years before her admission. According to Maneesha, her elder brother sold their father's apartment and then 'ran away with the money', while her mother stayed with her younger son and his wife and received her husband's pension. Maneesha used to have arguments with her sister-in-law, particularly if she went out to dance or if she spoke to any male outside the family. Her family did not approve of her engaging in this kind of behaviour. She admitted, though, that tensions might have been fuelled when she continued to visit her natal home after she had already been married. Particularly her brother and his wife told her repeatedly that this was not her house any more – as a married woman she now belonged to her husband's house. When she still came to visit her mother once more, her brother admitted her to the psychiatric hospital. According to Maneesha, he had the help of a local politician, who provided him with a jeep (and maybe also with political contacts) to admit her to Asha. During the interview, Maneesha called her brother a 'very bad man', her 'enemy' and a *harāmī* (bastard). Although Maneesha was his only sister, he had not come to visit her on Raksha Bandhan even once during the last four years. Maneesha was equally disappointed and angry with her husband, who refused to take her back home. According to Maneesha, her husband did not know that her brother planned to admit her to Asha. He came to visit her once a year and used to bring her soap, a toothbrush and underwear. Every time she saw him, he found excuses for not taking her home; for example, that she had refused to cook for him. Additionally, he was afraid that it would cost him too much if he looked after her at home. He was also afraid that he would not be able to handle her once she became excited or uncontrollable.

Maneesha repeatedly referred to her file when we asked her for details concerning her illness. We checked her file after the interview and found a note that mentioned the diagnosis 'paranoid delusions against family members'. A nurse's note described Maneesha as 'suspicious' and quoted her: 'My brother is on the battlefield with me.' Notes added by the psychiatric social worker at the time of Maneesha's admission mentioned that Maneesha reported to have a claim on her father's property but that her brothers were against her and consequently admitted her to Asha. I am not able to conclude if Maneesha's perceptions of her family were indeed 'delusional' or if what she said might have held some truth. Quite certainly, though, none of Maneesha's relatives accepted her or wanted to discharge her. The respective notes of the social worker stated that her brother refused to take any responsibility for her. He did not respond well to any of the letters the social worker had sent to him. The last time he had visited his sister was at the end of March 2008. Because contacting her brother had not worked out for the past two and a half years, the social worker eventually turned to Maneesha's husband, who had last visited her around a year before. Maneesha's file also mentioned that her case was discussed in front of the BOV in April 2011. She was not discharged at that time because her family was not ready to pay the hospital bills and take her home. When Rini and I spoke to Maneesha about her current situation, she started to cry. She knew that she could not discharge herself and that the BOV would not support a solo discharge. And even in the unlikely case that the committee would discharge her on her own, she was aware that she would not be able to pay the hospital bills.

'My Brother Is on The Battlefield with Me!': The Ambivalence of Kinship and Intimacy

Women's self-identities do not remain stable in the context of chronic illness: 'What is really at stake is the need to reclaim a sense of self in the face of an ongoing life trajectory of deprivation and challenge. . . . [P]atients strive to reconstitute their suffering as moral and creative agents' (Addlakha 2008: 36). Nisha Shakti Gore, whom I interviewed together with Kaveri at the beginning of October 2011, was from a popular neighbourhood in central Mumbai, where she lived with her husband. She was twenty-nine years old and hailed from a family of three sisters, who were all married, and one brother, who had remained unmarried. Her position in the ward was similar to the one Nikhat occupied (see Chapter 3). Nisha worked as a helper patient in the admission ward, was quite famous at Asha and had many friends. She had suffered from epileptic fits several times a day since her childhood and usually fell asleep afterwards. Her family had brought her to see various doctors, and they prayed at temples. Her brother, who was a computer engineer, took particular care of her. Unlike Nisha's sisters, who were all educated and working, Nisha left at twelfth grade. Nisha told us that her family, and her brother in particular, did not expect her to work. Some neighbours had suspected that she was affected by the elements of wind, fire and water and had recommended that she not leave the house. Nisha met her future husband at a concert. Both were from the same caste, and therefore their families agreed to the match, and the couple had a love marriage. Soon after the marriage, Nisha gave birth to a baby girl, but unfortunately she passed away. Nisha had been admitted to Asha three months previous, and she told us that the medication she had received was helping her and that the frequency of her fits had decreased remarkably. Her family used to bring a lot of food when they visited her: 'About my husband, don't even ask how much stuff he gets for me.' Nisha was sure that she would return to her husband's place soon: 'I am a married woman!' When we asked her if she had ever tried to run away from this place, she responded: 'My god! No, never! If I would do something like this, then my parents would be dishonoured by my behaviour in the community.' When we asked her what her expectations concerning her future were, she responded: 'I just want to live a happy, married life, have kids and take good care of them, not to give my husband any troubles or get sad myself. I just hope we both can live with each other in harmony, love and peace.' When we later had a look at Nisha's file, though, we discovered that her husband had divorced her. She had been treated at Asha before, for a two-year stretch, and was then discharged and went home to her natal family for a short period before she was readmitted again. The visitor cards in her file indicated that her father and her sister seemed to visit her regularly but obviously not her husband. Her file also included a letter from her father, written when she was admitted the last time. It stated that Nisha had run away from home for a whole month before she was finally found at a nearby train station. It was not clear if she had had her period yet (= if Nisha was pregnant), but that whatever the situation he was ready to take responsibility. In contrast to the woman who was portrayed in the file Nisha told a story that embodied the ideal of what an Indian woman should be: a woman that loves and cares for her husband and (future) children, that is loved and looked after by her brother and who respects and honours her parents. In this Nisha was creatively camouflaging how her life had departed from ideals and social norms during recent years and in doing so could perhaps reclaim a sense of self. During the interview, Nisha shared her plans with us to be discharged around Diwali, which was just two weeks away, and spend the holidays among her family. However, when I came back to Asha in January 2012 Nisha was still there.

In the beginning of a long-term illness episode, and when women felt supported by their families, they tended to collude with prevailing definitions of femininity and the female role. However, women's relations with and feelings surrounding their families varied, as illustrated by Maneesha's attitude, who openly expressed her anger, disappointment and hate towards her husband and brother, and transformed during their stay in the psychiatric hospital. Realizations concerning themselves and their future, dissolving relationships but also newly established and evolving relationships with the staff and copatients moulded women's narratives. Rucha Sonar, whom I met together with Rini in the beginning of August 2011, was thirty-eight years old, unmarried and had stayed in Asha for around two years. She told us that her family was originally from south, coastal Maharashtra and belonged to a caste that traditionally had the occupation of gold smiths. Rucha was very annoyed when Rini asked her about her 'mental problem' and why she was admitted to Asha. Rucha clarified that she was treated for the dizziness she used to experience at times. Rucha had three sisters and one brother. Her father died and her mother had become old and she therefore could not take care of Rucha any more. Rucha explained to us that her married brother already took care of their mother and therefore he could not take care of her as well. Since her admission, nobody of Rucha's family had come to see her in the hospital and her brother did not even send her any money on Raksha Bandhan. However, towards the end of our conversation, Rucha assured us that even though her family did not come to visit her often, she was certain that they still loved her. Even if the behaviour of her family seemed to indicate the contrary, Rucha's strong conviction provided her with an emotional anchor that prevented her from abandonment. Women in the hospital continuously struggled with the dissipation of love and the possible dissolution of relationships and had to make sense out of it in relation to their lives and selves.

In order to understand the whole dimension of intimate relationships and how women in Asha narrate and experience them, we have to take into consideration the fact that intimacy always entails ambivalence (Mitra and Nair 2011) and that attachment always comes with 'a certain agony' (Pinto 2014: 244). The ambivalence of intimacy, its potential to provide safety and accommodation and its capability to produce vulnerabilities and accommodate violence, is reflected in a dichotomous sociocultural discourse on marriage. The dominant popular discourse states that Indian marriages are almost unbreakable; divorces are rare, and Indian society is strong because of that. However, a fierce counter-discourse sees – particularly for women – oppression, control and dependency embedded in the institution of marriage (ibid.: 246). The sociocultural images of other kinship relations display similar ambivalences. For example, the relationship between parents and their children is highly idealized, and the cohesion and solidarity of family in general is stressed. In the respective counter-narratives, daughters are portrayed as having to put up with horrendous marriages that their families arranged for them, suffering abuse from their in-law families and as not supported and deserted by their parents. In reverse, there are said to be elderly people who have to live on the streets because the younger generation abandoned them or they are unmerciful regarding not taking proper care of their parents (Cohen 2000).

The narratives of women in the hospital drew on and at times played with the sociocultural ideals but also the potential nightmares that are inherent in kinship relations. They (over)idealized their husbands (e.g. Nisha, Rekha), praised their daughters' attributes as exemplary (e.g. Tasneem, Nisha) and blamed their parents for betraying them (e.g. Tasneem). Another culturally sacralised relationship that narratives of female inpatients often build on is the one between brother and sister. Brotherhood is socioculturally idealized and conceptualized as being about the backup and protection of women (Bennett 1989). The special connection between brothers and sisters is celebrated on Raksha Bandhan. The annually performed celebration, rooted in Hinduism, is centred around sisters tying a Rakhi, which symbolizes ritual protection, to the wrists of their brothers. The sister traditionally receives small gifts of money from her brother on this occasion. On the Raksha Bandhan celebration that took place at the beginning of August 2011, I observed many sisters tying the Rakhi to their brothers' wrists on the hospital premises. As reflected in Maneesha's and Rucha's narrative, the festival was of importance to many female inpatients at Asha. Both women mentioned that their brothers did not come to see them on Raksha Bandhan or send them any money. Rini and I observed another patient, Lata Jain, who was visited by her brother on this holiday and accordingly could tie the Rakhi to his wrist in the visiting room. Lata was thirty-nine years old and had been treated at Asha for ten years. Her brother, who was five years younger than her, told us that he visited his sister two times a month. Every four months he would discharge her and take her home. But usually after around fifteen days her symptoms would deteriorate again, and he had to bring her back to Asha. He explained to us that unfortunately he could not take Lata home permanently at the moment because his wife was pregnant, and Lata would need assistance with a lot of things; for example, going to the toilet. He brought Lata a variety of food and snacks: a 'Dairy Chocolate Collection', fruits, crackers, a soft drink and tea. While Lata took care of one treat after the other, her brother shared her story with us. When Lata was nineteen years old, she was married in a village in Rajasthan from where her family and community (Marwadi[8]) hailed. But after the marriage, Lata was maltreated by her in-laws. They tied her up during the night as they believed Lata to be possessed by a *bhūt*.[9] Additionally, there were rumours that her father-in-law had sexual relations with his daughters-in-law. While the wife of the older brother of Lata's husband apparently had managed to defend herself, in contrast Lata seemed to have endured his sexual assaults. Her mother, who came to know about the abuses when she visited her daughter, reported the case to the police. The mother's brother withdrew the report shortly after, though, because the in-law family started to threaten the whole family for reporting them to the police. Unfortunately, during this time, Lata's family did not have the financial and social means to be able to support her further. Their father's health deteriorated, and the financial situation was not stable because Lata's brother was still pursuing his studies. Therefore, the family had to send Lata back to her husband's house. But soon after she returned to her in-law family, the abuse started again: 'They treated her like an animal', the brother told us, shuddering. Around this time, Lata's mental health was poor, and she was treated in a governmental hospital in Mumbai at the beginning of the 1990s. The psychiatrist prescribed her ECT treatment, but it turned out that she was pregnant. The doctors did not want to risk abnormalities, and her unborn child was aborted. Two years later, Lata tried to commit suicide, and one year after her suicide attempt her husband filed for divorce. It took four more years until their separation was legally recognized and all disputes were settled between the families. The in-laws claimed that Lata had hidden her mental health problems at the time of marriage and achieved annulment of the alliance. During the time her brother was telling us her story, Lata had managed to finish all the snacks. Her brother then prepared to leave. Two attendants, who supervised the visiting room, asked him to sign the visitor book. He gave them ten rupees as a donation for the Ganpati celebrations that were about to take place within a few weeks. He told us how he had once donated mangos for all the patients in the female unit. One of the mango boxes he brought for the patients was stolen by a medical officer and he had to substitute it. Lata's brother was aware that corruption took place at Asha and knew about the bad conditions in the wards. 'One is happy if one's patient is alive – more you cannot expect,' was his pessimistic view of a hospital culture he had experienced for more than ten years. Nevertheless, he was convinced that he could help his sister by visiting her as often as possible because the hospital staff would treat patients better if their families visited regularly. He accompanied Lata up to the gate of the female section, where the attendants took over to take her back to the ward. Lata's brother waved a last goodbye as his sister disappeared out of sight.

When I discussed this encounter with Shubhada Maitra during an interview and implied that brothers could constitute an important sociocultural resource for some female inpatients, she responded with a counter-narrative:

> It is the question what the parents left behind. Even if it is a small amount, if the brother gets hold of the property, he may say, ok, I will get everything, but occasionally I may go and visit my sister, at least it keeps my conscience clear. I am sorry to say it like this. . . . Brothers could support their sisters in more concrete ways than just visit them in the hospital, because every person has the right to be free. (Interview with Shubhada Maitra, 2 January 2012).

In her comment Maitra draws the image of a self-centred, egoistic in contrast to a culturally idealized, caring brother. The matter of property that Maitra touches on brings to mind Maneesha's case and the brother who admitted her and declared her mentally ill to keep her hospitalized in order to prevent her from making any claim to the family property. However, Maneesha's narrative about her 'bastard' brother was not perceived as plausible and the anger that she expressed towards him was labelled 'mad' and accordingly noted down in her file as a suspected symptom by the psychiatric nurse.

The Gendered Fallout of Kinship: Imagining a Future beyond Family Ties

Psychiatric hospitals constitute a space where women's relationships vanish and break down in a great amount. Accordingly, Sarah Pinto (2011) comments that 'rather than enforcing normative configurations of "the family," [psychiatric] biomedicine grapples with the gendered fallout of kinship' (ibid.: 376). Therefore, contrary to social anthropologies traditional tendency to interpret kinship as being mainly about establishing and maintaining relations and affiliations it should theorize their dissolution and break down as well: '[K]inship seen as recombinant allows room for divorce and other dissolutions to be seen not solely as wrong, stigmatized, or posed against the (intact, Indian) family, but as part of the family's moving fibres' (ibid.: 255). Some time ago, Maneesha had met Prajakta, who was an external social worker, on the hospital premises. Prajakta told her about Tarasha, a community-based rehabilitation and recovery programme for women, and proposed that Maneesha join the programme in order to increase her chances of being discharged from Asha, getting a job and living independently. Even if family relationships had remarkably deteriorated, it was still hard for women at Asha to accept the prospect of a solo discharge in a context 'in which solo living is understood to constitute abandonment rather than independence, in spite of opportunity-expanding changes in lives and laws' (Pinto 2014: 30). Nevertheless, the dissolution, de-idealization or breakdown of kinship relations had the potential to open up space for the re-evaluation of expectations and (unconventional) imaginations concerning the future and intimate relationships. According to David Graeber (2015), 'the hidden reality of human life is the fact that the world doesn't just happen . . . – it exists because we all collectively produce it. We imagine things we'd like and then we bring them into being' (ibid.: 89). Take as an example the case of Asifa (see Chapter 3), who did not miss her husband or being married at all. Because of her experiences of abuse and violence in her natal family and by her husband, she hoped to marry a 'decent man' if she ever got married again. She further imagined a fulfilled life beyond family ties: once out of the hospital, she wanted to study Urdu. Before a maverick life can be considered worth living, though, it has to be imaginable.

The project Tarasha provided an alternative for some women who were otherwise destined to spend the rest of their lives at Asha. When Prajakta came to Asha, she made the rehabilitation programme a conversational topic among the women, and they began to imagine what a life outside the hospital could look like. For some women, for example Faiza (see Chapter 3), the programme was not enticing. Faiza held a respected and renowned position in her ward, and she told Prajakta that she would prefer to stay at Asha. Tarasha, a field action project of the Centre for Health and Mental Health, School of Social Work, Tata Institute of Social Sciences, Mumbai, was initiated by Shubhada Maitra in order to address core issues concerning the psychiatric treatment of female inpatients. For several years, there were no financial means to realize the project until a sponsor eventually turned up and the initiative finally started with four women, who were selected to be part of the project in 2011. The project addresses issues of 'Self, Shelter and Livelihoods' in the recovery process from a mental illness and particularly supports women who lack adequate family and social support and are 'long stay patients'. The project works from a rights-based perspective, assuming that '[w]omen recovering from mental disorders are entitled to an independent and a dignified life and cannot be institutionalised forever' (Tata Institute of Social Sciences n.d.). When I frequented the hospital in 2011, the project team was in the process of selecting suitable women to be discharged and rehabilitated. Prajakta regularly came to the hospital to speak with the women and to hold group sessions and discussions. Those women selected were women below forty-five years of age who had been at the hospital for a few years but not decades. 'We are ruling out too much chronicity, we don't want twenty-five, thirty years of mental illness, because that impairs to a certain amount, cognitive and emotional impairment are there,' Shubhada Maitra clarified during the interview. Women like Suman Vishwasrao Dere (see Chapter 3), who was sixty-seven years old and had been at Asha for thirty years, were therefore ruled out as potential participants. After the selection process, the project team initiated the women's discharge by the BOV and paid the hospital and treatment fees. Subsequently, the women moved into a hostel that was affiliated to the project and started to attend day-care centres and vocational training institutes. The project team also helped the women open bank accounts and procure *Aadhar* (identity) cards.

When I spoke to the superintendent, Dr Shukla, about Sarika N. Prakash's case (see Chapter 3) in January 2012, he considered her an 'ideal candidate for Tarasha'. It had come to light that her father would not discharge her and take her with him back to the US, and Sarika's husband had already left for South Africa. The superintendent suggested that it was in Sarika's best interests to learn how to be independent and make a success of it, as her family might otherwise disown her completely. When I came back to India more than a year later in March 2013, I surprisingly bumped into Sarika at the TISS campus. She was accompanied by Joyashree, one of the social workers attached to the Tarasha project. Sarika had been part of the second Tarasha batch that was discharged in November 2012, and her father financially supported her rehabilitation with a monthly donation to the project. Joyashree told me that even Faiza had recently spoken of her interest in taking part in the programme. Tarasha had gained a good reputation among the women in the hospital. 'It gives them perspective', explained Joyashree. Natalie Gies-Powroznik (2016: 18) followed up Sarika's story as part of her Master's degree research and describes in her work how Sarika started work as a receptionist in a restaurant in south Mumbai in 2014. She worked six days a week in shifts from noon to midnight or sometimes even longer. Soon after she had started working she also found a boyfriend. Her boyfriend and people at work did not know about her mental illness and the medication she took every day before and after work. She admitted to Natalie that she sometimes skipped the noon and afternoon doses or took them in the restaurant's cloakroom (ibid.: 33). Sarika was quite aware of the stigma that came with her mental illness: '. . . [I]t's part of my life, but I don't tell anyone. When I tell people, I can quit my job' (ibid.: 20). Similar to the other women who became part of the Tarasha programme, Sarika's long-term aim was to keep her job and thus eventually be able to find her own apartment. Her wish was to leave the hostel room that was rented by the project and that she had to share with six other women who were all once long-term patients at Asha.

If mental illness and gender is discussed at all in the Indian media, it mostly addresses the likely abandonment of women in mental hospitals and shelters : 'Mental illness is often neglected in India because of stigma and poor care. But women are the worst affected and are mostly abandoned by their families' (BBC News 2018). Even if a woman's position is certainly more vulnerable than a man's, Sarah Pinto nevertheless argues for using a language around the term 'abandonment' in psychiatry that is ethical and takes into account the complexities of kin life. She argues that the concept of 'dumped women' follows 'Michel Foucault in seeing the psychiatric patient, a central figure of modern power, and the asylum as part of a "disciplinary network" that depends on the family as "sovereign" object and agent of discipline' (Pinto 2009: 2). To address the 'new old problem of "dumped women"' (ibid.: 8), Pinto suggests deconstructing the cultural symbol and moral imaginary of the 'Indian family' and instead elaborating on the meaning intimacy, the body and life has for women. Social anthropology has to reflect on all the specific and fluctuating relationships that set the conditions for women in psychiatric hospitals: '. . . the stakes on "dissolution" (of marriage and mind) are set in specific legal structures that remain inaccessible to bioethical or social science languages that stop at "the family"' (ibid.: 9). How can the 'dissolutions' that determine Sarika's life be understood from a perspective that looks beyond traditional family structures? The relationship to her husband broke down in the course of her mental illness along with contact with her sons. Interestingly, the breakdown of this relationship was never discussed or morally elaborated on by Dr Shukla or the social workers. This may be reasoned by the fact that it was a 'love marriage' arranged by the couple and not supported by the young people's families. In this context, the alliance was probably considered as rather fragile, or at least more fragile than a traditionally arranged marriage would have been. The behaviour of Sarika's ex-husband, who left with both their sons without even informing her, seemed not to surprise or morally outrage people. In contrast, her father's behaviour was far more critically evaluated and commented on. Dr Shukla called him a 'nasty person' who refused to take over responsibility for his daughter. Why was the behaviour of Sarika's father judged so fiercely? At least he used to call Sarika regularly and was financially supporting her. The criticism of his behaviour stood in stark contrast to the silent acceptance of Sarika's husband's and his family's behaviour in deciding that Sarika would not be seeing her sons again and for whom it would have been far easier to come over to the hospital to take care of any formalities or paperwork. Pinto points out that divorce law in barring forms of support from ex-husbands or the in-law family 'further solidified dependence on natal kin rather than expanding the means for women to establish themselves independently' (ibid.: 6). Dr Shukla essentially criticized Sarika's father for refusing to occupy his socioculturally defined role as natal caretaker, and the reduction of care to financial and moral support via the phone equalled 'abandonment'. From his perspective, he left Sarika in the care (confinement) and custody (dependency) of Asha and therefore prevented her independence and freedom. The understanding and imaginations of what this exactly constituted were divergent, though. For Dr Shukla and other health professionals, freedom and independence meant a successful rehabilitation, preferably with a patient's family. Sarika's father had once respected his daughter's longing for freedom and independence when she had decided to run away with her husband and establish a family life on her own. For Sarika herself, freedom meant being able to avoid the stigma of mental illness. She decided to keep her past secret and conceal the fact that she was taking medication in order to be able to pass as a modern, middle-class and cosmopolitan woman who proudly maintains her job and has a boyfriend.

Gender is an influential sociocultural category when it comes to the institutional evaluation of narratives as well individual narrative practices. At the same time gender – as sociocultural stereotype and ideal – determines illness trajectories. Women who suffer from mental health problems are often disproportionally divorced and left by their families. While the narratives of these women and the entanglement of gender, sexuality and/or the breaching of sociocultural norms and expectations have received some attention (Wilce 1998; Davar 2001; Addlakha 2008; Pinto 2012), the narratives of 'mad' men are rarely analysed regarding any of these aspects. Rather, analysis is directed towards how the talk of people with a mental illness is generally categorized as 'mad', senseless and not worth listening to, while the male gender remains an unmarked category, for example, in asymmetric patient-practitioner relationships (see, for example, Wilce 1995: 944f.). Accordingly, the following two chapters focus on the enmeshment of male gender, sexuality and the legal context by focusing on a 'mad' and a 'queer' narrative that were both rendered unintelligible in the psychiatric sphere. Ramesh Krishna Doshi and Ajay Raj, the tellers of the narratives, both transgress sociocultural categories in their stories and break with socio-legal norms and values. Ramesh killed his mother during a psychotic episode, and Ajay does not want marriage and a heterosexual family life. These two examples illustrate that while men with a mental illness generally may be more privileged regarding the sociocultural resources that they are able to draw on, these also become exhausted at times and men are 'abandoned' too. Either it is because their mental illness is too disruptive and destroys family ties and cohesion or that they fall out of the kinship system because they do not comply with behavioural and gender 'norms'.

Notes

1. A simple, loose, often black, overgarment worn by some Muslim women.
2. Garment of clothing that covers the face. Worn by some Muslim women as part of a particular interpretation of hijab (modest dress).
3. In India the Hindu, Indian Christian, Muslim and Parsi Marriage Act apply to the respective communities. The Special Marriage Act applies to interreligious marriages.
4. A *maṅgalsūtra* (Marathi, from Sanskrit *maṅgala* = 'holy, auspicious' and *sūtra* = 'thread') is a necklace that the groom ties around the bride's neck during the Hindu marriage ceremony. The *maṅgalsūtra* clearly marks her as a married woman after the ceremony.
5. A *māṅglik* has a *maṅgal*, which means a bad omen, in one's horoscope.
6. The Mahadev Koli officially belong to the 'Other Backward Castes' (OBC) category, according to the Indian reservation policy.
7. The Chambar traditionally had the profession of cobblers and belong to the Dalit castes.
8. The Marwadi are an ethnolinguistic group that originates from the Marwar Shekhawati Jaipur region of Rajasthan and Haryana. They are known to be successful in business.
9. A *bhūt* (Hindi = ghost, bad spirit) is a common explanatory model for (mental) illnesses in South Asia (see H. Basu 2010b).

CHAPTER 6

'THIS HOSPITAL IS NOT GOOD'

WHAT A PSYCHIATRIC PATIENT CAN TELL US ABOUT PSYCHIATRIC CULTURE

> Ramesh (R) – This hospital is not good. I know. I have spent six and a half years here, so I know. Patients 'expire' here in ward number 11. In ward number 11, the sick ward. Patients die there.
>
> Akshay (A) – How do patients die?
>
> R – Because of 'heart attack'.
>
> A – Heart attack?
>
> R – Yes it's true. I have seen the dead body when they took it outside in the van. When they work, observe them. Patients die here. I don't know how they die, but patients die here. I think it's because of 'heart attack'. . . . I don't like this hospital. Because I saw a patient's dead body, ok, being taken away, after seeing this I understood that patients die here, that is what exactly happened to the patient.

Akshay and I met Ramesh Krishna Doshi at the beginning of September 2011 outside the criminal ward, which holds patients who either committed a crime during an acute phase of their mental illness or who fell mentally ill during their stay in prison. In the few sentences above, he quite well captured an atmosphere prevalent in the psychiatric institution that was determined by a lack of resources and the feeling of abandonment. I could relate well to Ramesh's description of the hospital as a place that has a tendency to break people and their hearts. However, during my research, I observed how voices of psychiatric patients like Ramesh were systematically silenced by being declared 'mad', 'nonsensical' and 'unintelligible'. From a social anthropological perspective, 'mad' narratives emerge as ways to experience and frame the world. Although narratives are not understood as accurate reports of personal experiences or social events, they nonetheless give us important insights into certain sociocultural processes connected with illness (Kleinman 1989). To reach these insights, however, we have to carefully reconstruct the situation in which the narrative was told, the discourse it may be part of and how we ourselves participated in producing it – for example as an interview partner (Csordas et al. 2010). In the following, I intend to show, by the narrative analysis that I employ, how Ramesh gives us access to a life world determined by the experience of suffering, structural violence and failure. His moral claims concerning psychiatric treatment and everyday life at Asha were mostly ignored though. This leads to another issue that I tackle in this chapter: 'mad' narratives differ in their properties – at times fundamentally – from conventional ones and therefore are often considered void of any social meaning. I argue, nonetheless, that they are all interpretable and understandable when appropriately contextualized socially, culturally and institutionally. Ramesh's case furthermore illustrates that 'mad' narratives themselves can serve as an effective tool in managing a life of unsoundness that has to be lived in an often-threatening institutional environment.

How Does it Feel?: Empathizing with the 'Mad'

Ramesh spoke so-called 'Bumbaiyya Hindi' – a kind of Hindi creole that mixes the pronunciation and words of several local languages. It is spoken in and around Mumbai, especially by people of the lower working class who grew up in Mumbai but whose parents are not originally from Maharashtra. During the interview, Ramesh also repeatedly used certain English terms (e.g. 'heart attack') and switched to English from time to time – particularly when conversationally turning towards me. Ramesh's dialect, use of language, long monologues and excited mood during our talk made his narrative less accessible than those of other patients I encountered in the hospital. On the one hand, he used so many familiar themes and symbols. On the other hand, he from time to time seemed to get lost in his monologues and in their idiosyncratic meanings. Indeed 'mad' stories tend to have a kind of ambivalent attractiveness for their recipients:

> Mad stories are evocative and metaphoric. They are full of symbols, but we think-that those symbols are used in very personal, even idiosyncratic ways. We consider them incoherent and incomprehensible. They are not 'rational' and do not represent any 'normal' logic. They do not fit into categories. They escape every classification, save that of 'psychotic stories' or 'mad stories'. They are matters out of place. They are viewed as signs of madness and therefore show how much we should value health and normality. Yet, mad stories are attractive. The many studies and literature on the topic which fill the shelves of bookstores and are so eagerly bought are the best proof of this attraction. (Van Dongen 2002: 25)

Psychiatry and neurolinguistic research developed several models to frame and categorize 'mad speech' (see Swartz 1994; Fine 1995; Kramer, Bryan and Frith 1998; Hensler 2009; Huang et al. 2009; McCabe 2009; Ryan, Woodyatt and Copeland 2010). The German authors Kindt and Schecker (1998) see a common reason for the unintelligibility of 'mad speech' in what they call *assoziative Überschwemmungen* (associative flooding), where a person is unable to suppress associations during the speech act. The associations instead 'break through' in the talk and transform the use of language, words and grammar in unconventional ways. 'Associative flooding' contributes to the impression that 'mad' narratives often seem to be full of symbols, secret messages and metaphors and to follow an unusual, mystic structure. Even if severe speech disorders seem to be absent in Ramesh's talk, it might be shaped by what clinical psychiatry denotes as a 'flight of ideas'. His speech lines up life events and associative ideas without following any real thread. Therefore, his narrative apparently lacks coherence. Nevertheless, Ramesh's talk always stuck to certain themes; namely, everyday life in the hospital, his family, employment and education and important biographic events.

Although social anthropologists share a method of interviewing with psychiatrists, they have a very different approach in interpreting and making sense of speech acts and life stories (Skultans and Cox 2000: 21) – they collect narratives 'in order to obtain information about cultural practices' (Van Dongen 2002: 28). Nevertheless, as Laurence J. Kirmayer stresses, 'empathy' provides an important tool in the clinician's as well as the social anthropologist's work (Kirmayer 2008). He defines empathy as understanding 'another's experience through feeling or thinking something similar oneself' (ibid.: 458). Empathy includes relatively simple mechanisms of imitation but also requires more complex cognitive functions and detailed knowledge of the sociocultural world of those with whom we empathize. The ability to empathize can give clinicians as well as social anthropologists an idea of 'the other's' experience. To achieve a close understanding of somebody else's feelings and experience, we have to imaginatively reconstruct and inhabit some portion of their world. This necessarily means decentring from our own habitual stance. Empathy is vulnerable to distortion by one's own personal associations and emotional responses, which may be projected onto the other or lead to biased interpretations (Braddock 2010). Empathic responses furthermore depend on accessing a system of associations governed by an 'affective logic' – a pattern of response that is partly 'hard-wired' and partly acquired – and additionally a 'social logic' – the meaning of specific situations, predicaments and scenarios, which is mostly acquired through learning the rules and practices of a social world. According to Kirmayer, failures of empathy occur either 'because our emotional logic does not fit' or 'because we lack the social background knowledge and experience to construct the correct model or elicit the right responses in a particular situation' (2008: 461). In the psychiatric context, difficulties of empathy occur 'because of altered logic, thought disorder, different affective logic, or psychic organization' (ibid.: 463). A theoretical understanding of psychopathology can enhance possibilities for empathy in the case of mental illnesses. In the ethnographic field, in contrast, social anthropologists have to face the challenge of understanding the experiences of people with different categories and concepts of self and emotion, who engage in different ways of constructing and interpreting life.

However, social anthropologists and clinicians both regularly struggle with the limits of their empathy. When we reach these, we experience people as alien, strange, bizarre and abnormal. Failures of empathy are inevitable and unavoidable. We can best counter these by acknowledging, exploring and reflecting on our limits. We have to assume that there are plenty of experiences that remain difficult to explicitly communicate (ibid.: 462). All means of communication – be it language, facial expressions, gestures and even the creation of a shared context that conveys tacit meanings or provokes parallel experiences – have their limits. As social anthropologists working with narratives, we continuously have to remind ourselves that '[s]tories don't give immediate access to experiences' (Van Dongen 2002: 28). In addition, particularly extraordinary experiences and severe suffering often escape words as well as empathy. Els van Dongen tries to put into words, to empathize with and to make sense of the experienced terror when 'psychotic people feel "touched" by others' (2004: 206). According to Van Dongen, it is a common psychotic experience when certain things that happen or are said are no longer kept at a distance from the body by the medium of language. Instead, speech becomes part of the body: 'Words and sense of touch fuse into one, and the relationship between psychotic people and others becomes lifeless' (ibid.). She tries to put this experience into words:

> For psychotic people metaphorical statements become 'literal inscriptions' whenever they refer to the body. That which others say about them or to them is, as far as the body is concerned, painful and destructive. It enters the body unbidden. The patient's body is not securely delimited, as ours is. It lies open and vulnerable to threatening actions and objects. (ibid.: 208f.)

Obviously, clinical tools and cultural models have their limits in helping us to empathize with certain experiences (see for Hacking 2009): 'there are always pockets of idiosyncratic, deviant, alien, and unique experience that arise in the private soliloquy of the theatre of the mind and may be enacted at the margins of culturally prescribed roles, rules, and practices' (Kirmayer 2008: 462). Additionally, empathic failure is likely to occur if one continuously encounters people that inhabit different worlds than one's own following different social logics. Therefore, Psychiatric clinicians entering inter- and transcultural encounters in their work have to be aware of and deal with empathic failures – as has the ethnographic researcher in a psychiatric setting in a different cultural context.

Empathic failures might be one reason that stories of atypical, deviant and resistant individuals are so often homogenized in ethnographic writing or buried in fieldnotes, even if to tell and unravel them might reveal important insights (Okely 1991). To find a balance between an integrated and contextualized representation of human lives, which are shaped by socio-cultural patterns and the diversity of human experience, is a common challenge faced by social anthropologists in ethnographic writing (cf. Gay y Blasco/Wardle 2009: 35). Empathizing with 'the mad', means to understand 'mad' people's worlds not merely as idiosyncratic, but as socially and culturally constructed (Sadowsky 2004).

A 'Mad' Narrative

According to Ramesh's file, which we were allowed to have a look at with his permission, he was thirty years old at the time of his first admission in 2005; his diagnosis was chronic schizophrenia, and he had already been suffering from this illness for approximately ten years at this point. One of the attendants shared with us that Ramesh killed his mother about six years ago when he had gone home for a 'leave of absence'. He was probably in a psychotic phase at that time, but not many details are known about what exactly happened. One of the two police men who had to be present in the criminal ward 24 hours a day told us that Ramesh sometimes got 'extraordinarily angry'. Additionally, he remarked that he was pig-headed: 'If you tell him [to do] something and if it is ok for him, only then he will complete the task, otherwise he won't listen to you.' He also mentioned that Ramesh was 'quite smart' and that 'he speaks English', which in India indicates education and earnt him a respect.

A – So what problem you faced before coming here?

R – There was no problem. I was admitted here. I am supposed to work, ok, where the money will come from? If I won't work, so where will the money come from? Madam [here he refers to me] is young; we all were young, so they told me, if you don't work, then we have to admit you in [Asha]. I said: Do it! I had to appear in court, and then I was admitted here. I don't know why I had to appear in court. I am no criminal.

A – That means you are from the 'civil ward'?

R – Yes. Civil.

A – Then here, in the sense . . . did you do something there [in the civil ward]? [Akshay implies here: Did you commit any crime?]

R – The Senior [attendant] here recognized me, so that the senior transferred me from there to here. I didn't do anything. The senior told, 'I came to know about him, he will work as a helper here.' I do the job of a helper here. . . .

A – And what type of work do you do here?

R – I bring food, I clean the ward. Because people stay here, so it has to be clean, ok, if it is dirty, it is not good, ok. If there is some patient who doesn't take bath, I bath him. Mummy and daddy expired.

A – When that happened? Six years back?

R – About six, seven years back. I was not working, ok, that is why they expired. Now, when I go outside, I will work.

Ramesh states that he was admitted to the hospital because he did not work and did not earn money. On another occasion, he mentioned that the (economic) 'atmosphere' at home was not good. He drank and then drove an auto rickshaw and was consequently admitted to the psychiatric hospital.

Ramesh narrates a story from the margins, and it is one of multiple struggles (Kleinman and Kleinman 1995). He tells us about a government institution that enacts control rather than providing care and cure: 'This hospital is not good.' Particularly 'mad' narratives have to be understood as embedded in institutional frameworks, its topography and ontology (Saris 1995: 39). Ramesh did not disclose to us that he was staying in the criminal ward. When the charge of murder against Ramesh was withdrawn some years before, an attendant wanted to escort him back to one of the general wards. But he was stopped by one of the nurses: 'Why are you bringing him here? He killed his mother!' According to the attendants, it would have been 'too dangerous' to carry out the interview in the ward itself because criminal patients often became violent or could try to run away. So Akshay, Ramesh and I sat in a nearby shed that was sometimes also used by visitors. One of the attendants commented: 'If a civil patient runs away, its ok, but if a criminal patient runs away, it will be a havoc.' He told us of an incident that occurred a year ago when a patient ran away at 4.00 AM. The attendants who were on duty at that time were held responsible and were all suspended for fifteen days.

Ramesh disclosed a shattered life and family that in his narrative he tried to cobble together the best way possible. He apparently belonged to a Hindu community, but during the interview he also mentioned that his mother was Muslim. Ramesh's father migrated from Karachi to Mumbai – probably during the time of the partition of India from Pakistan in 1947, a decision that Ramesh repeatedly rebuked during our conversation. Ramesh mentioned that his mother had died several years before. Shortly after, his father and brother also died, but he still had two living sisters. One of his sisters came to visit him from time to time, but she was not ready to take him back home. A note in Ramesh's file mentioned that she was afraid that he might kill her too. Ramesh did not reveal to Akshay and me that he killed his mother; he put the blame on his father. An attendant shared with us that he had never overheard Ramesh admitting to the murder of his mother and suggested that we had better not put too much trust in what a patient has to say in general: 'Patients lie all the time!'

Ramesh's story emanates from a schizophrenic mind. Ramesh indeed appeared as rather alien to Akshay and me; often his thought process was difficult to grasp. However, there was a thread of sympathy that bound us during our encounter and that guided us throughout the interview.

'They Have Made a Jail out of a Hospital': Talking about Psychiatric Culture

The criminal ward is known among patients as being a particularly 'bad ward' where the attendants' behaviour towards patients is more cruel and police officers are constantly present. Patients generally look down on patients admitted there. Therefore, Ramesh used to refer to himself as a 'civil patient' who belongs in the general wards, which was technically true, since the charge of murder against him had been withdrawn. For Ramesh, it was highly important that we did not identify him with the criminal ward: 'They took me to the court; I don't know why they took me to the court. I am no "criminal".'[1] When Akshay implies that he must have committed a crime to be in the criminal ward, Ramesh insists that he only works there as a 'helper', which meant having more status and certain rights. For example, he was allowed to move around more freely than other patients.

Ramesh commented on criminal patients' 'bullying behaviour' and repeatedly stressed how differently criminal patients behave and speak:

> R – See those are 'criminals', they talk a bit differently. The others who are 'civil' patients, they are somehow good. These 'criminals', what is this, sometimes they fight, sometimes they do other things. 'Criminals' what, they only want to eat, but they don't want to work. Their behaviour is just in the manner of 'criminals'. They eat a lot and if you say something to them, then they will pick a fight.

For Ramesh, 'the criminal' is an embodiment of immorality. Similar to how 'the mad' are compared to 'normal people', the 'criminal' is socially constructed as the antipode of a 'good citizen'. In the following, Ramesh describes how difficult it is to escape stigma after somebody is labelled a 'criminal'. Once admitted to jail, one has a similar fate to the 'mental patient' admitted to a psychiatric hospital. It is difficult and often not even desirable to come out again.

> A – So you mean they beat each other a lot, in this way?

> R – They are beating in the sense that they talk to each other as if they were fighting. Fighting . . . in the sense that they just want to quarrel. Because they have come from the central jail . . . . You know the situation there. Even in films they show the quarrelling of criminals. These people, they, to be saved from their crime, they want to save themselves now. Here they come to know about the psychology of this place, which is criminal. It is punishment, too. Even after discharge, the judge will declare 'they are criminal'. Because the judge is sitting in the committee [here he refers to the 'Board of Visitors', see Chapter 5], he will declare them criminal. They are finished, they have spent six, seven years here, still they don't want to go. To stay here, they have made the ward their home.

Ramesh was carving a desirable space for himself in the social order and hierarchy of the hospital with his stance on criminals as despicable. He perceived himself to be different from the others, even the civil patients, in manifold ways. Although he was very familiar with the hospital and its social structures, he claimed not to have any close friends.

> A – What about friends you have made here?
>
> R – The one who meets me, who helped me get admission to the college, I will go to his house. He must be engineer or officer somewhere. He knows me as his friend.
>
> A – But in this six, seven years you must have made friends here, so what about them?
>
> R – No, I interact with them just as [part of my] duty, as my work demands it. I am [interacting] as a patient, I am a [civil] patient! I have not made any friendship with anybody here.

Interestingly, for Ramesh, the statement 'I am a patient', which demarcates his status as a helper/civil patient in contrast to the 'criminals', has an empowering meaning in this ward at Asha. As it became clear in Chapter 3, in the other wards at Asha, it is common for a patient to insist that everybody else is 'a patient' or 'mental' but that they are 'normal' themselves. Particularly in institutions like the psychiatric hospital, in which family and friend networks are mostly absent, relationships with other patients can constitute an important social resource. However, for Ramesh to admit any social ties at Asha may have felt too threatening because of his weak ties with anyone outside of the hospital. Ramesh's statement that he did 'not make any friendship' at Asha also indicates that his experiences of social interaction in the hospital were determined by hierarchy and status roles. Interestingly, Ramesh first misunderstands Akshay and starts talking about his friend Jadhav outside the hospital. Ramesh referred to him repeatedly during our conversation. Apparently they studied together in college. Jadhav inspired Ramesh to change his field from commerce to engineering and helped him to get admitted as a student: 'He doesn't know that I am here. If he comes to know, he will come here to take me out.' Jadhav plays a crucial role in Ramesh's narrative. He mentions him in the context of deciding not to work in his 'father's field', in farming. He repeatedly links Jadhav with education, which Ramesh highly valued. Additionally, he mentioned some more friends later during our talk 'who stayed nearby' and who he claimed would visit him from time to time. However, an attendant later revealed to us that 'nobody comes to visit him'. On the visitor card in Ramesh's file, no other visitor but his sister was mentioned.

A – And do attendants harass you sometimes?

R – They beat with a stick.

A – With a stick.

R – Here at the back, down at the legs, like the police.

A – Police . . .

R – You know how the police beats – the attendants beat like them. Attendants should not beat like this. Because this is a hospital not a jail. They have made a jail out of a hospital.

Annika (An) – But it is a 'mental hospital', so . . .

R – Mental, we know that it is a mental hospital, we 'qualified' people, but for others, who are locked up,

> it is jail. At least 1,500 patients stay inside looked up. Inside there are four, five helpers who move around. They ask for money anyhow, 'Give two rupees, give ten rupees for tea.' They do like this – I have seen it. Helper people, ok, they also beat patients. If he asked to catch a patient, then they hold a patient and prepare them to get beaten up. Then here the stick, the stick here at the back. The reason why I don't intervene is, if I speak for the patient, then I won't be released. I would remain staying here. That's why I don't speak. These are no attendants, they are police. An attendant should be like a 'college student'. A 'college student' can do the work of an attendant for a doctor. But students of seventh/eighth SSC [Secondary School Certificate] cannot do it. Even SSC pass will not be able to do it. A student going to college can do the work of an attendant. He has the 'humanity', he has the *īsāniyat* [humanity], he would be able to do it.

For Ramesh, the similarities between the two 'total institutions' jail and hospital are striking in Asha's everyday routines. These include the brutality of the attendants, the constant presence of policemen and the judge in the Board of Visitors. Indeed, similar parallels can also be found historically. Until 1912, when 'mental hospitals' were formally declared 'medical institutions', the Inspector General of Prisons was in charge of these institutions. However, Ramesh's evaluation suggests that while the label may have changed, social structures and practices still resemble so called 'mental asylums' at the beginning of the twentieth century. Remarkably, Ramesh linkens attendants to the police. Police in India are infamous for being brutal, corrupt and unreliable. And Ramesh could indeed corroborate this.

> R – The police put me in the mental hospital the first time when I came here. Policemen are useless, the police here, ok, the Maharashtrian police is useless.
>
> A – Why?
>
> R – They bully people. They give slaps to the public. If they take somebody, ok, they slap him. And they

> abuse him, too. They abuse the name of one's mother. I have a friend . . . he told me, 'The police has beaten me'. So I said, 'Let's go and have a word with them'. Why to be scared, we are young chaps, come with me, I will go with you. He said 'no'.

Ramesh describes how physical violence ('they beat with a stick') and corruptive practices ('they ask for money') structure everyday interactions in the hospital. Besides holding his ground as a helper patient, Ramesh operates a second strategy to claim his superior status: he draws on his 'cultural capital', in Pierre Bourdieu's sense. This becomes apparent when he adopts a typical middle-class attitude in stressing the importance of education and uses the respective English terms 'college student', 'doctor', 'humanity'. The display of this habitus may have been further encouraged by the presence of Akshay and me, who were from educated families and hailed from a higher middle-class background. Furthermore, Ramesh established a link between us and himself by repeatedly referring to our common backdrop of 'being educated' (see above 'we "qualified" people'). Most people in Asha related my background in medical anthropology to something that was between psychiatry, psychology and social work. Ramesh advised us at one point in our conversation: 'Don't leave the "doctor field". Doctors are smarter (*hōshiyār*) than engineers.' This statement resonates with the ambivalent meaning that education had in Ramesh's life. He studied digital electronics but failed in his second year. One of the attendants even suggested that Ramesh's 'high education' was responsible for his 'excitement' when he was locked up in the ward. Because of this behaviour, the attendants decided to allow him to roam around outside the ward. This at least seemed to keep him quiet and calm.

Dying of a 'Heart Attack': Moral Claims of a Psychiatric Patient

> R – My mother was Muslim, she used to talk the same way you talk. If somebody talks like this, doctor or somebody else, I remember my mother. But I don't cry. I won't remember your face now. Mother told me, whenever you remember me be blessed. She used to

say, 'Don't assume that you go to die.' She used to say, if a young boy has to die, and when he has died, ok, his *ātmā* [spirit/soul] will stray. My mother used to say [this]. She told the truth. At times I hear voices in the ward. In ward number 11 and number 12 are voices: 'come here', 'come here'. I get scared. In the night I have heard it two, three times. I slept immediately. It is the truth; it is there in the ward. Those who stay in this ward, ok, those patients who 'expire' at a young age or who expire at an old age, their voices are there. The doctors know about it. He must hear the voices. . . .

A – How many patients die here?

R – Patients become very thin and ill; they don't eat. Because of food they become thin and get a heart attack. And some patients suffer from TB, become 'hollow' [*khōklā*] and die. There are TB patients here.

A – How many . . . in the sense . . .

R – I think around twenty/twenty-five TB patients stay there and [the] rest must be around thirty/forty ill patients. Those patients who are sleeping [not able to get up], are not fed by the nurses. They have to be fed by the nurses' hands, right, there are thirty/thirty-five patients, they have to be given and fed tablets. They don't feed them. I two, three times myself . . .

A – Why have you gone to the sick ward, what happened to you?

R – I was shivering like this, like this I was shivering, like this it started.

An – Fever?

R – Fever.

An – And what else was there?

R – When I went there, at that time, I didn't hear voices. Afterwards, they transferred me to Bhopatkar [an attendant], senior Bhopatkar's ward, ok, number 12, then the voices were there. This is the truth. From where do these voices come, I started to wonder,

> why are there voices at night? All the patients were sleeping on the beds, like this, this is the truth. We educated people don't believe in these things, but I believe this must be true. So all the patients are sleeping on the bed. They are not shaking like us, what sitting, however sitting, no, they were sleeping on their bed. Voices were there, 'come here', 'come here'. I was scared, I said stupid [*sālā*][2] 'medical science' does not believe this, we don't believe this, 'medical science' people, 'science students'. So why these voices are coming? I was scared, I chop-chop stood up and I wandered around in the night, until I chop-chop threw me on the bed's sheet and fell asleep. I was scared, I had not faced fear earlier, that was the first time that I was scared. This must be the truth. I am looking around, there is nobody, so whose voice is it?

Ramesh's mother provides an explanation why voices are audible in the wards; the concept that human beings who die before their time – before they have cleared an important stage in their life cycle, like marriage and having children, or who die a violent death – become ghosts is common all over the world. In India, too, the souls of some unfortunate individuals may remain in this world. Spirits or ghosts who trouble or even pose a potential threat to those left behind is a reality in many communities. Why were the *ātmās* at Asha not able to find peace? Ramesh provided a possible answer when he described patients becoming very thin and ill: 'they don't eat' and 'get a heart attack' while others 'become hollow and die'. He criticized the fact that patients are not taken care of properly – that is, 'are not fed by the nurses'. Their illness and death is often not caused by a physical disease, but neglect – social failure and moral corruptness. Additionally, Ramesh had observed how many bodies were not handed over to their families to be prepared for their last rites but instead were carried away in an anonymous van.

During the interview, I felt Ramesh's moral claims resonated with several of my fieldwork experiences. One day I joined a senior psychiatrists, Dr Kulkarni, on one of her daily rounds. As we left the female unit, we noticed an ambulance arrive. It was apparently carrying a single patient who had gone for an examination at the general hospital. Dr Kulkarni shared the patient's story with me: 'Half a year ago, she was diagnosed with cancer, a tumour is growing in her throat. We contacted her family and recommended that they should take care of her treatment. Her sister is a gynaecologist in a private hospital. But nothing has happened since then . . . I expect her to die during the coming days.' We reached the male unit, where the nurses presented the files of those patients who had to be examined or whose medication had to be reviewed. One of these was a helper patient, who had been at the hospital since 1988. During his stay he had developed a medical problem and was no longer able to walk. The costs for his treatment would amount to three thousand rupees (around fifty euros at that time). Dr Kulkarni asked the ward staff to check his old file for any contact details of his relatives. But his file could not be tracked down. So, who would pay for his treatment? Next, the nurses presented Dr Kulkarni with a death certificate that needed to be signed. When checking the document, the psychiatrist was taken aback and started to interrogate the nurses. The dead patient, a young man and 'MR ['Mental Retardation'] case', had been picked up by the police near a local train station in 2008 and did not know where he was from. About a month before I accompanied Dr Kulkarni, nurses and attendants had recognized that the patient suffered from a persistent cough. Accordingly, they added a remark in his file, but they neglected to inform a doctor and he was now dead. Nobody had come to know what finally killed him; Dr Kulkarni assumed that he must have been struck down by a tuberculosis infection. No further investigation was initiated, and no autopsy was performed; because the patient did not have any relatives, nobody was interested in the results. The patient's dead body was probably brought outside to one of the hospital vans and then interred anonymously. Dr Kulkarni then had to sign yet another death certificate. It was of a patient who was admitted to the civil hospital for treatment of his acute diarrhoea a few days previous. The day before, the civil hospital called to inform about his death. Nobody else other than the hospital staff came to know or was concerned about his fate. This patient, too, was left behind by his relatives.

'They have made a jail out of a hospital!' can be interpreted as inculpating the state for its failure to provide treatment for people and transform control into care. Psychiatric institutions should not be punishing patients and creating pain and suffering as retribution for what is perceived as a crime committed against the social order (Asad 1997). Nevertheless, Ramesh experienced Asha as unable to provide treatment, care or cure to its clients. They do not have the 'humanity' to do it, as Ramesh expresses it. This is why the hospital is 'not good'.

> R – Medicine is good, but you get sleepy because of it. Because of the tablets you get sleepy, there is little [effect on the] 'blood circulation'. It's just that you can sleep in the night. If I didn't sleep in the afternoon then I can sleep in the night. I do 'daily walking' in the afternoon here, so I am sleepy at night, that is because the thighs, so through walking the thighs, veins get full, blood goes properly to the brain. So I feel quite sleepy at night. See because I walk, there is good blood circulation to the brain, because of the walk. Then I am able to sleep in the night. After having food at 7:30, I go to sleep at 7:45. Medicine makes a difference as well as walking. The others, patients, stay awake in the night, too. *Bapre* [Oh dear!]! Sisters and all don't take the sleeping pills which they give to us. They don't eat the sleeping pills themselves, but they give them to us. Once I asked a sister whether she takes the pills. She said, 'Mental' [people] will take them, so why we should take them?' So I asked, 'Do we look like "mental" [people] or kids?' She told me '"Mental" [people] will take [these tablets], we don't take [them]'.

Ramesh correlates good mental health with good 'blood circulation to the brain', which I repeatedly heard during my research. The effectiveness of electroconvulsive therapy (ECT) was often explained by its ability to improve blood circulation to the patient's brain and therefore improve mental faculties. In his narrative, Ramesh presents medication as neither an instrument of cure nor of care. Rather, he portrays it as a tool of control and its consumption as something that marks people as 'mental' and 'patients'. Taking medication is experienced as an excluding and stigmatizing factor, which has been explored a lot in social anthropological literature (Rhodes 1984; Estroff 1985: 68; Saris 1995: 58).

As mentioned above, Ramesh's statement that patients at Asha die of heart attacks is not just the description of a mere medical disease but the identification of a 'sickness' in terms of neglect (Kleinman 1989: 621) prevalent in the hospital. 'Sickness' in Kleinman's sense, attaches cultural meaning to certain symptoms and diseases, often in connection with a moral judgement. People dying of a 'heart attack' in the hospital are not cared for but neglected. Ramesh's narrative metaphorically describes the suffering caused by structural violence prevalent in the psychiatric hospital. According to Paul Farmer (1997), to understand and explain suffering as a consequence of structural violence, we have to embed individual cases 'in the larger matrix of culture, history, and political economy' (ibid.: 272) and to take into account the various social axes like 'gender, ethnicity ("race"), and socioeconomic status' (ibid.: 274). What patients dying in Asha have in common 'is the experience of occupying the bottom rung of the social ladder' (ibid.: 263). During my fieldwork, I was asked by Dr Gambhire to visit her private clinic and see 'real patients'. She told me: 'These patients have a family who supports them. There you will learn far more about mental illness and how to treat it.' Dr Gambhire implies here that a 'real patient' – somebody who can be treated successfully and cured in the end – necessarily has to be backed by a social network. I have described elsewhere how the Indian concept of a person, which is not complete without their family and social relationships, shapes and determines psychiatric treatment in India (see Strauss 2011: 149f.). We can understand from the comment above that those who end up in the psychiatric hospital without a family's support are denied the status of (real) 'patients'. They are not granted a moral status as persons, which, at the same time, seems to mean that they lose their eligibility to be cured and cared for. They are, in a way, a lost cause and have already died their social death. Their physical death to follow seems to be only a matter of time.

Clearly, having a family that pays for one's treatment at Asha raises one's status and well-being in the ward. Only those patients whose hospital bill is paid regularly and who have a home in which they are looked after are able to get a 'leave of absence' and spend time outside Asha. As discussed, being female increases the risk of being abandoned by one's family. Equally, roadside destitutes picked up by the police and admitted to the psychiatric hospital occupy a particularly precarious position. The only possibility for improving one's situation in the ward without any family support is to try to climb the institutional ladder (see Chapter 3). Obviously, those not suffering from a severe impairment or a chronic mental illness are capable of doing so much more to improve their lot.

'Karachi is not Smart': Narrating the 'Mad' Way

While we may grant a certain kind of 'constructive power' to all kinds of narratives, 'mad' narratives construct reality in an even more fundamental, radical and magical way than 'non-mad' stories do. Ramesh's narrative creates its own world with its own rules and does not stop at describing experiences. He repeatedly refers to a solution for overcoming the suffering and structural violence in the hospital: better 'education' for the staff in order to facilitate 'humanity' and humane treatment of patients. Narratives, including 'mad' ones, are the effort of sociocultural beings to make meaning out of their experiences and surroundings by making use of terms and concepts already familiar to them. Gananath Obeyesekere (1990: xix) understands this 'process whereby symbolic forms existing on the cultural level get created and re-created through the minds of people' as the 'work of culture'. However, not all human minds make use of sociocultural patterns and symbols in the same way. For Els van Dongen (2004: 5), a person with psychosis turns out to be a wanderer through culture, creating a 'bricolage' reality from materials at hand. They 'roam the world of values, norms, ideas and beliefs, looking for whatever is sufficiently useful to give expression to their musings' (ibid.). Ramesh in his 'bricolage' adopts plenty of English terms and concepts, mimicking a middle-class habitus. English terminology from the medical and psychiatric discourse provides him with verbal tools that he uses in a creative bricolage to structure and interpret his institutional life. The words 'student', 'doctor', 'medical sciences' and 'heart attack' are powerful, almost magical entities because their meaning moves beyond the metaphorical. Els van Dongen claims 'mad' stories become odd not because they reveal hidden meanings but because they refer to too many meanings. This points to cultural reserves that we all take for granted and additionally reveals the 'inherent indeterminate and ambiguous meanings of symbols, myths, models and metaphors' (2002: 39). Van Dongen refers to the tellers of 'mad' stories as 'hermetic thinkers' for whom 'everything is meaningful' and who 'play "le jeu des ressemblances"' (ibid.). Their stories rest on core models, myths and metaphors of culture, which they use to make sense of their lives. This includes getting a handle on a shattered life and controlling the destructive powers of 'madness' and what seems to lie beyond human control: 'Culture, as a collective of stories, is used to practice magic' (ibid.: 42). Van Dongen understands magic here as 'the ability of words to effect things': 'Signs, symbols and myths are recycled, mixed, and put together in a way that alienates others, that has power to manipulate the course of events and the others' responsive actions' (ibid.). Ramesh in his narrative takes up the 'myth of education', understood as a conceptual part of a sociocultural discourse that claims education and rationality to be the way to a more human, 'modern' and 'civilized' Indian society (Quack 2012). As representatives of modernity, doctors and college students are assigned a salvific role in Ramesh's story. A high educational status can do away with the mischief of 'madness' and 'inhumanity' and the uncivilized behaviour of psychiatric patients and some of the staff at the hospital. Actually, Ramesh considers himself to be part of this magical sphere of salvation ('we educated people'), thereby detaching himself from the corrosive atmosphere of the place and the uncivilized behaviour of the criminal patients. Interestingly, terms and concepts that are granted magical powers in Ramesh's narrative serve as the exact opposite in the sociocultural discourse, as the antipodes of magical thinking. This becomes apparent when Ramesh narrates his experience of hearing voices in the sick ward. He is completely aware that the belief in straying souls belongs to what is labelled 'superstitious' and 'backward' thinking among the middle and higher classes of Indian society. The contradiction between the two powerful cultural protagonists in his narrative, 'educated people' (science) on the one hand and the 'voices of straying souls' (spirituality) on the other is obvious in the following statement: 'We educated people don't believe in these things, but I believe this must be true.' Eventually though, in this context, the voices win and overthrow their antipode 'rationality': 'The doctors know about it. He must hear the voices.' And 'I was scared, I said stupid medical science does not believe this, we don't believe this, medical science people, science students. So why are these voices coming?' Medical doctors do not generally occupy the role of saviours in Ramesh's story. At one point, he even criticized their behaviour as unethical and neglectful: 'What doctors do, they give tablets, take Maruthi car and go outside the gate. All the doctors, they don't tell person, you have to go home, no.' Instead of curing patients and sending them home, doctors just drug them. They try to spend as little time as possible on the hospital grounds, leaving around noon to provide services in their private clinics.

> R – 'Foreign countries' are smarter than Karachi. Karachi is not smart. My father came from Karachi, ok, Karachi is not smart. It seems to me that there is no agriculture in the Karachi sector. Here in Maharashtra there is agriculture, but there is no agriculture in Karachi. What the people who came here did, what my father did, I don't understand it. My mother, what she said to me, [she said] 'I am your mother.' So I said, 'I am your mother, then who is my father?', I asked. In the house daddy used to prepare the food, so, I asked, 'Who is daddy then?' Mother said, 'I am your mother.' Only then I understood that my father may not be smart. Daddy must have fought with somebody, he was beaten up. He had marks of a blade on the belly. Of the kind of blade which we use for shaving. Only then I understood, Karachi is not smart, the 'foreign country' and Maharashtra are smart. When I was also pulled by Jadhav, at that time I understood I shouldn't join the sector of my father. I will take my Hero Honda and I will go ahead. Nevertheless, I asked my father, that I want a Hero Honda. I felt bad, ok, because he was my father. So I said Hero Honda, he asked me, 'Which vehicle you may drive?', I said Hero Honda. He asked, 'Why no four wheeler?', I said 'Hero Honda,

> no four wheeler car!' So my father bought me a four wheeler, two wheeler Hero Honda. I did not come to know about the things that were discussed [at home], I don't know our family's story. Now, when I will go home, I will 'inquire', then I will come to know about where my father was staying, where mammy is from, how they came to Ulhasnagar. They didn't come to Thane, they didn't come to Mumbai, they didn't come to Bombay. How a man from Uttar Pradesh came here? My mother is smart, extremely 'talented'. Now I will 'inquire', then I will come to know. So how my mother died, why she died. Many people say, many friends come, ok, at times they say, your mother is dead. My mother is not in this world.
>
> A – Which friends come to visit you?
>
> R – There are two three friends, not from the college, those who stayed nearby, this people come. I don't understand how they [his parents] got married. Mummy died, ok, because of daddy. Because of daddy mummy died. . . .

Ramesh's narrative also illustrates the contagiousness and 'overuse' of magical symbols (words) that are typical for 'mad' stories (Van Dongen 2002: 39). When Ramesh spoke about his past and family history, he used the word *hōshiyār* (smart) extensively. His mother as well as being smart he furthermore denotes as 'talented' and intelligent, but he calls 'foreign countries' and the state 'Maharashtra' 'smart' as well. At another point in our conversation, he also described his sisters as 'smart'. However, his father was 'not smart' and the city, 'Karachi', where he came from, was not smart either. Obviously, his father had failed to make a good living in Mumbai; he was not in the right profession to become successful, and Ramesh distanced himself from agriculture. While Ramesh outlines a seemingly close and respectful relationship with his mother, he rather constructs his father as an anti-hero and loser. He even blames his father for the death of his mother: 'Because of daddy mummy died.' So the characteristics 'smart' and 'not smart' seem to be congruent with 'successful' and 'failure' and 'good' and 'evil' in Ramesh's narrative.

Ramesh employs the comprehensive term 'heart attack', that I interpreted as a fatal 'sickness' caused by moral failure above, extensively regarding his family background:

> A – What do you want to do once you go out?
>
> R – I will work.
>
> A – You will work, but which work will you do?
>
> R – I will work and manage, because now I don't even have parents, too.
>
> A – How your daddy expired?
>
> R – Daddy, because of 'heart attack'. Brother also died of 'heart attack'.
>
> A – And your mother?
>
> R – Mummy also of 'heart attack'. I have two sisters. But they don't come here. That means this hospital is not nice. They don't like it here. So they don't come here.

Though Ramesh experienced the failures of the hospital as well as the moral failure of family members when they did not fulfil their care obligations, he himself morally failed them. He remained unmarried, never brought home a daughter-in-law or founded a family: 'Now I reached the age of thirty-seven, thirty-eight so I won't marry now,' he shared with us. He failed to take care of his ageing parents, and his married sisters had to take care of him instead of him taking care of them as a 'good' brother would do. According to Ramesh, 'once in a year or two years' one of his sisters came to visit him, and the reason she did not visit him more often was because the hospital 'is not nice'. We could suspect, though, that his sisters actually did not like to visit him because their brother is 'not nice' – that actually they feared he might kill them too. The reversal of roles – the sisters taking care of their brother, and Ramesh's failure to perform his role as a caring, protecting brother – became prominent when one of his sisters visited him on Raksha Bandhan and he could not reciprocate her tying of the Rakhi with the traditional gift.

> An (Annika) [pointing to a thread tied around Ramesh's wrist] – Who gave this [to you]?

> R – My sister gave it, during Raksha Bandhan.
>
> A – Was she here?
>
> R – Yes she came here for Raksha Bandhan. . . . But she didn't take me home. . . .
>
> A – What did you give to her [in return]?
>
> R – I didn't have money. When I was at home I used to give money. I don't like to give gold and all that. I used to give money, five thousand, ten thousand.

Neither of Ramesh's sisters was interested in discharging him. Ramesh was well aware of the fact that a patient can only be discharged by a family member. Additionally, his sisters would need to pay the hospital bill and meet costs for the last six and a half years before they could take him home.

> R – My sisters married in good families. Both husbands are billionaires. They sit and eat [they do not have to work]. I don't understand why they don't come. But if nobody from my family comes, I can't get discharged from here. If nobody from my family comes, I can't get discharged. If nobody from my family comes, I can't get discharged.

According to Bruner (1991: 7), narratives always refer to particular happenings. A narrative's particularity 'achieves its emblematic status by its embeddedness in a story that is in some sense generic'. An example would be the experience of some kind of 'shock', which families of patients often mentioned to me in connection with the onset of a mental illness. This could be the death of the mother, conflicts with in-laws or problems in school. We find shock as the narrative's particularity embedded in an 'explanatory model' (EM) of illness, which commonly includes information about the aetiology of illness, time of onset of symptoms, pathophysiology, the course of sickness and the proper treatment (Kleinman 1989: 121). In Ramesh's story, the narrative's particularity is apparently the death of patients and several of his relatives. When he explains all these deaths with 'heart attack', he at first sight seems to adopt an EM that follows a similar logic to the ones that relate the onset of mental illness to an experience of 'shock'. However, 'heart attack' with the meaning of moral failure attached, does not explain primarily 'how' somebody died but rather 'why' and who is responsible for it. Therefore, Ramesh's narrative constructs the EM in an unconventional way as it does not explicitly refer to the experience of a certain social 'shock' that causes an illness that eventually leads to death. Rather, the meaning in Ramesh's narrative is constructed from the event of death: to have died of a 'heart' attack – the heart also being in India, a symbol for love, attachment and therefore social cohesion – reveals something about disturbed social relations that are responsible for the death. 'Heart attack', in his story, points to an unnatural and forceful death that was preceded by human-induced suffering. His story seems to be indifferent to the individual circumstances of each of the deaths – it is very unlikely that all persons died of a heart attack. Instead of revealing how all these people died, Ramesh's story literally exploits the ambiguous meaning of 'heart attack'. Explanatory models conventionally give reasons for certain events and experiences. In Ramesh's narrative, though, it is not the event that takes the centre stage but its emblematic meaning – a death caused by neglect/social failure or literally a 'broken heart'. In Ramesh's narrative this symbolism 'becomes flesh and blood' (Van Dongen 2002: 28). Van Dongen states that '[t]he problem that others have with these kinds of stories is that such things [e.g. dying of heart attack] are symbols for them, whereas they are reality for mad people' (ibid.). If we interpret Ramesh's story guided by conventional narrative principles, it appears to be odd and implausible. If we acknowledge that there are alternative narrative principles, though, the meaning of his 'mad' story finally becomes accessible. Ramesh's story, furthermore, by creatively transforming conventional narrative principles, impressively reveals the power of comprehensive terms and the subtle work of culture.

Performing Magic: The Constructive Power of 'Mad' Narratives

The moral categories of 'guilt' and 'human disaster' are present throughout Ramesh's narrative, but he creatively prevents them from becoming attached to his person. Through repeating certain elements and provoking emotional reactions in Akshay and me, his story becomes more than a mere act of lying or coping. As a constructive accomplishment, Ramesh's story challenges already existing and normative versions of reality. Van Dongen compares 'mad' people to tricksters – both work with morality and emotions but show excessive and compulsive behaviour (ibid.: 38). Tricksters as well as 'mad' people evoke strong and ambivalent feelings in others with their stories and actions. But the difference between them is that 'mad' people let 'others feel the stories they tell, because they do not stop to tell and because they perform so intrusively into others' space' (ibid.). According to the attendants, Ramesh is a liar and a trickster who does not reveal the truth about himself. Still, the tragedy of his life and being in the world is inescapably palpable in his narrative. According to Van Dongen, 'mad' people tend to tell their story compulsively and repeatedly because they have to practise 'double magic': they have to get control over and reverse the overwhelming powers of the 'healing' system as well as neutralize the destructive powers of 'madness'. Ramesh's story has the constructive power to transform his inferior position in the institution as a 'criminal patient' at the bottom rung of the ladder into an educated fellow who is superior to the uneducated attendants and nurses, whose actions and behaviours lack 'humanity'. In his narrative, he does not simply keep quiet about his fate, but he actively tries to solve the puzzle of his mother's death. Keeping his father responsible for deeds he himself committed could be interpreted as 'projection' and 'repression' from a psychological perspective. Ramesh avoids facing a reality in which he is guilty of murder and therefore responsible for becoming a psychiatric long-term patient while his life and family fall apart. His narrative enables Ramesh to master his past and survive in the present and can be understood as an attempt to convince himself of a possible future that is worth living.

> R – The attendant allows me to roam around. When you people were walking, I said 'Good Morning', at that time you were walking, I said 'Good Morning', I go outside, ok [He refers to when we met near the OPD in the morning]. These people also at times send me outside. Why is that? If they send me, I won't cre-

> ate a scandal [*kāṇḍ*]. Even if I get discharged, I won't create a scandal. To kill somebody, to take somebody's life, is unnecessary.

The last sentence takes up the crime of murder quite surprisingly at first sight. Though against the backdrop of Ramesh's past, his random and odd remark reveals something about himself: Even if he won't do it, killing somebody seems to at least be something that is on his mind. Throughout the narrative, he desperately avoids any direct connection between him and murder, therefore mentioning the pointlessness of killing to prove his innocuousness has the exact opposite effect. Moreover, the statement reverses the order of a common narrative structure. The last sentence cannot be the logical consequence of the previous one, but only the other way around: 'Killing somebody is unnecessary. [Therefore] I won't create [there is no sense in creating] a scandal when going out.' Nevertheless, this order would only make sense if Ramesh had spoken of his deed – something he obviously tried to avoid during our conversation. But as I stated above, the function or aim of Ramesh's narrative was certainly not to create a coherent account but to let words magically control and influence past, present and future.

Notes

1. Here he refers to the RO admission process, which requires the patient to be seen by a judge before they can be admitted to a psychiatric hospital involuntarily (see Chapter 4).
2. *sālā* (brother-in-law) is used as a curse word in colloquial language.

CHAPTER 7

BEING GAY AND FEELING FEMALE

QUEER VOICES FROM INDIAN PSYCHIATRY

I met Ajay Raj together with Dhaval in the admission ward in the male unit. Ajay told us that he was not treated well by the ward boys because they knew about him having 'gay sex'. Standing in front of us, he pulled his trousers down to show us a scar on the side of one of his legs that he claimed the ward boys were responsible for. Partly in English and partly in Hindi, Ajay shared with us that he was brought to Asha because he suffered from 'depression'. Not long into our conversation, I noticed Ajay's effeminate body movements. Dhaval commented later that Ajay 'moved like a woman'. He described the swaying of his head, especially, as being rather feminine. During our conversation, Ajay insisted that he was 'not a hijra' but later admitted that he had lived and worked for some time with the hijra community as a sex worker. An attendant sent Ajay to handle the distribution of medications, and so our conversation ended; Dhaval and I were invited to take part in the Raksha Bandhan celebrations that were about to take place in the ward afterwards. The Hindu festival traditionally celebrates the relationship between brother and sister, but nowadays it extends to almost all relations between men and women who are not related to each other as husband and wife (e.g. friends). All the patients in the ward were seated on blankets spread on the floor. The ward psychiatrist, Dr Gambhire, and the medical officer who had just finished their daily round sat down on chairs behind a table. Dhaval and I were given chairs to sit with them. On the table were Rakhis, which were tied to the wrists of patients one by one. The nurses, as the only female staff in the male unit, had organized the celebration.

As is usual on special occasions and on religious festivals, all patients received biscuits as a treat. After some time, Ajay also approached the table to receive his Rakhi. Immediately after the nurse had tied it to his wrist, he asked if he was allowed to tie one to the medical officer and Dhaval. As he was doing this, Dr Gambhire signalled for me to lean in close and then explained what was going on: 'Normally a Rakhi is tied by the sister to her brother. But this patient is gay. He wants to be a female. He has a "gender identity disorder".'

When I thought about this incident later that day, I was puzzled. Why had Dr Gambhire used the term 'gay' and 'gender identity disorder' apparently interchangeably? As far as I was familiar with these labels, being 'gay' and being 'transsexual' or 'transgender' constituted two exclusive psychiatric diagnoses and/or identity categories (either you are a male attracted to males OR a female in a masculine body attracted to males), respectively. But after this incident I wondered if the terms are used divergently in different (psychiatric) contexts. Psychiatry and medicine have often had a difficult relationship with the LGBTQ+ community. Intersexed and transgendered bodies and the 'sexually deviant mind' were once, and still are in some places, perceived as requiring treatment (Lang 2006). Queer bodies are inclined to be overlooked or rendered invisible, or if recognized, they are prone to be discriminated against or 'corrected' (Meer and Müller 2017). Queer persons' narratives tend to be silenced or ignored in everyday clinical life (Giffort and Underman 2016; Robertson 2017). In the following, I attempt to analyse Ajay's narrative and actions beyond the 'clinical gaze', which is merely interested in information about 'the nature' of his mental state, and instead try to frame his narrative about his experiences and life course in the context of the local queer landscape.

Sexuality and Queerness in Indian Psychiatry

In contrast to Western psychiatry, Indian scholars of psychiatry and psychology have never engaged in a vivid discussion on homosexuality or theorizing sexual orientation (Parekh 2003; Ranade 2009: 1). According to Arvind Narrain and Vinay Chandran, the medical discourse on sexuality in India is mainly informed by legal, religious and medical Western concepts that are 'heterosexist' and frame homosexuality as 'abnormal' (2005: 49). During the late 1970s, the first cases of 'transsexuality' were discussed in Indian psychiatry. Indian psychiatric literature predominantly discussed 'deviant' sexual or gender behaviour in terms of its treatment and correction – for example, 'aversion treatment' (e.g. giving electroshocks when exposing the patient to homoerotic stimuli) and other behaviour modification treatments that aimed at changing a patient's sexual behaviour (Sakthivel, Rangasami and Jayaraman 1979; Pradhan et al. 1982; Mehta and Deshpande 1983). So called 'conversion treatments' are still common to this day and are regularly utilized by Indian psychiatrists and psychologists. A qualitative study conducted by social scientist Ketki Ranade in 2009 in Mumbai and Pune found that half of forty interviewed health care professionals provided such treatments (Ranade 2009). They are usually sought by clients who are frustrated with their sexual desires and want to conform to social norms and family expectations, which include getting married and starting a family. This is a condition identified as 'ego-dystonic homosexuality' or homosexuality associated with feelings of alienation from or distress about one's sexual identity, and therefore perceived to be indicative of the need for conversion therapy methods (Narrain and Chandran 2005: 56). Examples of methods used are 'fantasy building', 'creative visualisation' and 'imagery' 'to help the person break this pleasurable association with same-sex contact and form a new association between sexual pleasure and opposite-sex contact' (Ranade 2009: 16). The primary assumption these techniques are based on is that homosexuality is a learnt or acquired behaviour wherein the person associates sexual pleasure with a person of the same sex. Narrain and Chandran, who conducted interviews with mental health professionals in Bangalore, reported the prevalence of similar aetiologies at the beginning of the twenty-first century among psychiatrists, psychologists and counsellors: they perceive homosexuality as resulting from growing up within a pathogenic family where the two sexes are rigorously separated, which finally leads to the formation of a homosexual orientation as linked to being trapped by people who are already homosexual (Narrain and Chandran 2005: 57; see also Parekh 2003: 156). These explanatory models match with the general sociocultural discourse that understands same-sex-desire as socially made rather than innate.

The psychiatrist Gurvinder Kalra (2012b) observed a paradigm shift from earlier behaviour modification techniques that claimed to 'cure' homosexuality to the use of antipsychotics and antidepressants 'under the pretext of helping the patient's depression or stress, possibly with the intention of reducing their overall sexual desire' (ibid.: 291). A common side effect of some psychotropic drugs is sexual dysfunction, which may include decreased libido, erectile dysfunction and ejaculatory disturbances in men. During psychiatric consultations in the OPD at Asha, too, I observed this strategy to medicate unwanted sexual desire. A young woman in her early twenties had complained about her high sexual desire. The psychiatrist explained to me that she had increased the dosage of her medication in order to decrease her libido; there were not many other options for treating a patient in her situation. She was not married yet, so medication could be used to control her urges.

Generally, sexual desire and its expression by inpatients was under constant surveillance at Asha and was strictly controlled. Nurses told us that they regularly checked female inpatients to make sure they were not inserting random items into their vaginas.[1] Maitra reports about same-sex couples in the female unit that were separated as soon as they displayed any public affection and were sometimes 'prescribed medication to control the excitable state' (2003: 55). When I was conducting fieldwork in a female ward, a female patient excitedly announced one day that she wanted to marry me because my appearance – fair skin and blond hair – was attractive to her. One of the nurses asked her half mockingly if she realized that I am a woman and that she therefore could never marry me. Male same-sex desire was a recurrent topic as well during my research. Aakil, a social work student from TISS, who was doing an internship at Asha at that time, came to know that men used to have sex during the night in one of the chronic wards. He told me that the men were regularly beaten up for their behaviour by the attendants in the mornings. In the private hospital, a social worker told me there had been two cases in which the infidelity of married men was conceptualized as a symptom of their 'antisocial personality disorder' and 'treated' accordingly during counselling sessions with their wives. In another case, sexual issues between a young married couple – their nonconsumption of marriage and the worries of the in-laws – led to the young wife being admitted because she apparently suffered from schizophrenia. Additionally, she shared with me that the leading psychiatrist had instructed her to never encourage female patients to consider divorce during counselling sessions. In the psychiatrist's opinion, a divorce was not a solution to family problems. The social worker, a divorced woman herself and a declared feminist, had a tough time reconciling her own stance with that of her boss on this topic.

All these examples show how psychiatric patients' sexual behaviour was morally evaluated in terms of appropriate sexual conduct. Particularly female 'uncontrolled' sexual behaviour taking place outside of heterosexual marriage was punished, suppressed or controlled. Other forms of sexuality like masturbation (see S.K. Ratnam, Chapter 4) were perceived as less problematic and were therefore tolerated. Sexual issues that influenced the social institution of marriage negatively, though, like its nonconsumption or (recognized) male infidelity, either became part of a mental disorder or were included in a treatment plan aimed at 'normalizing' the sexual relationship of the couple. Psychiatric diagnosis does not rely on any coherent theory of 'sexuality'. Rather, it categorizes and catalogues 'abnormal' and 'disordered' sexual and gendered behaviour and experiences (paraphilias, see Oosterhuis 2000). The 'normal' does not need any explanation or theorization as it is 'naturalized' (Narrain and Chandran 2005: 67). Unquestioned assumptions about what is 'normal' sexual behaviour and sexual attraction influenced how sexual health was approached by the medical staff at Asha. Dhaval and I once asked Dr Gambhire if condoms were provided or if any other measures were taken that encouraged patients to engage in safer sex, after Ajay had introduced us to his 'boyfriend' Nitin whom he had befriended in the ward. The psychiatrist responded that Ajay, who was HIV positive, had 'insight' into his sexual health status; implying that she expected him to abstain from sex with his boyfriend. Additionally, she was convinced that the other men in the ward had a 'normal' (= heterosexual) sexuality and therefore were not interested in any sexual interactions with Ajay or each other; an assumption that contradicted the reports of some attendants (see above).

Narrain and Chandra (2005) argue that psychiatric practice is inevitably entangled with moral and heterosexist ideas that are not appropriately reflected on. This has led the queer community to resist medical intervention and 'provide its own form of therapy' (ibid.: 67). Since the early 1990s, there has been an increasing number of queer and feminist campaigns (Menon 2007a: xiii) by the queer Indian diaspora (Roy 2007; Bacchetta 2007). In the 2000s, a branch of Indian queer and academic literature emerged that was predominantly swayed by queer theory, feminism and postcolonial studies (Vanita and Kidwai 2001; Vanita 2002, 2005; Narrain and Bhan 2005; Menon 2007a; Bose and Bhattacharyya 2007; Nayar 2007). Since the beginning of the twenty-first century, a number of psychiatrists, psychological counsellors and social workers have become actively involved in the LGBT rights movement in Mumbai. Among them is the psychiatrist Gurvinder Kalra, who is well-known in Mumbai's gay and transgender community (Kalra, Gupta and Bhugra 2010; Kalra 2012c). When I met him in March 2013, he described himself as specialized in the field of 'paraphilias' and as an active educator in the field of 'sex' and 'gender' for mental health professionals. He worked as a consulting psychiatrist at Humsafar Trust – an organization founded by the gay activist Ashok Row Kavi in 1994 with a focus on gay sexualities and sexual health in India. Additionally, he saw patients from the middle and upper socio-economic classes during his private consultation hours. According to Kalra, sexual orientation, gender and sex was not at that time regularly taught to medical practitioners in India. Therefore, he engaged in teaching trainees about homosexuality, gender identity disorder and how to deal with 'sexual variations' in clinical consultations. However, it was still very common among medical professionals to consider and treat homosexuality as a 'mental disorder'. Nevertheless, a number of authors started to speak against the medicalization and pathologization of alternate sexualities and asked psychiatry to break its fraternity with politics that failed to take a clear stance on decriminalizing and destigmatizing same sex relationships (Sathyanarayana Rao and Jacob 2012, 2014; Sathyanarayana Rao et al. 2016). More progressive psychiatrists actively promoted the exploration of health issues faced by queer patients (see Sathyanarayana Rao and Avasthi 2008; Kalra 2012c, 2012d; Verghese 2014). Furthermore, several authors looked at Indian culture and its impact on the experience of sexuality and sexual behaviour (Kalra and Bhugra 2010; Kalra 2012a; Chakraborty and Thakurata 2013; Mahajan et al. 2013). Finally, in March 2016, the Indian Psychiatric Society (IPS) under Dr G. Prasad Rao announced in a 'Position Statement on same-sex attraction, orientation, behaviour and life style' that it 'considers same-sex attraction, orientation and behaviour as normal variants of human sexuality' (IPS 2016) and recognizes that the social stigma and discrimination faced by people with same-sex orientation 'are a significant cause for their distress and calls for the provision of adequate mental health support'. Furthermore, the IPA took a clear political stance on LGBT rights in supporting 'the need to de-criminalise same-sex orientation and behaviour and to recognise LGBT rights to include human, civil and political rights' (IPS 2016). So queer voices finally started to be heard and supported in Indian psychiatry after years of being ignored. Additionally, an increasing number of counsellors and doctors seem to take a nonjudgemental position towards homosexuality in their clinical practice (Narrain/Chandran 2005: 64, Parekh 2003: 156).

Ganesh Jayaram was a researcher and counsellor at Humsafar Trust and had met Ajay when he worked as an outreach worker with the organization. Dhaval and I wanted to approach him to see if he could do anything to improve Ajay's situation, perhaps in terms of getting him discharged. We asked Dr Gambhire for her advice, and she asked us to hold off approaching Ganesh as she found Ajay to be 'absolutely not ok' and not fit for discharge. When we asked her for details, she told us: 'He tells us that he has a baby inside his belly.' When we met Ajay a short time later, he assured us that he had never said such a thing. And in his file, we could not find a note that confirmed he had been seen by Dr Gambhire recently. I cannot know for sure, but given she had previously associated Ajay's sexuality with having a gender identity disorder, the 'baby in his belly' could have been based on what she imagined a patient like Ajay would possibly say. Or maybe she just did not feel comfortable with me intervening in this situation or indeed perceived Ajay as not ready for counselling. Whatever the reason may have been, in her narrative Dr Gambhire was now constructing Ajay as a 'transsexual' man who was also 'mad' for imagining he had a full functioning female body. From this, it was obvious that Dr Gambhire's estimation of Ajay's behaviour was not based on any understanding of the hijra, who adopt a female-like appearance and habitus but are aware that they cannot procreate as women (Hall and O'Donovan 1996; Nanda 1999).

Dr Gambhire's perception of Ajay's behaviour and talk seemed foremost to have been shaped by sociocultural gender stereotypes and additionally by notions of the psychological categories of 'homosexuality' and 'gender identity disorder'. After fieldwork when I discussed during an interdisciplinary working group meeting our encounter with Ajay, a German psychiatrist commented that he could not possibly suffer from a 'gender identity disorder' because he seemed to be happy to have a penis and to engage in homosexual encounters. This statement – as Dr Gambhire's references to Ajay's behaviour do, too – illustrates how diagnosing always includes a process and clinical evaluation of narratives and actions. Additionally, what the psychiatrist implicitly referred to was Ajay's male 'gender identity' as it is outlined by the American Psychological Association:

> [g]*ender identity* and *sexual orientation* are not the same. *Sexual orientation* refers to an individual's enduring physical, romantic, and/or emotional attraction to another person, whereas *gender identity* refers to one's internal sense of being male, female, or something else. (APA 2011: 2)

To be a male-to-female transgender person and gay (male attracted to male) at the same time is ultimately impossible based on this distinction of gender identity from sexual orientation. A homosexual – 'gay' – orientation is categorized based on one's gender in reference to that of one's sexual or romantic partners. The – meanwhile both obsolete – psychiatric diagnoses 'Gender Identity Disorder' and 'Homosexuality' were based on particular assumptions of a person's inner experience of a 'sexual' self, on the one hand, and a 'gendered' one on the other. Ajay's 'doing gay sex' and 'feeling female' at the same time, do not match with these assumptions. His narrative and actions challenge and problematize the logics implicit in this categorization and therefore appears to be disruptive or simply 'queer'.

David Valentine (2007) makes the important point that 'gender' and 'sexuality' are not self-evident experiences or domains outside of language: 'Rather, they are linguistic tools which extract certain information, experiences, and feelings about ourselves and others from the stream of daily life for the purposes of making meaning about, and representing, ourselves and others' (ibid.: 31). Accordingly, the meaning of what exactly 'gay' denotes varies among those using the term in everyday life and as a self-identification. This Valentine realized when he encountered Fiona during his fieldwork in the United States. Fiona was a male-bodied person, claiming to be a woman but also 'gay' and therefore occupied 'the categories of *both* transgender *and* homosexual as equivalent categories of personhood' (ibid.: 4). Similarly to Ajay, for Fiona her 'gendered' life as a woman and her 'sexual' desire as a gay man did not pose ontological conflict. However, for the professionals that Fiona encountered in the diverse organizations and health facilities all around the city that constituted Valentine's ethnographic field, her view and understanding of her gendered and sexual identity was not an alternative categorization but a 'false' one. Similar to the German psychiatrist contemplating Ajay's case, they assumed that she would 'confuse' her 'transgender identity' with her 'homosexual desire' and therefore was 'not really' gay – in Ajay's case the psychiatrist assumed that Ajay did 'not really' want to be a woman. According to Valentine, these framings of Fiona's different experiences ignore the fact that they might be a result of class, racial or cultural inequalities that have left her outside certain conversations and historical developments. Similarly, Ajay's queer narrative in the midst of several socio-medico discourses represents a minority subject position in manifold ways: he self-identifies as gender-variant gay, is an inpatient in a psychiatric hospital, was admitted because his promiscuous lifestyle annoyed his neighbours and furthermore he belonged to a non-Western, non-middle-class queer community. In the following, I intend to show that a social anthropological analysis of his narrative has the potential to provide us with valuable insights about his queer experiences. It becomes apparent that Ajay's self-awareness and description is moulded on the one hand by globalized (psychiatric) categories that frame 'sex' and 'gender' but also by local terms, concepts and practices emerging from Mumbaikar queer activism and identity politics originally fuelled by HIV/AIDS interventions on the other. Similar to what Els van Dongen described for people with psychosis who wander through culture creating a 'bricolage' reality from materials at hand, Ajay wandered through the Mumbaikar landscape and created a 'queer bricolage' narrative (Van Dongen 2004: 5).

Ajay's Narrative: A Queer Bricolage

Ajay was thirty-two years old, and his paternal uncle (*chāchā*) had admitted him to Asha for the first time three years before, in November 2008. His mother also suffered from a mental illness and had disappeared ten years ago. Ajay's father had died some years before. His brother had suffered brain damage as a result of being in a train accident and was treated in a private facility in Mumbai. Ajay was diagnosed with depression (with manic episodes) and gender identity disorder. He was additionally found to be HIV positive by Humsafar Trust some years before. While Ajay's uncle had taken care of Ajay until he was admitted the last time around one month ago, he did not seem to want responsibility for Ajay any more. Ajay's brother, who was three years older than him, was in need of constant nursing care. Ajay's *chāchā* met the expenses for the brothers' treatments. One of Ajay's biggest wishes was to be able to pay for his brother's medical care one day.

Ganesh, the counsellor from Humsafar Trust who had worked together with Ajay, shared with us that people preferred to keep a distance from him, and nobody had been ready to support him when he was in trouble recently. Ajay's self-esteem appeared rather low; he had a tendency to take things personally and seemed to appreciate any attention he could get from others. When Dhaval and I asked him if he would like to be interviewed by us, his face lit up.

At the beginning of our conversation, Ajay told us about his family's background. His parents had migrated from Lucknow to Mumbai after their marriage. His father originally hailed from Pakistan. His father's family had chosen a girl who seemed to be a good match: she was educated, beautiful and came from a middle-class family who ran a shop that sold kurtis and pajamas.

After the marriage, Ajay's mother started behaving differently. Ajay told us how she would wander the street 'naked' and that 'she used to sleep under trucks, she used to sleep under buses'. Ajay also mentioned the maltreatment that he and his brother had to endure: she 'threw me from the first floor, my brother, me' and '[t]hen she poured kerosene oil in both our eyes'. After this incident, Ajay was operated on in a government hospital. His father was too poor to afford a divorce. He remembered that his mother tried to commit suicide once. She was treated in a hospital from time to time and was on regular medication. When Ajay was a teenager, his father migrated to South Africa. His brother had already moved out there and he followed him to get a job and earn money. He regularly sent a share of his salary to his *fūfā* (husband of father's sister), who handed it over to Ajay's brother. According to Ajay, his brother had regular fights with their neighbours and used to spend most of the money on alcohol and prostitutes. Subsequently, nothing was left to pay Ajay's school fees. He faced problems and harassment at school and finally had to quit; he was thus only educated until Senior KG (last year of kindergarten). Once he had dreamt of becoming a doctor. 'But my dream never became true,' Ajay said regretfully.

'Identified' as Gay: Queer Discourses in Mumbai

After leaving school, Ajay started to work in a textile mill. Here he was teased by his co-workers:

> A – . . . and there the Muslims tortured me a lot, that is why I left, they came to know that I am 'gay', so I move, ok, like girls would move, so that is how the Muslims came to know about it, so they started to tease me, they started to pass comments, they started to torture [me], they made fun of me, so out of that reason I stopped working there . . . .

Ajay experienced his body and how it was seen by others as gender-transgressing – as female rather than male. During our conversation, Ajay repeatedly described how people came to know about or 'recognized' (*pahachān hō ge*) him as being 'gay'. He rarely used the term 'gay' to describe what he identified as but to describe how he was seen and named by others. He used the English term 'gay' throughout our conversation.[2] He described how he was 'identified' as being gay by social workers at Humsafar Trust.

> A – I went to the loo, so to the loo gay people used to come.
>
> DJ – This loo is where?
>
> A – There is the Thane bus depot, isn't it, there in the bus depot is the loo, in west, there, where the Borivali-Bhiwandi bus is, S.T., S.T. Depot, in the loo there, they used to come there, so they identified me, they always came there . . . by meeting somebody else we had the impression, that we found our mother's stomach, in the sense our mother's lap, we had this impression, so we met with each other, had talks and thought that we are same, we are gay, so, like that the community came into being, after establishing the community we came to know about the NGO, they used to come there and teach us, we are legal, isn't it? Then automatically it started to come out of our mouths that we are gay. . . .
>
> DJ – When you people used to gather?
>
> A – We used to meet daily, in the evening, there was no particular time, any time we gathered, we met somebody and shared our feelings.
>
> DJ – When you came to know about it the first time? About the bus depot meetings?
>
> A – I just came to know like that in the loo during urinating, then there were 2–3 gay people from my area, they were from my area, they recognized that he must be gay, they called me, had a chat with me, greeted me, like that they used to recognize [me], in my area, ok, there were also some gay people.
>
> DJ – How the people from your area came to know about that you are gay?
>
> A – My walking was like that of girls, my talking was like that of girls, we were out of our society, we didn't stay with the straight people, the straight people

> would not accept us. If we came close to this people then this people would automatically recognize it.

Ajay describes certain nonverbal processes of reading, being read and recognized and the interpersonal construction of space that he experienced as protecting and comforting, just as a 'mother's lap'. The Thane bus depot, where Ajay encountered other 'gay people' and finally also social workers from Humsafar Trust, is a famous cruising place in the locality. Here men encounter men to engage in 'pleasure' or have *mastī* (fun) with each other (Khan 2001: 102). Public places – most commonly gardens, parks or public toilets – are particularly frequented by urban non-middle-class men who cannot afford private space such as owning a spacious flat or renting a hotel room to engage in same-sex sexual encounters (Al. Gupta 2005; Suresh 2011a). In a cultural context like India – where on the one hand society provides space for homosociality but open homosexual encounters and relationships are taboo and not tolerated on the other – men who seek sexual encounters with other men depend on nonverbal and furthermore necessarily ambivalent codes of communication.[3] These are supposed to be perceived by some but not others: 'As such the male-to-male body is constructed symbolically so that it may be read (or sometimes misread) through connections achieved in public' (Boyce 2007b: 404). When Ajay went to the public toilet the first time, he was not aware that 'gay people' used to meet in this place. Nevertheless, because of his body, its movements and his way of talking being read as female he was recognized as belonging 'to the line' (ibid.: 408) or to 'the community' as Ajay expressed it.

According to Shivananda Khan, it is common for men engaging in sex with other men to lead a double life away from a wife and children, so their sense of self is rather fluid and constructed differently in 'cruising' contexts. He cites an English-speaking man from Calcutta: '"Look, inside the park I am a gay. Once I leave the park and go to the streets that changes. Outside the park, I am a good Hindu, a married man with a good family"' (Khan 2001: 106). Unlike this man, Ajay did not succeed in consciously and unconsciously navigating these social complexities by being noticed in one context and remaining invisible in another; he was not read as 'gay' in one social context and as 'straight' in another. He experienced his sexual subjectivity as rather pervasive and the 'gay community' as separate from common people and mainstream society. Ganesh, the social worker from Humsafar Trust who worked with Ajay, remembered that 'He used to tell everybody that he is gay.' The overt articulation of his sexual identity suggests that it was an important pillar of who he is and how he wanted to be perceived by others. Moreover, him not 'passing' as straight in certain social contexts caused him to experience stigmatization and to not be 'accepted' as he is.

> DJ – For how many years have you been with Humsafar Trust? . . .
>
> A – For ten years . . .
>
> DJ – There they tested you.
>
> A – Yes.
>
> DJ – And they told you that you are positive?
>
> A – Yes, because . . . I stayed with TGs, ok, the TGs used to steal, the transgenders used to steal, they have stolen somebodies mobile, they have broken a chain and have taken it and they have stolen somebodies purse, they didn't like them. Because of that they told that I am positive. Out of that, you will leave their company, because the transgender will tell that you got aids, that is why you should not speak with us. We won't allow you to have sex, they will say that they will torture me everywhere. If you have sex with somebody we will tell that this guy is HIV positive, then all people will hate you, they will avoid you. Then, when they slowly do this, you will come to your own people.

Ajay experienced the screening for HIV not as a health intervention, but rather as a social one that addressed him being openly gay and part of a hijra ('transgender', 'TG') community. He took the test because his friends asked him to accompany them when he was still new to their 'gay community'. He interpreted this as a measure to separate him from the hijra community and bind him to 'his own people'. When Dhaval asked Ajay to specify what was meant by 'own people', it became apparent that Ajay distinguished between three 'gay' communities.

> DJ – Come to 'your own people'?
>
> A – To the gay people. Of us there are three, isn't it. One is 'kothi'. It's called 'kothi'. There is the 'Goda Trust', 'Udaan Trust' and a trust for transgender is there, it's of Lakshmi Narayan Tripathi and another trust is of gay people, of Ashok Row [Kavi].

'Kothi' is an identity category that was coined in the 1990s and denotes effeminate men, mostly from the working or lower middle classes, who are said to prefer being receptive when having sex with their often rather masculine and heterosexual-identified partners (often referred to as 'panthi'). Ajay refers to certain outreach initiatives within Humsafar Trust, founded by Ashok Row Kavi for 'gay people'. These evolved during the last three decades and are associated with the names of those that set them up. Lakshmi Narayan Tripathi, born in 1979 in Thane to a Brahmin family, came to know about Ashok Row Kavi's activism during the early 1990s, and was the only 'homosexual' known in Mumbai at that time. She remembers in an interview published in 'Project Bolo'[4] that she was often called a '*chakka*' (six, Kannada expression for hijra), 'hijra' or 'homo' during her childhood. During that time 'it was only "gay". There was no "kothi", nothing, nothing! And it was, "Oh, sister!", "Hello, sister!" and all these things, you know?' In the mid-1990s, there was an explosion of queer spaces. In Mumbai, the 'Humsafar Friday Meetings' were a welcome space where gay men gathered every week and talked about being 'gay'. Alok Gupta (2005), who came out during these meetings, remembers them as follows:

> The discussions were in English, of course, and shuttled between the social, the political, or sometimes something that was fun and frivolous. I also used the Internet, and read gay books in English from the Humsafar library. This led to an immediate identification with the global gay identity. (ibid.: 124)

Because the regulars at the meetings were keen on having a different space away from activism and Humsafar Trust's primary focus was on health and HIV, a parallel support group called Gay Bombay was formed. There were similar developments in other big metropolitan cities in India like Bangalore, Delhi and Kolkata, and these meetings were almost exclusively frequented by urban middle-class gay- and bisexual-identified men. During this period, outreach to people from the lower middle and working classes as well as to lesbians, hijras or other effeminate communities like kothis was negligible (ibid.: 127). In this context, 'Udaan' – meaning 'a flight' (in the hope of liberty) – was cofounded by Goda Bai as a support and advocacy group for MSM ('Men having Sex with Men')-identified men from lower middle- and working-class backgrounds in 1992.

The integration of the lower middle and working class and kothis and hijras into queer organizations happened predominantly in the context of outreach work on HIV (ibid.). Hijras and kothis were employed in large numbers by MSM-focused organizations all over the country as 'peer-educators' and 'outreach workers'. In this context also Ajay received a job with a small monthly payment at Humsafar Trust.

> A – We distributed condoms in the loo. We took the condoms from the government hospital. We gave them a letter and took a box filled with condoms. We gave it to the people of our community [for free], and for the straight people there were outlets, these people spent five rupees, took it, and went.

Alok Gupta cites Goda, who commented on these developments: '"No gay man would go and distribute condoms at the toilets at railway stations. You need kothis to do that"' (ibid.). With these developments, kothis and hijras became more and more integrated in the organizational structures, claimed more and more distinct spaces for meetings and support groups and demanded independent recognition as sexual minorities and partners in the queer movement.

Mumbaikar queer identity politics are palpable throughout Ajay's narrative.

> DJ – What is the meaning of 'kothi'?
>
> A – 'Kothi' has a meaning, but this I also don't know so well. They say that 'kothi' is the code word for us people, the meaning is just 'kothi'. The Udaan Trust

> says we are kothis, so. Kothi people go and live with the hijras. That is 'kothi'. But in the society they are not accepted, so they go to the hijras and live there, wear a sari . . . They speak of them as the Udaanvalas, as Goda's.
>
> DJ – So which kind of work does Udaan do.
>
> A – HIV, Aids, they work with positive people, they work only with kothis.
>
> DJ – So that is the 'community identity'? It's the feeling of all your, your . . . that is why the 'gay community' does not feel that you should go to the 'transgender community'. That is why they scared you. So you didn't go.
>
> A – Yes, yes . . . yes.

Dhaval brought up the English term 'community identity' in order to describe Ajay's relation to the Udaan Trust and the category 'kothi'. Ajay, when denoting 'kothi' as a '"code word" for us people' additionally illustrates that the 'call to recognize oneself' in the framework of a certain sexual identity in the Mumbaikar queer discourse is not necessarily about the adoption of an 'ontology of personhood that is permanent' (Khanna 2007: 179) but rather about becoming a member of a certain community. Akshay Khanna (2005) suggests that the basis of postcolonial constitutions and of progressive politics in India is the imagination of 'Indian society' 'into neat and pre-existing, natural "communities"' (ibid. : 99), with each having a natural leader that represents the community's interests. Khanna argues that the disjuncture between the representation of sexual identities and perceptions of self that necessarily occurs in queer groups, especially those that have arisen in response to the HIV/AIDS epidemic and have evolved from NGOs, is '"systematically" managed through local configurations of power' (ibid. 2007: 180).

> For example, some NGOs have strict rules of conduct for their 'employees' – one may not participate in meetings except as a 'representative' of the organization or one may not attend meetings at all. There are

> dynamics of merit, efficiency and capability within organizations and in the queer movement, in general, only people who have 'command' over English, for example, are sent to certain meetings or seminars where interactions are in English. What this could mean is that those who speak in idioms that fit well with the understanding of the NGO head gain access to locations of speech and participation, at the cost of those who do not 'make sense' or who provide a challenge to the dominant framing. (ibid.)

Ajay, who confessed in our conversation that 'kothi' has a meaning 'but this I also don't know so well' certainly is not somebody who 'makes sense' and therefore had no access to positions of speech and negotiation.

Differentiating between 'Gay' and 'Transgender'

The local construction and representation of identities is only one side of the coin, though. As Paul Boyce (2007a: 178) points out, besides illuminating how identity categories are constructed in local discourses, social anthropology should additionally scrutinize how men who use the term 'kothi' understand their (sexual) subjectivity in order to disrupt simplistic perspectives on the cultural coherence of the category. Ajay, besides marking 'kothi' as a 'community label', also commented: 'Kothi people go and live with the hijras.' While the central demarcation discourse in the context of the competition for international funds for HIV prevention programmes was majorly based on the category 'gay' as opposed to 'kothi', Ajay's definition points to another categorical opposition: 'kothi' and 'hijra'– the latter also referred to as 'transgender' (TG):

> DJ – Where you used to roam with the TGs?
>
> A – In Shilphata I did 'business' together with them . . .
>
> DJ – What kind of?
>
> A – I did 'body business' [*jism kā dhandā* = prostitution], selling of the body.
>
> DJ – You also used to dress like they do?

> A – Yes, that I like. . . .
>
> DJ – Who came there?
>
> A – Truck drivers came. . . .
>
> DJ – One *customer* in one night?
>
> A – It takes half an hour, we take them to the 'business place'. . . .
>
> DJ – You were with the 'transgenders', that is why after that Humsafar people scared you? Why you left them?
>
> A – Because I am HIV positive, so they came to my house and tortured me.
>
> DJ – Who?
>
> A – Hijras [*chakke lōg*] came and tortured me, they started saying that if you do the business then we people will become *positive*, don't come there to do business with us. . . .
>
> DJ – So that is why they all came to the house and started saying, don't send him, that is why you left?
>
> A – Yes, then they also stole so I even feared them more. There was one good friend of mine, Shetti, he was also like us [a kothi], they hit him on the neck and threw him in a stepwell.
>
> DJ – Why?
>
> A – Somebody committed a theft and he was charged with it.

Ajay had joined the hijras/TGs to earn a living. Similarly, Gayatri Reddy (2005a: 56) reports from her fieldwork in Hyderabad that some kothis used to join hijra communities to do sex work. When Ajay used to 'do business with the TGs' he earned 400–500 to 2,000–3,000 and sometimes even five thousand rupees per night, which is quite an amount. When he started to work with Humsafar Trust later, he received a monthly salary of 1,500 rupees, which is remarkably less, particularly if one has to make a living in an expensive city like Mumbai. Apparently, the hijra community ostracized Ajay when he tested HIV positive and this is what brought him to join the gay community. The hijra are a community with an elaborated kinship network and a unique identity. They live a life full of rituals, symbols and cultural meaning, described in detail in Serena Nanda's (1999) ethnography 'The Hijras of India'. Nanda demonstrates in her work how the hijra function as a religious cult as well as a 'caste'– a community organized around a traditional occupation. The hijras' traditional role in society was to function as cultural performers at homes where a male child was born or at marriages. Ajay pointed out the difference between TGs and gays: while the former only 'do sex for business', the latter, gays like himself, do sex work but have sex for pleasure too and frequent cruising places like the public toilet at the bus depot. Ajay also used to pick up sex partners on the local trains[5] while working:

> DJ – What were your working timings in Humsafar recently?
>
> A – It was 'part time'. From four to eleven in the night.
>
> DJ – So what you did before that?
>
> A – I had sex.
>
> DJ – In the morning?
>
> A – Not in the morning, sometimes during work.
>
> DJ – At work? In between four and eleven?
>
> A [laughing] – Yes. I went there for work. In the train I 'did closing' [looked out for somebody], in the train, after 'doing the closing' [attracting somebody] in the train I took them home.

Indeed, hijras – with renunciation being an important pillar of their self-identity – are labelled and understand themselves as 'asexual', 'impotent' and/or 'physically impaired' and therefore as people who do not engage in sexual activities (Nanda 1986). In reality, however, many hijras have to earn their living doing sex work and enjoy a certain reputation as sex workers. They are perceived as being able to work in places like 'the truck line', also mentioned by Ajay above, which is perceived as too dangerous for female sex workers. Furthermore, having sex with a hijra does not threaten a man's male status. It is even said that one should try having sex with a hijra at least once in life

(Reddy 2005a: 50). One hijra that Nanda portrays in her ethnography claims the advantage of being a hijra is 'not contracting diseases' like female prostitutes, who 'have all sorts of diseases because they go to all sorts of men' (ibid.). However, the highest HIV infection rates are found among *nirvān*[6] hijras (Row Kavi 2007: 397). By ostracizing Ajay when they came to know about his HIV infection, the hijras may have indeed believed they were protecting their reputation as unique and safe providers of sexual services. Their sexual practice – being all *gāṇḍūs*[7] (meaning 'one who uses his ass') – their preference for 'real men' (who perform the act of penetration during intercourse) as sexual partners – and perceiving themselves as 'female like' is what seems to unite hijras and kothis as being members of one 'family' (Reddy 2005a: 46). So even if, as Ajay points out, there might be certain tensions and disagreements between the hijra/TG community and kothis at times, they nevertheless seem to have a strong bond. Reddy states that hijras in Hyderabad did not want to interact with and had the biggest contempt for a group called 'AC/DCs' or 'double deckers', who could be either a penetrating or penetrated partner in a sexual encounter. This moral categorization hints to the act of penetration as a relevant axis of gender differentiation (ibid.: 72).

> DJ – What is the difference between gay and transgender?
>
> A – Transgenders let their, ok, penis [*ling*] get cut off, and after it has been cut, where the urine comes out, ok, there they make a small hole. And they fit 'silicon' here [pointing to his chest]. They grow from the 'injections', they do a 'laser treatment', transgenders do it. And we gays, we live in the 'reality'. If we have to tell someone, we will say that we are just like that, we just have sex, we don't cut our cock, because god made us like that, we just tell it like that, that we are gay. Those people [TGs] don't live openly, they have to earn money. They created a source for earning money.

While in Reddy's account the hijras take pride in their visible performance of gender transgression and explicitly deride non-cross-dressed kothis for their shame-ridden, invisible and/or secret lives (ibid.: 261), Ajay perceives TGs as not 'living in reality' in not openly admitting any sexual desire and claiming to have sex only to earn a living. He furthermore refers to the emasculation ritual or *nirvān* traditionally undergone by hijras as the major difference between gay and transgender people: somebody who is gay would not cut off his penis. The *nirvān* ritual is described by Serena Nanda as a symbolic identification of rebirth that transforms an impotent male into a spiritually potent hijra (Nanda 1999: 24). Impotence can be transformed into the power of generativity through the ideal of *tapasya*, the practice of asceticism. Sexual desire is seen as a distraction from spiritual purpose, with sexual activity that involves a loss of semen resulting in a loss of spiritual energy. The penis and testicles are completely separated from the body. After the cut is made, the blood gushes out and nothing is done to stem the flow: it is considered to be the male part that a person should be drained of. A small stick is put into the urethra to keep it open, which creates the hole Ajay refers to above. He further refers to other medical interventions, namely 'silicone' breast implants, hormone 'injections' and probably facial hair removal by 'laser treatment'. These clearly did not belong to traditional hijra practices in the 1980s, when, according to Nanda, hijras used to wear a 'padded bra' and 'pluck[ed] out their facial hair so that their skin remains smooth like a woman's' (1999: 17). Moreover, Ajay's use of the term 'transgender' or 'TG' instead of 'hijra' indicates a conflation of the different identity categories. Indeed, in India's urban centres there is a growing number of 'transgenders' who do not identify as part of the hijra community. Their self-understanding is rather modelled on the Western category of transgender as 'transient' or 'genderfluid'. They mostly belong to the upper and elite middle classes and may opt for sex reassignment surgeries and a legal sex change (Gupta and Murarka 2009; Windzio 2014). Gurvinder Kalra told me that he encountered hijras who preferred not to undergo the *nirvān* ritual 'because of its crudeness'. In order to be allowed 'to go under a surgeon's knife', as Kalra expressed it, they needed to consult him as a psychiatrist to certify their 'gender identity disorder' (Kalra 2012a: 124).

> DJ – You liked to wear this kind of dress [a sari, like hijras wear it]?

A – There are 'hormones' in my body, ok, in my, the male ones are much, and female are less, in our body the hormones got less. In yours the male ones are more and female less.

DJ – And in yours?

A – In my are the male ones less, and the female ones more.

DJ – Ok.

A –When I was small, ok, what mum did, she made me to wear dresses for girls. She gave me rings for the feet and an anklet. She took a lot of small items and gave to us children. See, we are like females. So from the inside automatic I was female, she took a lot of small things and gave them, toys . . . . The body was male, the feeling was female.

DJ – Like that it started that you used to wear this dress?

A – There is the feeling, Mammi, when I was small she made me wear a girls dress, so after growing up, we feel like this like it gives friendship, if it is thirty-first, in our building we celebrate New Year, outside there is the Ganapati festival, so I feel automatically that I should dress in girl's clothes.

DJ – You like that.

A – Yes, I like that, to be like a female.

DJ – You don't like the Rakhi?

A – I like it.

DJ – But where is yours?

A – I am female, ok, so I tie it, like it is tied, tied on them, on the doctors.

DJ – That is why you took it off?

A – I didn't get one tied. No, no. Not at all. I tied it to the doctor and to you, too, please don't tie it to me, because we people understand ourselves as female, ok.

Ajay mentioned 'hormonal imbalances' as well as childhood experiences, when his mother cross-dressed him, as responsible for him being 'like a female' and his 'female feelings' and implicitly for being gay (being attracted to men instead of women). In his narrative, he borrowed the biological concept 'sex hormones', which are biochemical influences on the development of gonads, sexual characteristics and sexual functions, including the female menstrual cycle. If and how sex hormones are connected to gender identity and expression, sexual attraction and to sexual behaviour has not yet been fully understood scientifically; certainly sex hormones are not the exclusive factor determining sexual attraction. Nonetheless, in Ajay's narrative and explanatory model he states that sex hormones are directly linked to his feeling 'female from the inside' and 'like a female'. The explanation for how he became who he is, though, is neither a physical nor biological one: his mother made him like this. According to Ajay, he grew up wearing female dresses, jewellery and playing with girls' toys. This perception of 'being made' female is in accordance with explanatory models from the literature about hijras and kothis. It is often stated that they are 'spoiled' as a consequence of their first sexual experiences with a man as a receptive partner, which prevents further heterosexual/penetrative intercourse (Nanda 1999: 116; Reddy 2005a: 46). This could either point to a belief that this sexual act 'weakens' their sexual organ and makes them impotent or that they are only able to subsequently enjoy anal sex after the incident.

Paul Boyce (2007b: 408) mentions that the seduction of a man in Kolkata is often described as *pakkī korechhi*, literally 'I have done knowledge'. The phrase refers to the seducer introducing the seducee to sex between men and making him aware of its existence. What is remarkable about this expression is that it 'emphasizes the correspondence between "knowing" and "sexuality", literally stressing that (homo)sexual subjects are produced by their being made aware of a particular sexual context' (ibid.). Similarly, Ajay is the way he is because he was 'made aware' of girls' clothing and being 'female like' by his mother. In Western discourse, there are activists who explicitly argue that being gay, lesbian or transgender is not a 'life choice'. Sexual orientation is characterized as 'innate' and to a certain extent as unchangeable and unswayable. The argument that people cannot be made homosexual by others counters conservative voices that claim that a legalization of same-sex relationships and gay marriage would result in more gay people. Furthermore, when sexual orientation and gender identity is understood as 'innate', to render someone's identity as morally wrong or prohibit them legally becomes a violation of human rights. Aside from the influence during his upbringing that Ajay's mother had on him 'feeling female', he describes his 'being female from the inside' as physically (hormonally) imprinted as well.

Reddy describes kothis – and hijras – as perceiving themselves not as women but rather as 'effeminate' men who adopt the receptive (female) role during intercourse and engage in 'female'-classified activities and tasks (Reddy 2005a: 74). Similarly, Ajay did not want the Rakhi to be tied to his wrist but preferred to tie it 'female-like' to other males. During my fieldwork, I came across an article in a newspaper that described a case of 'forced marriage'. When the husband came to know that his wife was forced into the alliance by her parents after she had secretly married her boyfriend, he asked her to tie him a Rakhi. The Rakhi served as a symbol that he had not entered a husband-wife relationship with her and that his parents accepted her as their daughter.[8] This gesture enabled the young woman to remain honourable during her stay with the family before she finally returned to the boyfriend she had married. The story epitomizes how the tying of the Rakhi is borrowed from its ritual context and used symbolically to classify a relationship as nonsexual. Ajay similarly borrows the tying of the Rakhi to classify himself as 'not male' ('please don't tie it to me'),[9] but 'rather female' ('because we people understand ourselves as female').

'We Also Have the Right to Live': Stigma, Assault and Competing Moral Discourses

> DJ – How do you perceive yourself? As a woman or a man?
>
> A – I am gay.
>
> DJ – If you go by train, do you go by male or by female compartment?
>
> A – In both we suffer, nobody created a jail, nobody a compartment [for us].

Ajay felt lonely and out of place, belonging to nobody and nowhere in particular. The themes of loneliness and stigmatization dominated the last part of our conversation and were closely connected to his mental troubles, which were diagnosed as 'depression':

> DJ – What troubled you? You say that you have a mental disorder, what does that mean?
>
> A – Loneliness eats me.
>
> DJ – That means, in which way?
>
> A – In the sense that I stay alone, so many things go through my mind, different thoughts, as 'Why I am like that?', why the society does not give me respect, I pay the maintenance tax to the society, so the respect that others get, why I don't get this respect, this thoughts eat my mind a lot, and if I go to my community, my community people also fight.
>
> DJ – What else do you think? What do you feel about that?
>
> A – I go into depression, I feel lonely.
>
> DJ – So what do you do then?
>
> A – I go to my community and sit there, then in my community people also keep fighting with each other, so then where should I go?
>
> DJ – So there is no peace?
>
> A – And I am openly gay, so the building people look at me for fucking. And everybody realized that I am gay, because I work in an NGO, so everybody came to know about it, that I am gay. That is why everybody looks at me for having sex. . . . where I live, there I want to live peacefully. And if I do something wrong, then to stay in society will be less easy. Outside I can do anything, but wherever I stay I should stay 'straight'. Prostitutes also do sex outside, but in their backyard they live that normally that nobody calls them a prostitute.

Ajay associates his 'mental disorder', 'going into depression' with the feelings of loneliness and brooding due to a lack of 'respect' or even open contempt he faces in his neighbourhood. Reddy points out the great significance 'respect' (*izzat*) has for hijras in Hyderabad. Respect operates as 'a complex qualitative currency of moral worth' (Reddy 2005b: 261) and is closely bound to the 'local moral world' of the hijra community; for example, a hijra is expected to wear only women's clothing, grow their hair long, pluck out their beards rather than shave and learn the hijra lexicon and body language. Gaining respect and status in their own community can serve as an antipode and counterweight to the stigma and ostracism they experience from 'respectable' society. In contrast, Ajay is not part of a community that constitutes its own coherent 'local moral world'. The hijra community excluded him out of fear that his HIV infection might threaten their reputation. The kothi community cannot support him morally because it operates away from mainstream society rather than providing an alternative 'moral economy'.

Ajay does not succeed in navigating the complexities of the 'moral economy' of the neighbourhood he lives in and pass as 'straight'. Instead, he behaves 'openly gay'. He brought home other men to have sex with them instead of doing it 'outside' in places designated for such encounters (e.g. parks and public toilets). In the end, Ajay's openly deviant behaviour led to his admission to Asha. Furthermore, his behaviour caused stigmatization. Ajay experienced a 'spoiled identity' (Goffman 1986) as a consequence of others' deprecatory reaction towards him. Ajay did not cover up the stigma and he did not separate his public life from his 'secret life'[10] of being gay. Ajay compares his situation to that of a sex worker, of whom society equally expects not to 'contaminate' family and community with their 'dirty work'.[11] The two spheres of community and secret life were conflated when Ajay eventually joined Humsafar Trust. Eventually everybody came to know about him being 'gay'. Apparently, he was approached for sex by some of his neighbours. Ajay himself did not like that 'because where I live, there I want to live peacefully'. Here the modern and open 'gay culture', as proposed by activist Ashok Row Kavi, clashes with 'shame culture' (Narrain 2004: 45) and the local moral world order of Ajay's neighbourhood. In the community where his house is located as well as in the gay community, Ajay longs to be a 'respected' member; unfortunately, and perhaps because of his 'shameless' behaviour, he does not accomplish this in either context.

When Dhaval asked Ajay if he had ever been in a relationship with a man, implying if he had ever entered a long-term commitment or fallen in love with somebody, Ajay recalled a story of his friend, Muskan, who had severely suffered in a romantic relationship.

> A – I have never maintained any relation. My friend had one, then all became a mess. Muskan, she was a TG, she loved somebody, and he 'committed blood', he murdered, she brought him from jail, again and again, today she became poor herself, that is why I don't maintain any relation. . . .
>
> DJ – Why not? Things like relationships happen, don't they?
>
> A – No, in America they are there, in India they aren't, Indian culture doesn't believe in this thing. The Hindu culture. It is against the whole thing. Religious leaders are against this thing, they say that this thing is wrong. There was Ramdev Baba, he was against us, he told that where their blood is used it will create gay [*samlingī*] children, so don't use their blood anywhere. So the religious leaders are against us, but if they torture us, then where the religious leaders go?
>
> DJ – How do you feel about that, that they are all against [you]?
>
> A – It is wrong, isn't it, because we have also come into this world and which sin we committed? Like it is the right of people in society to live, like that they also should allow us to live, isn't it, like it is our entitlement, we also have a life to live, we also have some rights.
>
> DJ – So, you think that if it was made legal, then . . .
>
> A – If it was made legal, it does not just work like that, it's very difficult, if there is a child, then straight people are tied to each other by attachment. We cannot give birth to children, so how any attachment can remain between a couple? That is why we keep changing our partner, for sex.

The case of Muskan, who seems to have sacrificed a lot for her lover and in the end 'became poor herself', served as a discouraging example for Ajay to ever enter into a romantic relationship that is driven by infatuation. Arranged alliances tend to follow certain social conventions concerning gender, caste and age. Additionally, Indian culture 'doesn't believe', as Ajay expresses it, in same-sex alliances. Here he particularly refers to Hinduism and Hindu religious leaders. One example is the yogi guru Swami Ramdev, who, according to Ajay, uses the explanatory model of 'innate' homosexuality to warn against its possible inheritance. In 2009 he filed a petition with the Supreme Court of India to oppose the Delhi High Court ruling on decriminalization and claimed that homosexuality could be 'cured' by yoga (Nelson 2009). Ajay took America and the West as a counter-example in which open same-sex relations and (romantic) long-term relationships are socially approved. Ajay repeatedly stressed that gay people should also have rights. The national law and Section 377 IPC are criticized by queer activists as violating their rights to privacy, dignity, health, equality, non-discrimination and freedom of expression (Menon 2007b; Baxti 2011; Al. Gupta 2011; Dutta 2011; Puri 2013). Ajay did not believe, though, that the abolishment of Section 377 would lead to 'gay' people falling into the relationship patterns of 'straight' people. A long-term alliance seemed not to make sense for him if it did not pursue the aim of procreation. Kishori Nayar, a counsellor working for Humsafar Trust, told me that she had encountered same-sex couples who frame marriage as equally conservative and traditional as most straight people in India. Most marry to make sure that they are entitled to get their part of the property in case of a divorce or so that there is somebody to take care of them during old age. Alternate sexualities, gender and intimacies are certainly seen as against mainstream society and their values, but queer lives and communities also reproduce certain gender stereotypes and follow social norms that are upheld by the very society they are ostracized by (Mitra and Nair 2011).

For Ajay, being gay seemed to be predominantly about having sex with those people whom he physically desired. The lack of social institutionalization of same-sex intimacies, particularly in certain contexts like cruising and prostitution, can lead to a depersonalization of sexual encounters (Khan 2001: 110). Where same-sex encounters mostly take place in public, foreplay, personal choice, privacy and individuality tend to be minimalized. Sex in these contexts may be experienced as a matter of urgent (sexual) release or 'discharge'. The lack of intimacy and acceptance and the experience of loneliness and abuse in Ajay's life became tremendously evident towards the end of our conversation.

> A – What is there right now? My life is over.
>
> DJ – Why is it over?
>
> A – What is there right now? The society doesn't accept me, relatives don't accept me, there is no acceptance from anybody. And I was made crazy and kept [here] – what should I do? The ward boys keep beating me, they insult me badly, they keep saying bad words, why god gave us this burden of nature? They tie the hands and undress and beat a lot, with hands, with this they beat, with this, with this [makes a gesture with his elbow].
>
> DJ – What you have just shown to us, your injury, how you got injured?
>
> A – Those who did sex with me and broke my hip, the ones from the building. They gave sleeping tablets in the food, they broke the lock, they came and used to fuck me, they fucked me, and the building boys did it to me, too. By force. . . .
>
> DJ – So how you have gotten the injury you showed to us?
>
> A – This . . . I went by train and jumped from it.
>
> DJ – Why?
>
> A – I tried to commit suicide.

Reddy (2007: 314) mentions that she 'heard innumerable accounts of suicide attempts by kothis' during her fieldwork, all on account of the suffering they experienced due to the physical and emotional abuse of their 'husbands' or rejection by their families and society in general. Sex for men outside heterosexual marriage is not only conceptualized as play (*khel*) or fun (*mastī*) but can also be a social 'power arena' in a 'do-or-be-done-to world' (Cohen 2007: 214). The act of sexual penetration here is a definer of 'phallic power' (Khan 2001: 107). Vaginal and anal penetration become a marker of 'manliness', while the penetrated, or literally 'fucked' one, will be seen as 'not man', the one who 'has to take it', the one 'it is done to'. The penetrated other here is not framed as an object of 'love' or 'desire' but as somebody who in an act of bodily violence of social difference 'must take his desire through you or be taken by yours' (Cohen 2007: 215). In this sociocultural logic of penetration, those men who like to have anal sex become associated with the female gender, who are naturally destined to be unchangeably penetrated and 'done to' in sexual intercourse. Janina Geist reports from her fieldwork in Delhi that because kothis are associated with the female and a feminine appearance, they commonly experience sexual harassment and assault by men in public. The counsellor Kishori mentioned that many of her clients who live in same-sex relationships report emotional abuse, exploitation and a lack of sexual satisfaction. Some of them identify as kothi and just perform oral or receptive anal sex with their partners although they want to engage in penetration – to articulate one's sexual needs and desires is generally not very common and mostly taboo. Even hijras, who are feared for their belligerent, aggressive style in public, rather tend to identify with women on the issue of 'domestic abuse' (Reddy 2005a: 51). Reddy mentions that the hijras she encountered saw themselves as relatively helpless when faced with regular violence from their 'husbands'. When she suggested that they could or should resist this behaviour and retaliate, they reacted rather depreciatively.

Indian feminist authors suggest a general connection between a higher incident of so called 'common mental illnesses' like depression in women and their subordinate role and the structural, physical and emotional violence they have to endure on an everyday basis (Davar 1995, 1999, 2001). This seems to apply to a certain extent to kothis and hijras as well. Therefore, Ajay's story of loneliness and suffering is typical rather than exceptional. Generally, Ajay occupies a very ambivalent sociocultural space. He transgresses psychological (gay/transgender) and gender categories (male/female), he navigates diverse and at times contradicting urban spaces (truck line/his neighbourhood/NGO/cruising places/psychiatric hospital) and negotiates and tries to fit in with the different communities associated with these places (hijras and transgenders/neighbours/queer activists/gays and kothis/fellow patients and hospital staff). And finally, he has to balance and bear the tensions of the metropolitan sphere: the promises that come with striving for a 'modern' lifestyle – new concepts of ('gay') masculinity on the one hand and moral and social obligations rooted in the cultural value system on the other (Srivastava 2004). The development of a 'modern' gay culture became possible in the context of liberalization and globalization of the economy in the early 1990s, which 'facilitated the emergence of an increasingly wealthy upper middle and middle class populace who not only had access to previously out-of-reach objects and narratives but who could, for the first time, also afford them' (Reddy 2004: 158). Those who identify as gay and hail from the upper middle class do not usually construct their identities on the penetrative/receptive, female/male and sexual/asexual axes as kothis and hijras do, but they rather understand 'their sexuality' as opposed to 'heterosexuality'. Therefore, membership is not defined by kinship or certain gendered practices as cross-dressing but rather through a commitment to gay identification, political liberation and the awareness of the global queer discourse (ibid. 2005a: 64; Hall 2005). Individuals like Ajay construct themselves within the meaning and subject positions of the hijra/kothi model while also drawing on certain aspects of 'modern sexuality' and 'being gay'.

> DJ – As you are being a gay, what has to happen in society, what do you think?
>
> A – As you have the right to live in society, we also have to be granted the same. Because we too have the right to life in this society because god created us.

Ajay insists on not being discriminated against for having sex with men. However, he did not claim his right to have an equitable, romantic same-sex relationship. Ajay rather relates the latter to the West, as it does not match with sociocultural and moral contexts in India (Kuku 2013). Although Ajay learned to speak decent English in the NGO context and adopted certain concepts for himself from the queer discourse, he definitely did not fully embrace middle-class culture and its habitus.

As Janina Geist (2014) reports from her fieldwork, becoming older poses a challenge for many kothis. Not matching the idealized image of the young and attractive any longer, many kothis face a loss of self-worth and abandonment by their lovers. Earning a reasonable living by doing sex work becomes more difficult. Kothis who lead a double life as married husbands navigate this transition more easily. Those who do not may finally decide to become a full member of the hijra community and consequently become accommodated in their kinship and social network (Reddy 2005a: 53). Ajay could not imagine a future for himself at the time of our conversation. His father had died, and the relationship with his uncle was damaged. He had accused him of stealing his father's money that he had left for him before leaving to South Africa. Additionally, Ajay was worried for his brother, who was not treated well at the hospital. He planned to work further with Humsafar Trust and hoped to somehow survive on his meagre salary.

Queer Categories and Building a Moral Self

In queer activist literature, the propagation of rights for hijras, aravanis or alis[12] either works by deliberately relating these local identity categories to global medical and psychiatric terms like 'transsexuals' and 'transgender' (Sukthankar 2005; Govindan and Vasudevan 2011) or by actively rejecting and questioning these (Chakravorty 2007; Suresh 2011b). While the Indian queer movement rejects some Western (and medical) concepts like 'homosexual', others like queer, lesbian and gay are accepted and are widely used (Geist 2008: 11; see also Ramakrishnan 2007). While in the West alternative sexualities were theorized as paraphilias in the psychiatric discourse from the end of the nineteenth century (Oosterhuis 2000), in India identification and labelling happened predominantly in the context of the medical and public health discourse that evolved around HIV prevention and intervention programmes (Cohen 2005; Row Kavi 2007; Boellstorff 2011; Strauss 2022). This discourse, mainly carried by internationally connected NGOs and by the Indian elite and higher middle class, additionally gave rise to a new moral discourse that draws on the globalized value of 'human rights'

(Khanna 2005, 2007). In contrast, Indian psychiatric practice is rather oriented towards local moral discourses that draw on sociocultural norms and values. Mental health professionals who are educated according to Western standards and with a good proficiency in English sooner or later go abroad to advance their careers,[13] and psychiatrists and sexologists who stay back in India, running private clinics or practices, depend on their reputation within local communities or on attracting non-residential Indians (NRIs) by drawing on traditional moral codes (Srivastava 2004: 366).

Both the global and local moral discourse are palpable in Ajay's narrative. Narratives are depicted as 'moral laboratories' by Cheryl Mattingly (2013: 303): 'Self-narratives are created as we – in terror – try to defend our own actions . . . .' She argues that through the 'processes of interrogation', which narratives often revolve around, our 'moral selves' are born. According to Mattingly, particularly in moments of crisis narrative experiments can serve as a catalyst for moral transformations in everyday life. Constitutive of Ajay's 'moral self' that he lined out in his narrative is his positioning within a certain community (kothi), but he also draws lines of demarcation concerning certain (identity) categories (hijra/TG; 'straight people'). He did this by drawing on several moral codes from medical, religious, local as well as queer discourses. By using his actual, unbearable situation as a negative backdrop, Ajay narratively tried to imagine and create a liveable world for himself while in conversation with Dhaval and me. Although at the same time, he described his life as 'over', which indicates that his moral self felt weak, exhausted and hopeless.

Ajay's narrative had an emotional and moral impact on me (Stodulka 2015), which was a driving factor in asking Ganesh to accompany us to Asha. Probably I hoped that he might help to address and relieve Ajay's feelings of hopelessness. When Ganesh eventually came to Asha to meet Ajay, he had a very pragmatic way of evaluating the situation of his former colleague. As a former social work student of TISS, he was familiar with Asha and even knew some of the social workers who worked there. He evaluated Ajay's situation as 'not so bad after all', as he at least was provided with food and shelter and did not have to live on the streets. Additionally, he was accommodated in the admission ward – here nurses are present 24 hours a day in contrast to the 'chronic wards', where attendants alone are in charge.

When I, together with another social work student, had started to speak up for Ajay, I experienced a fierce pushback from the side of the social workers. According to one of the senior social workers, Gadge madam, who was in charge of Ajay's ward, he actually received loads of attention because 'we fell for his attention seeking behaviour'. After Ganesh had dropped by the social workers' office during his visit, he shared with me that the social workers had inquired about the role I had played in Ajay's case and how they eventually commented: 'These foreigners always want to change everything.'

The last time I heard from Ajay was in March 2013, when I visited Humsafar Trust. I met Ganesh again, who told me that Ajay had been discharged from Asha and that he used to call by the office from time to time – the last time was on 14 February, to wish everybody a nice Valentine's Day. The 'festival of love' serves as another sociocultural concept that signifies and to a certain extent also models intimate relationships; it has gained increasing nationwide popularity in recent decades, though its meanings may differ significantly depending on local contexts and discourses (Brosius 2013).

Notes

1. They mentioned that they had removed bed sheets and in one case even a sparrow from a woman's vagina.
2. The only exception was when we discussed with him the attitude of Hindu religious leaders towards same-sex behaviour. At this point he used the Hindi term *samlingī*.
3. The emergence of the internet, of dating platforms and online gay communities and the increasing affordability of smartphones for non-middle-class Indians have increased the possibility of finding sexual partners. On dating platforms, it may be more important to be able to name and describe one's sexual desires and preferences (Geist 2013).
4. An 'Indian LGBT Oral History Project' produced by Humsafar Trust in association with Solaris Pictures and supported by UNDP (India) (see http://www.projectbolo.com/).
5. According to Kishori Nayar, a counsellor from Humsafar Trust, the local trains are well known as cruising places in Mumbai. Men particularly meet in compartments called 'Twobytwo', which are located close to the ladies' compartment.

6. *nirvān* hijras are hijras who have undergone the emasculation ritual, which includes castration and penectomy.
7. The pejorative term is used by hijras either in abusive, derogatory contexts, or in humorous, self-denigratory ones (Reddy 2005a: 64).
8. The tying of the Rakhi symbolically excludes the husband-wife relationship as this is sexual and is not a relationship that is perceived as sacred like the brother-sister relationship (see Bennett 1989).
9. He removed the Rakhi from his wrist shortly after the nurses had tied it to him.
10. 'Secret life' refers to the fact that kothis, unlike hijras, do not wear female attire in public or during the day. Furthermore, Kothis often have wives and children who do not know about their 'second life'.
11. A common expression in Hindi for sex work, see Asifa's case in Chapter 2.
12. *Aravani* or *ali* are further local terms for hijra.
13. Gurvinder Kalra, for example, received his working visa for Australia and moved there with his family a year after I met and interviewed him in his flat in south Mumbai in March 2013.

CONCLUSION

LISTENING TO 'MAD' NARRATIVES

Particularly in the psychiatric context, narratives tend to be unstable and even unintelligible. Bureaucratic-psychiatric institutions frame narratives of illness experiences and provide a framework in which one's mental health problems can be expressed and articulated. The colonial establishments of mental asylums and the modern psychiatric movement, respectively, brought with them a rational and disciplined behaviour, consciousness and habitus (H. Basu 2009, 2018: 134; Quack 2014). Therefore, narratives can have dire medical or legal consequences, as I illustrated with the case studies of Hemant and Tasneem (Pinto 2014: 30). Psychiatric practice scrutinizes narratives and tries to distinguish between 'sane' and 'mad' talks. In the local psychiatric culture of Asha, this categorization was crucial in the context of deciding if a patient was 'fit for discharge'. Asha's bureaucratic and biomedical approach to the 'management of madness' provides mental health professionals with 'an agenda of questions and procedural routines that prevent them from hearing patients' deepest concerns' (Wilce 1995: 947). The procedural reshaping of mental health complaints – or their dismissal if they do not comply with the organizational standards – is one of the discursive means that sustains the institution's hierarchies of power and social order. It is not by the ill means of individual staff members that people experience negligence, maltreatment or are even killed in public medical institutions. Bureaucratic systems appear so brutal at times because they are organized and regulated by rules that serve to uphold a social order. The principles that determine the social practices in Asha do not aim at maximizing the well-being of individual persons but at managing 'madness' in a time- and resource-efficient way.

Psychiatric institutions that are organized by means of bureaucratic principles operate by categorizing and treating their clients according to a classificatory and organizational system that they – in order to uphold it – have to continuously clean and purify of ambivalent things and beings.

As became apparent in previous chapters, narratives served patients in creating inhabitable worlds and liveable futures, reinforcing, breaking and at times playing with kinship roles and expectations. Nevertheless, voices of psychiatric patients run the permanent risk of being silenced by practitioners if their words are pathologized and declared as mere symptoms (ibid.). In this way, moral claims concerning psychiatric treatment are systemically overheard and not taken up by professionals in the context of ethical contemplations or debates (Brodwin 2013: 131). Damian E.M. Milton (2016) states regarding 'autism' that a dominance of the 'theory of mind' or the 'mentalising' theory leads to 'the framing of the social interaction difficulties autistic people face as primarily located within the brain/mind of the autistic person' (ibid.). He points out, though, that this is a problem experienced by both parties, 'a breakdown in reciprocity and communication between two differently disposed "social actors"' (ibid.). What Milton (2012) calls a 'double empathy problem' we can also observe in the case of 'mad' narratives: While their tellers are labelled as unintelligible and unable to follow and anticipate conventional narrative principles, their listeners do not bother or at least struggle to understand 'mad' narrative principles, too. A lack of empathy and contextualization often leads to the dehumanization of 'mad' stories and a loss of status of their tellers, who are not perceived as full moral persons (Van Dongen 2002: 33). Additionally, in the psychiatric context, 'mad' narratives tend to be ripped apart in the bureaucratic and diagnostic process. Clinicians taking a clinical interview primarily aim at gaining insights into the nature of the 'patient's illness'. Interviewing in clinical settings is often framed as a standardized survey instrument that produces reliable 'facts' to assess a patient's symptoms.

During my research, I accompanied Dr Kulkarni when she carried out mental status examinations in the male admission ward. I observed how she asked a patient, a young man, what time it was. He hesitated and looked at his left wrist. Dr Kulkarni commented: 'He seems to have visual hallucinations. He is not aware he is not wearing a watch.' She had immediately categorized his behaviour as symptomatic. Analysing the encounter between patient and psychiatrist, I reflected on the fact that the patient had just been admitted to Asha – less than a few hours ago – and may have forgotten that he had removed his watch as part of the procedure of changing into a patient uniform. Or was he even sarcastically proposing how it would even be possible for him to tell her the time without a watch? This was not the only incident I witnessed the 'psychiatric gaze' in operation. What follows is a description of further examinations in my fieldnotes:

> Then the boy with 'MR' ['Mental Retardation']. Seeing his posture, she [Dr Kulkarni] suggests psychosis (> psychotic mannerism). Every behaviour is psychiatrically classified. One patient reports that he watches a lot of TV (> mild grandiosity). With another she gets a 'praecox feeling', a feeling of being excluded from his world. Again another patient is attributed 'inadequate affect' because he answers to her questions calmly and does not challenge her, how she expresses it (> 'other people would demand and start fighting'). It is not cross-checked whether other things could explain the psychiatrist's impression. The patients are only looked upon with psychiatric goggles, with the 'symptom scanner'. Everything is interpreted as a symptom. [Dr Kulkarni] doesn't explain the patient's 'exited' and 'highly irritable' state yesterday [but calm today] with his admission to a mental hospital, but with the fast effect of Clozapine that he had taken up this morning. (Fieldnotes 17 August 2011)

My observations illustrate how the clinical framing of the interview situation as an encounter between the 'symptomatic' patient and the psychiatrist, who embodies the interpretive authority, might lead to a decontextualization of speech acts and behaviour. A scarcity of time and the pressure for a 'fast diagnosis', as is usually the case in public hospitals and in the Indian context generally (Nunley 1992), might additionally amplify these dynamics. Meaning-making processes tend to become monocausal and stereotypic. Every speech act, posture and habitus is a potential symptom under the psychiatric gaze and interpreted accordingly. Therefore, Thomas Csordas et al. (2010: 30) proposed that clinical interviews should be seen as 'speech events' and not be understood as a screening tool for symptoms. Speech events are jointly constructed by interviewers and respondents, and the meanings of questions and answers are contextually grounded. Therefore analysis and interpretation would be based on a theory of discourse and meaning rather than on a psychiatric catalogue of symptoms and disorders (Mishler 1986). This approach transforms the 'symptomatic patient' whose behaviour and speech seems to be predominately determined by a biochemically unbalanced brain into a sociocultural being who continuously interacts with their environment (Van Dongen 2002: 33).

Analysing 'mad' narratives and experiences in the context in which they emerged can give us important insights into sociocultural and therefore 'fundamental human processes' (Jenkins 2004). Rosenhan (1973) criticised psychiatric diagnosis because it 'locates the sources of aberration within the individual and only rarely within the complex of stimuli that surrounds him' (ibid.: 253). People who face mental health issues might perceive the world differently, but are by no means detached from their surroundings; they react emotionally and adjust to their respective environments behaviourally (Corin 1990, Kring/Germans 2004). It would be wrong to assume that 'mad' narratives just break with conventions and are therefore 'crazy' and 'alien' because they do not follow any structure or principle. We cannot reduce 'mad' narratives to unstructured and senseless mumbling. Even if people with mental illnesses are talking in an unconventional way, we have to concede that they equally construct a reality guided by certain psychological and cultural principles, shaped by social encounters and institutional contexts. Elizabeth B. Purcell (2016) in her article 'Disability, Narrative, and Moral Status' responds to arguments that state that persons with severe cognitive impairments should not enjoy the full moral status or dignity of other 'cognitively-able' humans. She suggests instead that the social ability and the capacity to narrate should be grounds for achieving the full moral status:

'Telling stories is a particular function of *what humans do*. It is something we learn at a very young age and is initiated by those around us. It is how we understand ourselves in time and in relation to others' (ibid.). Purcell argues that many, if not all narratives are socially dependent and co-authored with others. Therefore, a human's 'narrative capacity' does not have to be fully realized by themselves. It can include social relationships that enable us to tell our story and encompass its meanings. This applies even if, for example, our episodic memory is not fully functional because we suffer from a disability that means we are not able to construct a story on our own. 'In other words, what gives us moral relevance is not what can be determined by the performance of tasks or a high IQ; to the contrary, it is the story we live that enables us to flourish' (ibid.). I tried to show in this ethnography that there is not only one way to narrate but a variety of ways and levels of narration. All of them are meaningful and have the potential to co-construct social reality. This includes 'mad' narratives, and if we follow Purcell's argument, their narrators should be heard and granted full moral status. It would be inappropriate to see the labelling of these stories as 'unintelligible' and 'alien' as a consequence of 'othering' and 'stigmatization'. 'Mad' narratives are shaped by experiences that are at times fundamentally different from conventional ones, in that they are not only the product of divergent mental or neurological processes but of what is an 'institutionalized' life.

Institutional Changes

Asha belongs to a group of bureaucratic institutions that are perceived as colonial artifacts in the process of abolishment and therefore about to disappear from the Indian psychiatric landscape (H. Basu 2018). This does not mean the disappearance of bureaucratic psychiatric organizations altogether, though. Indeed, it seems that bureaucracy looms in a new guise in private psychiatry. In contrast to Asha, which was spatially organized according to racial and caste structures and where the wards' functions are divided according to diagnostic and treatment categories, the wards in the private hospital were ranked according to socio-economic class structures: clients were asked to choose between an admission to the normal, second, first and deluxe (VIP) ward. While the spatial organization of the governmental hospital follows the logic of sociocultural hierarchies, the organization of the wards in the private hospital is market-based. The times I frequented the private psychiatric department the social worker was commonly busy with taking care of paper work and making sure that all patients' files contained the legally necessary consent forms. On one occasion, she was preparing for an inspection of the department by a committee of reputed mental health professionals delegated by the state government in the context of the renewal of the official licence, which is necessary when one wants to operate a psychiatric nursing home. In the clinical everyday practices of the hospital, however, paperwork played only a very minor role. Consent forms for the administering of ECT, for example, were often signed by the patient after he/she had already received several treatments. In contrast, bureaucracy in the private institution did not so much structure, manage and organize the delivery of mental health care but rather aimed at controlling and monitoring the private hospital's provision of psychiatric services according to the guidelines outlined in the Indian Mental Health Act 1987. David Graeber (2015) argues that bureaucracy increases under neoliberal market conditions and that our so-called era of 'postbureaucratic organization' is actually a period of 'total bureaucratisation'.

In order to analyse bureaucratic institutions, Laura Bear and Nayanika Mathur (2015) suggest focusing on the 'public good' – the utopian goals bureaucracies exist for, rest their legitimacy on and 'attempt to materialize [as] this contract between citizens and institutions' (ibid.: 19). Mental health activists refer to exactly this contract between citizens and the state when they criticize the 'indifference' and the insufficiency of psychiatric treatment and care that is delivered to patients in psychiatric hospitals. Equally, several activists criticized the quality of psychiatric treatment in the private sector. During my stay in Mumbai, private psychiatric services were accused of inappropriate and non-scientifically proven propagation of ECT treatment as a cure for nearly every psychiatric illness and for charging patients for ineffective psychotherapy sessions that were held while patients were still severely symptomatic or suffering from memory loss as an adverse effect of ECT treatment. The activists doubted that the measures were administered in order to improve the patients' well-being but suspected doctors of being mainly interested in boosting the department's revenue. In general, private psychiatric facilities were perceived as business-oriented, serving and satisfying the demands and expectations of their clients, namely the patients' families, while public hospitals were often seen as a waste of time and characterized by a lack of human and material resources (Barua 2005). Irrespective of the kind of hospital, mental health institutions were generally experienced as not having the understanding to cure individual mental illnesses as its primary objective. Rather, the bureaucratic infrastructure was suspected of predominantly serving the well-being of the psychiatric institution and to preserve pre-existing structures.

Shortly after I finished my fieldwork at Asha, bureaucratic structures and patient rights were legally reformed in a Mental Healthcare Bill, finally passed as the Mental Health Care Act 2017 on 7 April. It received mixed responses from mental health professionals (Kala 2013; Dhar 2013; Antony 2014). The Act seeks to fulfil India's international obligation in line with the UN 'Convention on Rights of Persons with Disabilities' to create a rights-based framework for persons with mental health issues. Patients can now challenge the decision of a doctor to admit them by contacting the 'Mental Health Review Board', which has replaced the abolished BOV (Sachan 2013). Additionally, a person with a mental illness now has the right to make an advance directive that states how he/she wants to be treated for their illness and who his/her nominated representative shall be. It is mandatory for every medical officer and psychiatrist to provide treatment to an individual as per the advance directive – where this cannot be provided – for example, where the patient lacks free will, information or capacity – the Mental Health Review Board has to be consulted. Whereas the Act of 1987 provided general protections against indignant or cruel treatment, Chapter V of the new Act provides a more detailed charter of rights for persons with mental illnesses. How these rights are implemented or are going to be implemented in clinical practice, though, has yet to be evaluated. New policies do not necessarily mean new realities, as the example of community psychiatry and the earlier national strategy of integrating mental health within existing primary care services illustrates. According to Jain and Jadhav (2008), it was a bureaucratic and culturally incongruent top-down endeavour in which rural community voices were edited out. The same thing might happen to patients claiming their rights – if the lack of resources and hierarchical power structures within families and mental health institutions are not also addressed at the same time.

Imaginations of Future Psychiatric Cultures

Intellectuals and social scientists like Bhargavi V. Davar (2014) criticize Indian psychiatry for its lack of reflection on 'the colonial basis of mental health practices in India, or on the question of community choices and alternatives' (ibid.: 277). Indian psychiatrists in their 'early reliance on Western knowledge, as well as their reluctance to challenge it' (Bayetti, Jadhav and Deshpande 2017) promote a psychiatric approach that aims at disciplining thinking and controlling behaviour and emotions. It stresses the importance of a steady intake of medication, regular work and taking responsibility for oneself and others (H. Basu 2018: 132). Some anthropologists and medical scientists are against relying on biomedical psychiatric services exclusively and suggest embracing India's traditional healing sites as an equivalent source in the national mental health system (Raguram et al. 2002; Sax 2014). Other authors want Indian psychiatry to break with its colonial past and thus no longer be perceived through 'the prism of Western science' (A.R. Basu 2005: 127). In this way it can develop its own 'theoretical concepts of Indian psychiatry' (ibid.: 129). Innovative and critical reflexive research methods that in particular were developed in applied anthropology, autoethnography and collaborative 'experimental' ethnography and knowledge production (Estalella and Criado 2018) could facilitate the ethical development of psychiatry and mental health services and thus go beyond the 'scaling up' of services available in the global north (Mills and Fernando 2014: 196). A collaborative approach enables an independent development of frameworks that are '"home-grown" within the local contexts from which distress emerges' (ibid.) and owned and sustained by people whom local facilities are supposed to serve.

During the last two decades, a number of nongovernmental organizations (NGOs) have taken up the task of enhancing psychiatric services by implementing rehabilitation, counselling or therapeutic measures and advancing research (Patel and Thara 2003; Patel and Varghese 2004). The Banyan Academy of Leadership in Mental Health (BALM) and the Bapu Trust have a promising approach in the area of innovative and interdisciplinary research and education.[1] The BALM developed together with mental health professionals an innovative series of short, annual courses on social science theory and methods applied to mental health in South Asia, which include clinically applied anthropology and cultural psychiatry (Derges et al. 2012). A localized development and critical reflection of methods, curricula and knowledge and the establishment of collaborative interdisciplinary and international partnerships can advance the evolvement of a culturally sensitive psychiatric practice. Social anthropology and especially medical anthropology can inspire and assist in this process with its localized approach and taking into account the particular. Additionally, a symmetric approach to illness narratives of patients – individual, biographical narratives – will give them greater importance during clinical encounters and diagnostic processes. Instead of contrasting personal (illness) experiences with medical (disease) categories, an innovative psychiatric practice could embrace the concept of 'cultural biology' (Kirmayer 2006) and simply integrate illness and disease narratives. The Cultural Formulation Interview (CFI) can be understood as an endeavour in this direction. The CFI is a semi-structured interview included in Section III 'Emerging Measures and Models' of the DSM-5 and is composed of sixteen questions 'that clinicians may use to obtain information during a mental health assessment about the impact of culture on key aspects of an individual's clinical presentation and care' (American Psychiatric Association 2013: 750). The CFI has been developed by an international consortium of mental health care providers. Nevertheless, as a clinical tool, the CFI needs local acknowledgement, training and awareness as its implementation and utility faces different challenges and barriers respective of the sociocultural context (Aggarwal et al. 2013; Paralikar et al. 2015; Stege and Yarris 2017). Anyway, the CFI is only one piece of the puzzle when it comes to implementing sociocultural sensitivity and empathy in psychiatric and clinical practice. Practitioners are only able to develop 'cultural competence' when it is additionally included in their training and medical curricula and it is embodied and embraced professionally (Adeponle et al. 2015; Mills et al. 2017). Medical sciences can benefit from social anthropology's self-reflexive lens here: psychiatric and medical education has to become aware of their sociocultural imprinting, and medical narratives have to become more culturally sensitive and integrative. If medicine is not able to take this 'reflexive turn', illness narratives will likely remain 'the Other' in clinical encounters and psychiatric practice and research will continue to mean to 'act upon' instead of 'doing with' people (Van Dongen 2000: 138).

Note

1. For more information about The Banyan Academy of Leadership in Mental Health, visit https://balm.in/. For information about the Bapu Trust, visit https://baputrust.com.

REFERENCES

Abu-Lughod, Lila. 1991. 'Writing Against Culture', in Richard Fox (ed.), *Recapturing Anthropology: Working in Present*. Santa Fe, NM: School of American Research Press, pp. 137–62.

Addlakha, Renu. 2001. 'The Lay and Medical Diagnoses of Psychiatric Disorder and the Normative Construction of Femininity', in Bhargavi V. Davar (ed.), *Mental Health from a Gender Perspective*. New Delhi: Sage, pp. 313–33.

——. 2007. 'Gender, Subjectivity and Sexual Identity: How Young People with Disabilities Conceptualise the Body, Sex and Marriage in Urban India'. *Working papers eSocialSciences* (id: 2075): 1–31. Retrieved 16 May 2019 from http://www.esocialsciences.org/Download/repec Download.aspx?fname = Document11862009330.9677851.pdf&fcategory = Articles&AId = 2075&fref = repec.

——. 2008. *Deconstructing Mental Illness: An Ethnography of Psychiatry, Women, and the Family*. New Delhi: Zubaan.

Adeponle, Ademola B., Danielle Groleau and Laurence J. Kirmayer. 2015. 'Clinician Reasoning in the Use of Cultural Formulation to Resolve Uncertainty in the Diagnosis of Psychosis', *Culture, Medicine, and Psychiatry* 39: 16–42.

Agarwal, A.K., Andrade Chittaranjan and M. Venkataswamy Reddy. 1992. 'The Practice of ECT in India: Issues Relating to the Administration of ECT', *Indian Journal of Psychiatry* 34(4): 285–97.

Agarwal, S.P. (ed.). 2004. *Mental Health: An Indian Perspective 1946–2003*. New Delhi: Elsevier.

Aggarwal, Neil Krishnan, et al. 2013. 'Barriers to Implementing the DSM-5 Cultural Formulation Interview: A Qualitative Study', *Culture, Medicine, and Psychiatry* 37(3): 505–33.

American Anthropological Association (AAA). 2011 [1998]. 'Code of Ethics', in Antonius C.G.M. Robben and Jeffrey A. Sluka (eds), *Ethnographic Fieldwork: An Anthropological Reader*. Oxford: Blackwell Publishing, pp. 325–30.

American Psychiatric Association. 2013. *Diagnostic and Statistical Manual of Mental Disorders - DSM-5 - Fifth Edition*. Arlington, VA: American Psychiatric Association.

American Psychological Association (APA). 2011. 'Answers to Your Questions about Transgender People, Gender Identity, and Gender Expression'. Retrieved 1 July 2017 from http://www.apa.org/topics/lgbt/transgender.aspx.

Andrade, Chittaranjan. 2003. 'Unmodified ECT: Ethical Issues', *Indian Journal of Medical Ethics* 11(1): 9–10.

——. 2007. 'Letter to the Editor: Patients and Electroconvulsive Therapy. Knowledge or Attitudes?', *Indian Journal of Psychiatry* 49(2): 145.

Andrade, Chittaranjan, A.K. Agarwal and Venkatswamy M. Reddy. 1993. 'The Practice of ECT in India II: The Practical Administration of ECT', *Indian Journal of Psychiatry* 35(2): 81–86.

Andrade, Chittaranjan, et al. 2000. 'Musculoskeletal Morbidity with Unmodified ECT May Be Less Than Earlier Believed', *Indian Journal of Psychiatry* 42(2): 156–62.

Anspach, Renee R. 2011. 'Preface', in P.J. McGann and David Hutson (eds), *Sociology of Diagnosis* (12 Advances in Medical Sociology). Bradford: Emerald Group Publishing Limited, pp. xiii–xxvii.

Antony, James T. 2014. 'The Mental Health Care Bill 2013: A Disaster in the Offing?', *Indian Journal of Psychiatry* 56(1): 3–7.

Appell, G.N. 1978. *Ethical Dilemmas in Anthropological Inquiry – A Case Book*. Waltham, MA: Crossroads Press.

Asad, Talal. 1979. 'Anthropology and the Analysis of Ideology', *Man (N.S.)* 14: 607–27.

——. 1997. 'On Torture, or Cruel, Inhuman, and Degrading Treatment', in Arthur Kleinman, Veena Das and Margaret M. Lock (eds), *Social Suffering*. Berkeley, CA: University of California Press, pp. 285–308.

Bacchetta, Paola. 2007. 'Rescaling Transnational "Queerdom": Lesbian and "Lesbian" Identitary-Positionalities in Delhi in the 1980s', in Nivedita Menon (ed.), *Sexualities*. New Delhi: Women Unlimited, pp. 103–27.

Bahri, Deepika. 2017. *Postcolonial Biology: Psyche and Flesh After Empire*. Minneapolis: University of Minnesota Press.

Bandyopadhyay, Mahuya. 2010. *Everyday Life in a Prison: Confinement, Surveillance, Resistance*. New Delhi: Orient Blackswan.

Barua, Nupur. 2005. 'How to Develop a Pro-Poor Private Health Sector in India?', *Global Forum for Health Research* 9. Retrieved 22 December 2018 from http://www.hum.au.dk/hsre/Docs/Paper_GF9_NupurBarua.pdf.

Basu, Amit Ranjan. 2005. 'Historicizing Indian Psychiatry', *Indian Journal of Psychiatry* 4(2): 126–29.

Basu, Helene. 2008. '"Schmutzige Methoden": Geisteskrank durch Besessenheit und schwarze Magie in Gujarat/Indien', in Martin Vöhler and Angelika Malinar (eds), *Un/Reinheit: Konzepte und Erfahrungsmodi im Kulturvergleich*. Munchen: Fink Verlag, pp. 47–66.

——. 2009. 'Contested Practices of Control: Psychiatric and Religious Mental Health Care in India', *Curare* 1 + 2(32): 28–39.

——. 2010a. 'Besessenheitskrankheit und Psychiatriereform in der indischen Moderne', in Dorothea E. Schulz and Jochen Seebode (eds),

Spiegel und Prisma: Ethnologie zwischen postkolonialer Kritik und Deutung der eigenen Gesellschaft. Hamburg: Argument Verlag, pp. 195–209.

——. 2010b. 'Possession', in Knut A. Jacobsen et al. (eds), *Brill's Encyclopedia of Hinduism*. Leiden: Brill, pp. 416–26.

——. 2011. 'Darstellungen der Psychiatrie in indischen Filmen', *Zeitschrift für Ethnologie* 136: 69–92.

——. 2014. 'Dava and Dua: Ritual Healing of Madness', in Harish Naraindas, Johannes Quack and William S. Sax (eds), *Asymmetrical Conversations – Contestations, Circumventions, and the Blurring of Therapeutic Boundaries*. New York: Berghahn, pp. 162–99.

——. 2018. 'Säkulare Konversion zur Psychiatrie? Gesundheitshandeln in Filmen der indischen Mental Health Bewegung', in Wolfgang Drews, Ulrich Pfister and Martina Wagner-Egelhaaf (eds), *Religion und Entscheiden*. Wurzburg: Ergon, pp. 119–40.

Baxti, Upendra. 2011. 'Dignity in and with NAZ', in Arvind Narrain and Alok Gupta (eds), *Law Like Love: Queer Perspectives on Law*. New Delhi: Yoda Press, pp. 231–51.

Bayetti, Clément; Jadhav, Sushrut and Sumeet Jain. 2016. 'The Re-covering Self: A Critique of the Recovery-Based Approach in India's Mental Health Care', *Disability and the Global South* 3(1): 889–909.

Bayetti, Clément, Sushrut Jadhav and Smita N. Deshpande. 2017. 'How Do Psychiatrists in India Construct their Professional Identity? A Critical Literature Review', *Indian Journal of Psychiatry* 59(1): 26–37.

Bayetti, Clément, Sushrut Jadhav and Sumeet Jain. 2019. 'Mapping Mental Well-Being in India: Initial Reflections on the Role of Psychiatric Spaces', *Puruṣārta* (Collection Puruṣārta. Éditions de l'École des hautes études en sciences sociales) 36: 133–77.

BBC News. 2018. 'The Indian Women Abandoned Because of Mental Illness', 16 October. Retrieved 5 March 2019 from https://www.bbc.com/news/world-asia-india-45861899.

Bear, Laura, and Nayanika Mathur. 2015. 'Introduction. Remaking the Public Good: A New Anthropology of Bureaucracy', *The Cambridge Journal of Anthropology* 33(1): 18–34.

Beatty, Andrew. 2010. 'How Did it Feel for You? Emotion, Narrative, and the Limits of Ethnography', *American Anthropologist* 122(3): 430–43.

Behar, Ruth. 1997. *The Vulnerable Observer: Anthropology that Breaks Your Heart*. Boston, MA: Beacon Press.

Bell, Kirsten. 2014. 'Resisting Commensurability: Against Informed Consent as an Anthropological Virtue', *American Anthropologist* 116(3): 511–21.

Bennett, Lynn. 1989. *Dangerous Wives and Sacred Sisters: Social and Symbolic Roles of High-Caste Women in Nepal*. New York and Oxford: Columbia University Press.

Berger, Peter. 2010. 'Assessing the Relevance and Effects of "Key Emotional Episodes" for the Fieldwork Process', in Dimitrina Spencer and James Davies (eds), *Anthropological Fieldwork: A Relational Process*. Newcastle: Cambridge Scholars, pp. 119–43.

Berger, Peter L., and Thomas Luckmann. 1990 [1966]. *The Social Construction of Reality: A Treatise in the Sociology of Knowledge*. New York: Anchor Books.

Bhugra, Dinesh. 2006. *Mad Tales from Bollywood: Portrayal of Mental Illness in Conventional Hindi Cinema*. Hove and New York: Psychology Press.

Boellstorff, Tom. 2011. 'But Do Not Identify as Gay: A Proleptic Genealogy of the MSM Category', *Cultural Anthropology* 26(2): 287–312.

Bose, Brinda, and Subhabrata Bhattacharyya (eds). 2007. *The Phobic and the Erotic: The Politics of Sexualities in Contemporary India*. London: Seagull.

Bourdieu, Pierre. 2002. *Outline of a Theory of Practice* (Cambridge studies in social anthropology 16). Cambridge: Cambridge University Press.

Bourdieu, Pierre, and Loïc J.D. Wacquant. 1992. *An Invitation to Reflexive Sociology*. Chicago, IL: University of Chicago Press.

Boyce, Paul. 2007a. '"Conceiving Kothis": Men Who Have Sex with Men in India and the Cultural Subject of HIV Prevention', *Medical Anthropology Cross-Cultural Studies in Health and Illness* 26(2): 175–203.

——. 2007b. '(Dis)locating Male-to-Male Sexualities in Calcutta: Subject, Space and Perception', in Brinda Bose and Subhabrata Bhattacharyya (eds), *The Phobic and the Erotic: The Politics of Sexualities in Contemporary India*. London: Seagull, pp. 399–416.

Braddock, Louise. 2010. 'Emotions, Interpretation and the Psychoanalytic Countertransference', in Dimitrina Spencer and James Davies (eds), *Anthropological Fieldwork: A Relational Process*. Newcastle: Cambridge Scholars, pp. 204–28.

Brodwin, Paul. 2013. *Everyday Ethics: Voices from the Front Line of Community Psychiatry*. Berkeley, CA: University of California Press.

——. 2014. 'The Ethics of Ambivalence and the Practice of Constraint in US Psychiatry', *Culture, Medicine and Psychiatry* 38: 527–49.

Brodwin, Paul, and Livia Velpry. 2014. 'The Practice of Constraint in Psychiatry: Emergent Forms of Care and Control', *Culture, Medicine, and Psychiatry* 38: 524–26.

Brosius, Christiane. 2013. 'Love Attacks: Romance and Media Voyeurism in the Public Domain', in Sanjay Srivastava (ed.), *Sexuality Studies*. New Delhi: Oxford University Press, pp. 255–86.

Bruner, Jerome. 1991. 'The Narrative Construction of Reality', *Critical Inquiry* 18(1): 1–21.

Callahan, Sidney. 1988. 'The Role of Emotion in Ethical Decision Making', *The Hastings Centre Report* 18(3): 9–14.

Campbell, John. 2000. 'Narrative and Method in the Anthropology of Medicine – Crossing Bridges', in John Lee Cox and Vieda Skultans (eds), *Anthropological Approaches to Psychological Medicine*. London: Jessica Kingsley, pp. 105–22.

Caudill, William. 1958. *The Psychiatric Hospital as a Small Society*. Cambridge, MA: Harvard University Press.

Chakraborty, Kaustav, and Rajarshi Guha Thakurata. 2013. 'Indian Concepts on Sexuality', *Indian Journal of Psychiatry* 55: 250–55.

Chakravorty, Bhaswati. 2007. 'Rights for the Third Gender: Problems of Identity and Recognition', in Brinda Bose and Subhabrata Bhattacharyya (eds), *The Phobic and the Erotic: The Politics of Sexualities in Contemporary India*. London: Seagull, pp. 369–90.

Chandra, Prabha S., et al. 2003. 'A Cry from the Darkness', *Psychiatry* 4(66): 323–34.

Chavan, B.S., et al. 2006. 'ECT: Knowledge and Attitude Among Patients and Their Relatives', *Indian Journal of Psychiatry* 48: 34–38.

Cheney, Ann M., Steve Sullivan and Kathleen Grubbs. 2018. 'The Morality of Disordered Eating and Recovery in Southern Italy', *Medical Anthropology Quarterly* 32(3): 443–57.

Clifford, James, and George E. Marcus (eds). 2010. *Writing Culture: The Poetics and Politics of Ethnography*. Berkeley, CA: University of California Press.

Cohen, Lawrence. 1995. 'The Pleasures of Castration', in Paul R. Abramson (ed.), *Sexual Nature, Sexual Culture*. Chicago, IL: University of Chicago Press, pp. 276–304.

——. 2000. *No Aging in India: Alzheimer's, The Bad Family, and Other Modern Things*. Berkeley, CA: University of California Press.

——. 2005. 'The Kothi Wars: AIDS Cosmopolitanism and the Morality of Classification', in Vincanne Adams and Stacy Leigh Pigg (eds), *Sex in Development: Science, Sexuality, and Morality in Global Perspective*. Durham, NC: Duke University Press: pp. 269–303.

——. 2007. 'Holi in Banaras and the "Mahaland" of Modernity', in Nivedita Menon (ed.), *Sexualities*. New Delhi: Women Unlimited, pp. 197–223.

Corin, Ellen E. 1990. 'Facts and Meaning in Psychiatry: An Anthropological Approach to the Lifeworld of Schizophrenics', *Culture, Medicine and Psychiatry* 14: 153–88.

Cortazzi, Martin. 2013. 'Narrative Analysis in Ethnography', in Paul Atkinson et al. (eds), *Handbook of Ethnography*. Los Angeles: SAGE, pp. 384–94.

Csordas, Thomas J. 1990. 'Embodiment as a Paradigm for Anthropology', *ETHOS* 18: 5–47.

Csordas, Thomas J., et al. 2010. 'Ways of Asking, Ways of Telling: A Methodological Comparison of Ethnographic and Research Diagnostic Interviews', *Culture, Medicine, and Psychiatry* 34: 29–55.

Das, Veena. 2001. 'Stigma, Contagion, Defect: Issues in the Anthropology of Public Health'. *Stigma and Global Health: Developing a Research Agenda, 2001; September 5–7, Bethesda, Maryland*. Retrieved 12 March 2014 from http://www.stigmaconference.nih.gov/FinalDasPaper.htm.

Davar, Bhargavi V. 1995. 'Mental Illness among Indian Women', *Economic and Political Weekly* 30(45): 2879–86.

——. 1999. *Mental Health of Indian Women: A Feminist Agenda*. New Delhi: Sage.

——. 2012. 'Legal Frameworks For and Against Persons with Psychosocial Disabilities', *Economic & Political Weekly* XLVII(52): 123–31.

——. 2014. 'Globalizing Psychiatry and the Case of "Vanishing" Alternatives in a Neocolonial State', *Disability and the Global South* 1(2): 266–84.
Davar, Bhargavi V. (ed.). 2001. *Mental Health from a Gender Perspective*. New Delhi: Sage.
Davar, Bhargavi V., and Madhura Lohokare. 2008. 'Recovering from Psychosocial Traumas: The Place of Dargahs in Maharashtra', *Economic and Political Weekly* XLIV(16): 60–68.
Davenport, Nancy H.M. 2011. 'Medical Residents' Use of Narrative Templates in Storytelling and Diagnosis', *Social Science & Medicine* 73: 873–81.
Davies, James Peter, and Dimitrina Spencer (eds). 2010. *Emotions in the Field: The Psychology and Anthropology of Fieldwork Experience*. Stanford, CA: Stanford University Press.
Derges, Jane, et al. 2012. 'Challenges of Teaching Clinically Applied Anthropology and Cultural Psychiatry in India: An Evolving Partnership between a UK University and an Indian NGO', *Teaching Anthropology* 2(2): 3–14.
Devereux, Georges. 1998. *Angst und Methode in den Verhaltenswissenschaften*. Frankfurt am Main: Suhrkamp.
Dhar, Aarti. 2013. 'Cabinet Clears Mental Health Care Bill', *The Hindu*, 14 June. Retrieved 10 October 2018 from http://www.thehindu.com/news/national/cabinet-clears-mental-health-care-bill/article4812291.ece.
Dilger, Hansjörg, Susann Huschke and Dominik Mattes. 2014. 'Ethics, Epistemology, and Engagement: Encountering Values in Medical Anthropology', *Medical Anthropology* 34(1): 1–10.
Douglas, Mary. 1984. *Purity and Danger: An Analysis of the Concepts of Pollution and Taboo*. London: ARK Paperbacks.
Durkheim, Émile, and Marcel Mauss. 1963. *Primitive Classification*. Chicago, IL: University of Chicago Press.
Dutta, Aniruddha. 2011. 'Section 377 and the Retroactive Consolidation of "Homophobia"', in Arvind Narrain and Alok Gupta (eds), *Law like Love: Queer Perspectives on Law*. New Delhi: Yoda Press, pp. 162–73.
Ecks, Stefan. 2014. *Eating Drugs: Psychopharmaceutical Pluralism in India*. New York: New York University Press.
Ecks, Stefan, and Soumita Basu. 2009. 'The Unlicensed Lives of Antidepressants in India: Generic Drugs, Unqualified Practitioners, and Floating Prescriptions', *Transcultural Psychiatry* 46: 86–106.
——. 2014. '"We Always Live in Fear": Antidepressants Prescriptions by Unlicensed Doctors in India', *Culture, Medicine, and Psychiatry* 38: 197–216.
Elder-Vass, Dave. 2012. *The Reality of Social Construction*. Cambridge: Cambridge University Press.
Ernst, Waltraud. 1991. *Mad Tales from the Raj: The European Insane in British India, 1800–1858*. London and New York: Routledge.
——. 2007. 'Madness and Colonial Spaces: British India, c. 1800–1947', in Leslie Elizabeth Topp, James E. Moran and Jonathan Andrews (eds), *Madness, Architecture and the Built Environment: Psychiatric Spaces in His-*

torical Context – Conference Entitled 'Space, Psyche and Psychiatry'. New York and London: Routledge, pp. 215–38.

Estalella, Adolfo, and Tomás Sánchez Criado. 2018. *Experimental Collaborations: Ethnography Through Fieldwork Devices* (EASA Series, Volume 34). New York: Berghahn.

Estroff, Sue E. 1985. *Making it Crazy: An Ethnography of Psychiatric Clients in an American Community*. Berkeley, CA: University of California Press.

Fabrega, Horacio Jr. 2009. *History of Mental Illness in India: A Cultural Psychiatry Retrospective* (Dominik Wujastyk and Kenneth G. Zysk (eds), Indian Medical Tradition X). Delhi: Motilal Banarsidass.

Fainzang, Sylvie. 2014. 'Anthropology, Ethical Dissonance, and the Construction of the Object', *Medical Anthropology* 34(1): 11–23.

Farmer, Paul. 1997. 'On Suffering and Structural Violence: A View from Below', in Arthur Kleinman, Veena Das and Margaret M. Lock (eds), *Social Suffering*. Berkeley, CA: University of California Press, pp. 261–83.

Fengler, Christa, and Thomas Fengler. 1984. *Alltag in der Anstalt*. Rehburg-Loccum: Psychiatrie-Verl.

Fine, Jonathan. 1995. 'Towards Understanding and Studying Cohesion in Schizophrenic Speech', *Applied Psycholinguistics* 16(1): 25–41.

Foucault, Michel. 1994. *The Birth of the Clinic: An Archaeology of Medical Perception*. New York: Vintage.

Freud, Sigmund. 1960. *Totem and Taboo*. London: Routledge and Kegan Paul.

Gaines, Atwood D. 1992. 'From DSM-I to III-R: Voices of Self, Mastery and the Other: A Cultural Constructivist Reading of U.S. Psychiatric Classification', *Social Science & Medicine* 35(1): 3–24.

Gandevia, Katy Y. 1993. 'Community Mental Health: A Historical Overview of Past and Present Interventions', in Purnima Mane and Katy Y. Gandevia (eds), *Mental Health in India: Issues and Concerns*. Bombay: Tata Institute of Social Sciences, pp. 144–71.

Gangadhar, B.N., Vivek H. Phutane and Jagadisha Thirthalli. 2010. 'Research on Electroconvulsive Therapy in India: An Overview', *Indian Journal of Psychiatry* 52(7): 362–65.

Ganju, Vijay. 2000. 'The Mental Health System in India', *International Journal of Law and Psychiatry* 23(3–4): 393–402.

Gardner, John, and Clare Williams. 2015. 'Corporal Diagnostic Spaces: Clinicians' use of Space and Bodies During Diagnosis', *Sociology of Health and Illness* 37(5): 765–81.

Gay y Blasco, Paloma, and Huon Wardle. 2009. *How to Read Ethnography*. London: Routledge.

Geertz, Clifford. 2006. *The Interpretation of Cultures: Selected Essays*. New York: Basic.

Geist, Janina. 2008. *Queer in Indien – Selbst- und Fremdkonstruktionen indischer Queers in Politik, Gesellschaft und Medien unter besonderer Berücksichtigung des Internets*. Unveröffentlichte Magisterarbeit. Munchen: Institut für Ethnologie und Afrikanistik, Ludwig-Maximilians-Universität.

——. 2013. 'Queering Cyberspace in New Delhi: Negotiating Femininity, Masculinity and Thirdness', in Adam L. Brackin and Natacha Guyot (eds), *Stories in Post-Human Cultures*. Oxford: Interdisciplinary Press, pp. 119–32.

——. 2014. 'Queer Urban Spaces in New Delhi: Negotiating Femininity, Masculinity and Thirdness from a Kothi Perspektive', in Silke Förschler, Rebekka Habermas and Nikola Roßbach (eds), *Verorten – Verhandeln – Verkörpern: Interdisziplinäre Analysen zu Raum und Geschlecht*. Bielefeld: Transcript, pp. 85–116.

Gies-Powroznik, Natalie. 2016. *Madness and Mental Health in South Asian Settings*. Arbeitspapiere zur Ethnologie/Working Papers in Social Anthropology. Munster: Institut für Ethnologie: Masterarbeit am Institut für Ethnologie der Westfälischen Wilhelms-Universität 2015.

Giffort, Danielle M., and Kelly Underman. 2016. 'The Relationship Between Medical Education and Trans Health Disparities: A Call to Research', *Sociology Compass* 10: 999–1013.

Godderis, Rebecca. 2011. 'From Talk to Action: Mapping the Diagnostic Process in Psychiatry', in P.J. McGann and David Hutson (eds), *Sociology of Diagnosis*. Bradford: Emerald Group Publishing Limited, pp. 133–52.

Goffman, Erving. 1968. *Asylums: Essays on the Social Situation of Mental Patients and Other Inmates*. Harmondsworth, Middlesex: Penguin.

——. 1986. *Stigma: Notes on the Management of Spoiled Identity*. New York: Simon & Schuster.

Govindan, Padma, and Aniruddhan Vasudevan. 2011. 'The Razor's Edge of Oppositionality: Exploring the Politics of Rights-based Activism by Transgender Women in Tamil Nadu', in Arvind Narrain and Alok Gupta (eds), *Law like Love: Queer Perspectives on Law*. New Delhi: Yoda Press, pp. 67–83.

Graeber, David. 2015. *The Utopia of Rules: On Technology, Stupidity, and the Secret Joys of Bureaucracy*. Brooklyn: Melville House.

Gremillion, Helen. 2001. *Feeding Anorexia: Gender and Power at a Treatment Center*. Durham, NC: Duke University Press.

Gupta, Akhil. 2012. *Red Tape: Bureaucracy, Structural Violence, and Poverty in India*. Durham, NC: Duke University Press.

Gupta, Alok. 2005. 'Englishpur Ki Kothi: Class Dynamics in the Queer Movement in India', in Arvind Narrain and Gautam Bhan (eds), *Because I Have a Voice: Queer Politics in India*. New Delhi: Yoda Press, pp. 123–42.

——. 2011. 'The Presumption of Sodomy: Section 377 in India and Beyond', in Arvind Narrain and Alok Gupta (eds), *Law like Love: Queer Perspectives on Law*. New Delhi: Yoda Press, pp. 115–61.

Gupta, Richie, and Anil Murarka. 2009. 'Treating Transsexuals in India: History, Prerequisites for Surgery and Legal Issues', *Indian Journal of Plastic Surgery* 42(2): 226–33.

Hacking, Ian. 1986. 'Making Up People', in Thomas C. Heller, Morton Sosna and David E. Wellbery (eds), *Reconstructing Individualism: Auton-*

omy, Individuality, and the Self in Western Thought. Stanford, CA: Stanford University Press, pp. 222–36.

——. 2007. 'Kinds of People: Moving Targets', *Proceedings of the British Academy* 151: 285–318.

——. 2009. 'Autistic Autobiography', *Philosophic Transactions of the Royal Society B* 364: 1467–73.

Hak, Tony. 1998. '"There Are Clear Delusions": The Production of a Factual Account', *Human Studies* 21: 419–36.

Hall, Kira. 2005. 'Intertextual Sexuality: Parodies of Class, Identity, and Desire in Liminal Delhi', *Journal of Linguistic Anthropology* 15(1): 125–44.

Hall, Kira, and Veronica O'Donovan. 1996. 'Shifting Gender Positions among Hindi-Speaking Hijras', in Victoria L. Bergvall (ed.), *Rethinking Language and Gender Research – Theory and Practice*. London: Longman, pp. 228–66.

Handelman, Don. 1978. 'Introduction: A Recognition of Bureaucracy', in Don Handelman and Elliot Leyton (eds), *Bureaucracy and World View: Studies in the Logic of Official Interpretation*. St. John's: Institute of Social and Economic Research, Memorial University of Newfoundland, pp. 1–14.

——. 1998. *Models and Mirrors: Towards an Anthropology of Public Events*. New York: Berghahn.

Hausen, Karin. 1976. 'Die Polarisierung der "Geschlechtscharaktere": Eine Spiegelung der Dissoziation von Erwerbs- und Familienleben', in Werner Conze (eds), *Sozialgeschichte der Familie in der Neuzeit Europas*. Stuttgart: Klett, pp. 363–93.

Heckert, Carina. 2016. 'When Care is a "Systematic Route of Torture": Conceptualizing the Violence of Medical Negligence in Resource-Poor Settings', *Culture, Medicine, and Psychiatry* 40(4): 687–706.

Hensler, Mira Manuela. 2009. *Sind konkretistische Denkstörungen eine homogene Entität? – Untersuchungen zum Verständnis nicht-wörtlicher Sprache bei schizophrenen Patienten*. Inaugural-Dissertation zur Erlangung des Doktorgrades der Medizin. Tubingen: Medizinische Fakultät der Eberhard-Karls-Universität zu Tubingen. Retrieved 17 May 2016 from https://publikationen.uni-tuebingen.de/xmlui/bitstream/handle/10900/45461/pdf/schizophrenieundsprache.pdf?sequence=1.

Herdt, Gilbert H. ed. 1996. *Third Sex, Third Gender – Beyond Sexual Dimorphism in Culture and History*. New York: Zone Books.

Herzfeld, Michael. 1993. *The Social Production of Indifference – Exploring the Symbolic Roots of Western Bureaucracy*. Chicago, IL: University of Chicago Press.

Hinton, E. Devon, and Laurence L. Kirmayer. 2017. 'The Flexibility Hypothesis of Healing', *Culture, Medicine, and Psychiatry* 41(3): 3–34.

Hirschauer, Stefan. 1993. *Die soziale Konstruktion der Transsexualität – Über die Medizin und den Geschlechtswechsel*. Frankfurt am Main: Suhrkamp.

Hollan, Douglas. 2016. 'Psychoanalysis and Ethnography', *ETHOS* 44(4): 507–21.

Hollin, Gregory. 2017. 'Autistic Heterogeneity: Linking Uncertainties and Indeterminacies', *Science as Culture* 262: 209–31.

Huang, Jia, et al. 2009. 'An Exploratory Study of the Influence of Conversation Prosody on Emotion and Intention Identification in Schizophrenia', *Brain Research* 1281: 58–63.

Hull, Matthew S. 2012a. *Government of Paper: The Materiality of Bureaucracy in Urban Pakistan*. Berkeley, CA: University of California Press.

——. 2012b. 'Documents and Bureaucracy', *Annual Review of Anthropology* 41(1): 251–67.

Huschke, Susanne. 2014. 'Giving Back: Activist Research with Undocumented Migrants in Berlin', *Medical Anthropology* 34(1): 54–69.

Indian Psychiatric Society (IPS). 2016. 'The Indian Psychiatry Society's Position on Same-Sex Attraction, Orientation, Behaviour and Lifestyle'. Gurgaon, Haryana: 7 March.

Irvine, Janice M. 2005. *Disorders of Desire: Sexuality and Gender in Modern American Sexology*. Philadelphia, PA: Temple University Press.

Ivan Crozier. (ed.). 2008. *Sexual Inversion: A Critical Edition: Havelock Ellis and John Addington Symonds (1897)*. Basingstoke: Palgrave Macmillan.

Jackson, Jean E. 2005. 'Stigma, Liminality, and Chronic Pain: Mind-Body Borderlands', *American Ethnologist* 32(3): 332–53.

Jackson, Michael. 2010. 'From Anxiety to Method in Anthropological Fieldwork: An Appraisal of Georges Devereux's Enduring Ideas', in James Davies and Dimitrina Spencer (eds), *Emotions in the Field: The Psychology and Anthropology of Fieldwork Experience*. Stanford, CA: Stanford University Press, pp. 35–54.

Jadhav, Sushrut. 1994. 'Folk Appropriation of ECT in South India', *Psychiatric Bulletin* 18(3): 180.

——. 2004. 'Dhāt Syndrome: A Re-evaluation', *Psychiatry* 3(4): 14–16.

Jain, Sumeet, and Sushruth Jadhav. 2009. 'Pills that Swallow Policy: Clinical Ethnography of a Community Mental Health Program in Northern India', *Transcultural Psychiatry* 1(46): 60–85.

——. 2008. 'A Cultural Critique of Community Psychiatry in India'. *International Journal of Health Services* 38(3): 561–84.

Jenkins, Janis Hunter. 2004. 'Schizophrenia as a Paradigm Case for Understanding Fundamental Human Processes', in Janis Hunter Jenkins and Robert John Barrett (eds), *Schizophrenia, Culture, and Subjectivity: The Edge of Experience*. Cambridge: University Press, pp. 29–61.

——. 2015. *Extraordinary Conditions: Culture and Experience in Mental Illness*. Oakland, CA: University of California Press.

Jutel, Annemarie Goldstein. 2011. *Putting a Name to It: Diagnosis in Contemporary Society*. Baltimore, MD: Johns Hopkins University Press.

Jutel, Annemarie Goldstein, and Kevin Dew. 2014. *Social Issues in Diagnosis: An Introduction for Students and Clinicians*. Baltimore, MD: Johns Hopkins University Press.

Kala, A.K. 2004. 'Private Sector Psychiatry: Phenomenal Growth and Persistent Myths', in S.P. Agarwal (ed.), *Mental Health: An Indian Perspective 1946–2003*. New Delhi: Elsevier, pp. 161–65.

Kala, Anirudh. 2013. 'Time to Face New Realities: Mental Health Care Bill – 2013', *Indian Journal of Psychiatry* 55: 216–19.

Kalra, Gurvinder. 2012a. 'Hijras: The Unique Transgender Culture of India', *International Journal of Culture and Mental Health* 5(2): 121–26.

——. 2012b. 'Pathologising Alternate Sexuality: Shifting Psychiatric Practices and a Need for Ethical Norms and Reforms', *Indian Journal of Medical Ethics* IX(4): 291–92.

——. 2012c. 'A Psychiatrist's Role in "Coming Out" Process: Context and Controversies Post-377', *Indian Journal of Psychiatry* 54(1): 69–72.

——. 2012d. 'Letters to Editor: Breaking the Ice: IJP on Homosexuality', *Indian Journal of Psychiatry* 54(3): 299–300.

Kalra, Gurvinder, and Dinesh Bhugra. 2010. 'Migration and Sexuality', *International Journal of Culture and Mental Health* 3(2): 117–25.

Kalra, Gurvinder, Susham Gupta and Dinesh Bhugra. 2010. 'Sexual Variation in India: A View from the West', *Indian Journal of Psychiatry* 52(7): 264–68.

Kapur, R. L. 2004. 'The Story of Community Mental Health in India', in S.P. Agarwal (ed.), *Mental Health: An Indian Perspective 1946–2003*. New Delhi: Elsevier, pp. 92–100.

Khan, Shivananda. 2001. 'Culture, Sexualities, and Identities', *Journal of Homosexuality* 40(3–4): 99–115.

Khanna, Akshay. 2005. 'Beyond "Sexuality" (?)', in Arvind Narrain and Gautam Bhan (eds), *Because I Have a Voice: Queer Politics in India*. New Delhi: Yoda Press, pp. 89–104.

——. 2007. 'Us "Sexuality Types": A Critical Engagement with the Postcoloniality of Sexuality', in Brinda Bose and Subhabrata Bhattacharyya (eds), *The Phobic and the Erotic: The Politics of Sexualities in Contemporary India*. London: Seagull, pp. 159–200.

Khare, R.S. 1976. *The Hindu Hearth and Home*. New Delhi: Vikas.

Kindt, H., and M. Schecker. 1998. 'Sprache und Schizophrenie'. *Working Papers in Neurolinguistics and Neuroscience* 3 (Neuro 3). Retrieved 28 November 2012 from http://www.neurolabor.de/work3.htm.

Kirmayer, Laurence J. 2006. 'Beyond the "New Cross-cultural Psychiatry": Cultural Biology, Discursive Psychology and the Ironies of Globalization', *Transcultural Psychiatry* 43(1): 126–44.

——. 2008. 'Empathy and Alterity in Cultural Psychiatry', *ETHOS* 36(4): 457–74.

Kleinman, Arthur. 1977. 'Depression, Somatization and the "New Cross-Cultural Psychiatry"', *Social Science & Medicine* 11: 3–10.

——. 1989. *The Illness Narratives: Suffering, Healing, and the Human Condition*. New York: Basic.

Kleinman, Arthur, and Anne E. Becker. 1998. 'Sociosomatics: The Contributions of Anthropology to Psychosomatic Medicine', *Psychosomatic Medicine* 60: 389–93.

Kleinman, Arthur, and Joan Kleinman. 1995. 'Suffering and its Transformations', in Arthur Kleinman (ed.), *Writing at the Margin: Discourse between Anthropology and Medicine*. Berkeley, CA: University of California Press, pp. 95–119.

Kramer, Sarah, Karen L. Bryan and Christopher D. Frith. 1998. 'A Framework for Assessing Communication in Mental Illness', *International Journal for Language & Communication Disorder* 33: 164–69.

Kring, Ann M., and Marja K. Germans. 2004. 'Subjective Experience of Emotion in Schizophrenia', in Janis Hunter Jenkins and Robert John Barrett (eds), *Schizophrenia, Culture, and Subjectivity: The Edge of Experience*. Cambridge: Cambridge University Press, pp. 329–48.

Kuku, Diepiriye. 2013. 'Queering Subjectivities: On the Praxis of Outing Gender, Race, and Class in Ethnographic Fieldwork', in Sanjay Srivastava (ed.), *Sexuality Studies*. New Delhi: Oxford University Press, pp. 161–83.

Kutchins, Herb, and Stuart A. Kirk. 1997. *Making Us Crazy: DSM: The Psychiatric Bible and the Creation of Mental Disorders*. New York: Free Press.

Lambek, Michael. 2010. *Ordinary Ethics: Anthropology, Language, and Action*. New York: Fordham University Press.

Lang, Claudia. 2006. *Intersexualität: Menschen zwischen den Geschlechtern*. Frankfurt and New York: Campus Verlag.

Lang, Claudia, and Eva Jansen. 2013. 'The Ayurvedic Appropriation of Depression. Biomedicalizing Ayurvedic Psychiatry', *Medical Anthropology* 32(1): 25–45.

Latour, Bruno. 1994. *We Have Never Been Modern*. Cambridge, MA: Harvard University Press.

——. 2010. *On the Modern Cult of the Factish Gods*. Durham, NC: Duke University Press.

Latour, Bruno, and Steve Woolgar. 1986. *Laboratory Life: The Construction of Scientific Facts*. Princeton, NJ: Princeton University Press.

Lawlor, Mary C., and Olga Solomon. 2017. 'A Phenomenological Approach to the Cultivation of Expertise: Emergent Understandings of Autism', *ETHOS* 45(2): 232–49.

Lederman, Rena. 2013. 'Ethics: Practices, Principles, and Comparative Perspectives', in James G. Carrier and Deborah B. Gewertz (eds), *The Handbook of Sociocultural Anthropology*. London: Bloomsbury, pp. 588–611.

Lévi-Strauss, Claude. 1997. *Le cru et le cuit*. Paris: Plon.

Levy-Bruhl, Lucien. 1966. *How Natives Think*. New York: Washington Square Press.

Linska, Marion. 2015. 'Personale Feld-Reflexion: Überlegungen und Leitfaden zur Einbeziehung von Selbstfürsorge, Emotion und Selbstreflexion in den Feldforschungsprozess anhand phänomenologischer Methoden der Existenzanalyse', *Curare* 38(1 + 2): 73–86.

Linska, Marion, and Annika Strauss. 2015. 'Selbstreflexion im Kontext medizinethnologischer Langzeitforschung. Einleitung', *Curare (Selbstreflexion im Kontext medizinethnologischer Langzeitforschung/Self-reflection in the Context of Long-term Field Research Medical Anthropology)* 38(1 + 2): 9–24.

Lipsky, Michael. 1980. *Street-level Bureaucracy – Dilemmas of the Individual in Public Services*. New York: Russell Sage Foundation.

Littlewood, Roland. 2000. 'Psychiatry's Culture', in John Lee Cox and Vieda Skultans (eds), *Anthropological Approaches to Psychological Medicine*. London: Jessica Kingsley, pp. 66–93.

Long, Debbi, Cynthia L. Hunter and Sjaak van der Geest. 2008. 'When the Field is a Ward or a Clinic: Hospital Ethnography', *Anthropology & Medicine* 15(2): 71–78.

Lorimer, Francine. 2010. 'Using Emotion as a Form of Knowledge in a Psychiatric Fieldwork Setting', in James Davies and Dimitrina Spencer (eds), *Emotions in the Field: The Psychology and Anthropology of Fieldwork Experience*. Stanford, CA: Stanford University Press, pp. 98–126.

Lucas, Rod. 2004. 'In and Out of Culture: Ethnographic Means to Interpreting Schizophrenia', in Janis Hunter Jenkins and Robert John Barrett (eds), *Schizophrenia, Culture, and Subjectivity: The Edge of Experience*. Cambridge: University Press, pp. 146–63.

Luhrmann, Tanya M. 2000. *Of Two Minds: The Growing Disorder in American Psychiatry*. New York: Knopf.

Madden, Raymond. 2011. *Being Ethnographic: A Guide to the Theory and Practice of Ethnography*. London: Sage.

Mahajan, Priyanka Thukral, et al. 2013. 'Indian Religious Concepts on Sexuality and Marriage', *Indian Journal of Psychiatry* 55: 256–62.

Maitra, Shubhada. 2003. *Status of Women in Mental Hospitals in Maharashtra. A Report*. Unpublished Report. Mumbai: Department of Medical & Psychiatric Social Work, Tata Institute of Social Sciences, Prepared for Maharashtra State Commission for Women.

Mak, Geertje. 2004. 'Das vergeschlechtlichte Selbst als Nebenprodukt der medizinischen Geschlechter-Konstruktion – Hermaphroditen in klinischen Begegnungen im 19. Jahrhundert', in Stefan Micheler (ed.), *Kontakte – Freundschaften – Partnerschaften*. Hamburg: Männerschwarm Skript Verlag, pp. 95–109.

Marcus, George E. 1994. 'On Ideologies of Reflexivity in Contemporary Efforts to Remake the Human Sciences', *Poetics Today* 15(3): 383–404.

Marriot, McKim. 1968. 'Caste Ranking and Food Transactions: A Matrix Analysis', in Milton Singer and Bernhard S. Cohn (eds), *Structure and Change in Indian Society*. Chicago, IL: Aldine, pp. 133–71.

———. 1976. 'Hindu Transactions: Diversity Without Dualism', in Bruce Kapferer (ed.), *Transaction and Meaning: Directions in the Anthropology of Exchange and Symbolic Behaviour*. Philadelphia: Institute for the Study of Human Issues, pp. 109–42.

Mattingly, Cheryl. 2013. 'Moral Selves and Moral Scenes: Narrative Experiments in Everyday Life', *ETHOS* 78(3): 301–27.

Mauss, Marcel. 1973. 'Techniques of the Body', *Economy and Society* 2(1): 70–88.

McCabe, Rosemarie. 2009. 'Specifying Interactional Markers of Schizophrenia in Clinical Consultations', in Ivan Leudar and Alan Costall (eds), *Against Theory of Mind*. New York: Palgrave Macmillan, pp. 108–25.

Meer, Talia, and Alex Müller. 2017. '"They Treat Us Like We're Not There": Queer Bodies and the Social Production of Healthcare Spaces', *Health & Place* 45: 92–98.

Mehta, M., and S. Nimgaonkar Deshpande. 1983. 'Homosexuality: A Study of Treatment and Outcome', *Indian Journal of Psychiatry* 25(3): 235–38.

Menon, Nivedita. 2007a. 'Introduction', in ibid. (ed.), *Sexualities*. New Delhi: Women Unlimited, pp. xiii–lx.

——. 2007b. 'Section 377: How Natural is Normal?', in Brinda Bose and Subhabrata Bhattacharyya (eds), *The Phobic and the Erotic: The Politics of Sexualities in Contemporary India*. London: Seagull, pp. 339–41.

Mental Health Act. 1987. Mental Health Act 1987 with the State Mental Health Rules, 1990 and the Central Mental Health Authority Rules, 1990. Allahabal, U.P., India: Law Publishers.

Mills, China, and Suman Fernando. 2014. 'Globalising, Mental Health or Pathologising the Global South? Mapping the Ethics', *Theory and Practice of Global Mental Health* 1(2): 188–202.

Mills, James. 2001. 'The History of Modern Psychiatry in India, 1858–1947', *History of Psychiatry* xii: 431–58.

Mills, Stacia, et al. 2017. 'Training on the DSM-5 Cultural Formulation Interview Improves Cultural Competence in General Psychiatry Residents: A Pilot Study', *Transcultural Psychiatry* 54(2): 179–91.

Milton, Damian E.M. 2012. 'On the Ontological Status of Autism: The "Double Empathy Problem"', *Disability and Society* 27 (6): 883–87.

——. 2016. *Aut-ethnography: Working from the 'Inside-out'*. Retrieved 2 March 2016 from https://theautismanthropologist.wordpress.com/tag/aut-ethnography/.

Mishler, Elliot G. 1986. *Research Interviewing: Context and Narrative*. Cambridge, MA: Harvard University Press.

Mitra, Nishi, and Pooja Nair. 2011. 'In Conversation: Negotiating Femininity and Intimacies in Our Lives', in Samita Sen, Ranjita Biswas and Nandita Dhawan (eds), *Intimate Others: Marriage and Sexualities in India*. Kolkata: Stree, pp. 436–65.

MJ. 2016. '9 Indian Doctors Who Claim to Have a Cure for Homosexuality'. gaysi. The Gay Desi, 28 May. Retrieved 10 April 2019 from http://gaysifamily.com/2016/05/28/9-indian-doctors-claim-cure-homosexuality/.

Mukharji, Projit Bihari. 2009. *Nationalizing the Body, the Medical Market, Print and Daktari Medicine*. London: Anthem Press.

Myers, Neely, Anne Laurenzo, and Tali Ziv. 2016. '"No One Ever Even Asked Me that Before": Autobiographical Power, Social Defeat, and Recovery among African Americans with Lived Experiences of Psychosis', *Medical Anthropology Quarterly* 30(3): 395–413.

Nadig, Maja, et al. 2009. 'Einführung in eine ethnopsychoanalytische Deutungswerkstatt mit Beiträgen von vier Psychoanalytikern zu Kulturschock und Chaos', in Gerhard Schneider and Hans-Jürgen Eilts (eds), *Klinische Psychoanalyse heute: Forschungsfelder und Perspektiven. Herbst-*

tagung 2008. Deutsche Psychoanalytische Vereinigung, Bad Homburg, 19. bis 22. November 2008, pp. 419–29.

Nagaraja, D., and Pratima Murthy (eds). 2008. *Mental Health Care and Human Rights*. New Delhi: National Human Rights Commission.

Nakamura, Karen. 2013. *A Disability of the Soul: An Ethnography of Schizophrenia and Mental Illness in Contemporary Japan*. Ithaca, NY: Cornell University Press.

Nanda, Serena. 1986. 'The Hijras of India', *Journal of Homosexuality* 11(3–4): 35–54.

——. 1996. 'Hijras: An Alternative Sex and Gender Role in India', in Gilbert H. Herdt (ed.), *Third Sex, Third Gender: Beyond Sexual Dimorphism in Culture and History*. New York: Zone Books, pp. 373–417.

——. 1999. *Neither Man nor Woman: The Hijras of India* (second edition). Belmont, CA: Wadsworth.

Naraindas, Harish, Johannes Quack and William S. Sax. 2014. 'Introduction: Entangled Epistemes', in ibid. (eds), *Asymmetrical Conversations: Contestations, Circumventions, and the Blurring of Therapeutic Boundaries*. New York: Berghahn, pp. 1–25.

Narrain, Arvind. 2004. *Queer: 'Despised Sexuality', Law and Social Change*. Bangalore: Books for Change.

Narrain, Arvind, and Gautam Bhan. 2005. 'Introduction', in Arvind Narrain and Gautam Bhan (eds), *Because I Have a Voice: Queer Politics in India*. New Delhi: Yoda Press, pp. 1–30.

Narrain, Arvind, and Vinay Chandran. 2005. '"It's Not My Job to Tell You That's Okay to Be Gay": Queer Politics and Legal Reform in India', in Arvind Narrain and Gautam Bhan (eds), *Because I Have a Voice: Queer Politics in India*. New Delhi: Yoda Press, pp. 49–69.

Nayar, Pramod K. 2007. 'Queering Culture Studies: Notes towards a Framework', in Brinda Bose and Subhabrata Bhattacharyya (eds), *The Phobic and the Erotic: The Politics of Sexualities in Contemporary India*. London: Seagull, pp. 117–48.

Nelson, Dean. 2009. 'Hindu Guru Claims Homosexuality Can Be "Cured" by Yoga', *Telegraph*, 8 July. Retrieved 1 June 2019 from https://www.telegraph.co.uk/news/worldnews/asia/india/5780028/Hindu-guru-claims-homosexuality-can-be-cured-by-yoga.html.

Nichter, Mark. 1980. 'The Layperson's Perception of Medicine as Perspective into the Utilization of Multiple Therapy Systems in the Indian Context', *Social Science & Medicine* (14B): 225–33.

——. 1981. 'Idioms of Distress: Alternatives in the Expression of Psychosocial Distress: A Case Study from South India', *Culture, Medicine and Psychiatry* 5: 379–408.

Nuckolls, Charles W. 1992. 'Notes on a Defrocked Priest: Comparing South Indian Shamanic and American Psychiatric Diagnosis', in Atwood D. Gaines (ed.), *Ethnopsychiatry: The Cultural Construction of Professional and Folk Psychiatries*. Albany: State University of New York Press, pp. 69–84.

Nunley, Michael. 1992. 'The Mind Doctor's Dharma: On the Social Construction of Hospital Psychiatry in Eastern Uttar Pradesh, India', Ph.D. dissertation. San Francisco and Berkeley, CA: University of California.
——. 1996. 'Why Psychiatrists in India Prescribe so Many Drugs', *Culture, Medicine and Psychiatry* 20: 165–97.
——. 1998. 'The Involvement of Families in Indian Psychiatry', *Culture, Medicine and Psychiatry* 22(3): 317–53.
Obeyesekere, Gananath. 1990. *The Work of Culture: Symbolic Transformation in Psychoanalysis and Anthropology*. Chicago, IL: University of Chicago Press.
Okely, Judith. 1991. 'Defiant Moments: Gender, Resistance and Individuals', *Man, New Series* 26(1): 3–22.
——. 1996. 'The Self and Scientism', in Judith Okely, *Own or Other Culture*. London: Routledge, pp. 27–44.
Oosterhuis, Harry. 2000. *Stepchildren of Nature: Krafft-Ebing, Psychiatry, and the Making of Sexual Identity*. Chicago, IL: University of Chicago Press.
Orsini, Gisella. 2017. '"Hunger Hurts, but Starving Works": The Moral Conversion to Eating Disorders', *Culture, Medicine, and Psychiatry* 41: 111–41.
Paralikar, Vasudeo P., et al. 2015. 'Clinical Value of the Cultural Formulation Interview in Pune, India', *Indian Journal of Psychiatry* 57(1): 59–67.
Parekh, Suresh. 2003. 'Homosexuality in India: The Light at the End of the Tunnel', *Journal of Gay & Lesbian Psychotherapy* 7(1/2): 145–63.
Parkin, David I985. 'Introduction', in David Parkin, *The Anthropology of Evil*. Oxford, UK: Blackwell, pp. 1-25.
Parsons, Talcott. 1951. *The Social System*. London: Routledge & Kegan Paul.
Patel, Vikram, and R. Thara. (ed.). 2003. *Meeting the Mental Health Needs of Developing Countries*. New Delhi: Sage.
Patel, Vikram, and Mathew Varghese. 2004. 'NGOs and Mental Health: Search for Synergy', in S.P. Agarwal (ed.), *Mental Health: An Indian Perspective 1946–2003*. New Delhi: Elsevier, pp. 145–51.
Patel, Vikram, et al. 1999. 'Women, Poverty and Common Mental Disorders in Four Restructuring Societies', *Social Sciences and Medicine* (49): 1461–71.
Pathare, Soumitra. 2003. 'Beyond ECT: Priorities in Mental Health Care in India', *Indian Journal of Medical Ethics* 11(1): 11–12.
Perrin, Jennifer S., et al. 2012. 'Electroconvulsive Therapy Reduces Frontal Cortical Connectivity in Severe Depressive Disorder', *Proceedings of the National Academy of Sciences of the United States of America* 109(14): 5464–68.
Pink, Sarah. 2009. *Doing Sensory Ethnography*. Los Angeles: Sage.
Pinto, Sarah. 2009. 'Crises of Commitment: Ethics of Intimacy, Kin, and Confinement in Global Psychiatry', *Medical Anthropology: Cross Cultural Studies in Health and Illness* 28(1): 1–10.
——. 2011. 'Rational Love, Relational Medicine. Psychiatry and the Accumulation of Precarious Kinship', *Culture, Medicine and Psychiatry* 35: 376–95.

——. 2012. 'The Limits of Diagnosis: Sex, Law, and Psychiatry in a Case of Contested Marriage', *ETHOS* 40(2): 119–41.

——. 2014. *Daughters of Parvati: Women and Madness in Contemporary India*. Philadelphia, PA: University of Pennsylvania Press.

——. 2015. '"The Tools of Your Chants and Spells": Stories of Madwomen and Indian Practical Healing', *Medical Anthropology* 35(3): 263–77.

Pradhan, P.V., K.S. Ayyar and V.N. Bagadia. 1982. 'Homosexuality: Treatment by Behaviour Modification', *Indian Journal of Psychiatry* 24(1): 80–83.

Purcell, Elizabeth B. 2016. 'Disability, Narrative, and Moral Status', *Disability Studies Quarterly* 36(1). Retrieved 11 December 2022 from https://dsq-sds.org/index.php/dsq/article/view/4375/4207.

Puri, Jyoti. 2013. 'Decriminalization as Deregulation? Logics of Sodomy Law and the State', in Sanjay Srivastava (ed.), *Sexuality Studies*. New Delhi: Oxford University Press, pp. 141–60.

Quack, Johannes. 2012. *Disenchanting India: Organized Rationalism and Criticism of Religion in India*. Oxford: Oxford University Press.

——. 2014. 'Porous Dividuals: Complying to the Demands of a Healing Temple (Balaji) and a Psychiatric Out-Patient Department (OPD)', in Harish Naraindas, Johannes Quack and William S. Sax (eds), *Asymmetrical Conversations: Contestations, Circumventions, and the Blurring of Therapeutic Boundaries*. New York: Berghahn, pp. 56–84.

Raguram, R. et al. 2002. 'Traditional Community Resources for Mental Health: A Report of Temple Healing from India', *British Medical Journal* 325: 38–40.

Rajagopal, R. et al. 2012. 'Knowledge, Experience & Attitudes Concerning Electroconvulsive Therapy Among Patients & Their Relatives', *Indian Journal of Medical Research* 135(2): 201–10.

Ramakrishnan, L. 2007. 'Putting the "B" Back in LGBT: Bisexuality, Queer Politics and HIV/AIDS Discourse', in Brinda Bose and Subhabrata Bhattacharyya (eds), *The Phobic and the Erotic: The Politics of Sexualities in Contemporary India*. London: Seagull, pp. 291–300.

Ranade, Ketki. 2009. *Medical Response to Male Same-Sex Sexuality in Western India: An Exploration of "Conversion Treatments" for Homosexuality*. New Delhi: Population Council.

Rapport, Nigel. 2004. 'The Narratives as Fieldwork Technique: Processual Ethnography for a World in Motion', in Amit Vered (ed.), *Constructing the Field: Ethnographic Fieldwork in the Contemporary World*. London: Routledge, pp. 71–95.

Reddy, Gayatri. 2004. 'Crossing "Lines" of Subjectivity: The Negotiation of Sexual Identity in Hyderabad, India', in Sanjay Srivastava (ed.), *Sexual Sites, Seminal Attitudes: Sexualities, Masculinities and Culture in South Asia*. New Delhi: SAGE, pp. 147–64.

——. 2005a. *With Respect to Sex: Negotiating Hijra Identity in South India*. Chicago, IL: University of Chicago Press.

——. 2005b. 'Geographies of Contagion: Hijras, Kothis, and the Politics of Sexual Marginality in Hyderabad', *Anthropology & Medicine* 12(3): 255–70.

——. 2007. 'Sexual Differences and Their Discontents: Shifting Contexts of 'Thirdness' in Hyderabad', in Brinda Bose and Subhabrata Bhattacharyya (eds), *The Phobic and the Erotic: The Politics of Sexualities in Contemporary India*. London: Seagull, pp. 301–22.

Rhodes, Lorna Amarasingham. 1984. '"This Will Clear Your Mind": The Use of Metaphors for Medication in Psychiatric Settings', *Culture, Medicine and Psychiatry* 8: 49–70.

——. 1986. 'The Anthropologist as Institutional Analyst', *ETHOS* 14(2): 204–17.

——. 1991. *Emptying Beds: The Work of an Emergency Psychiatric Unit*. Berkeley, CA: University of California Press.

——. 2004. *Total Confinement: Madness and Reason in the Maximum Security Prison*. Berkeley, CA: University of California Press.

Richardson, Laurel. 1995. 'Narrative and Sociology', in John Van Maanen (ed.), *Representation in Ethnography*. Thousand Oaks: Sage, pp. 198–221.

Ricoeur, Paul. 1974. *The Conflict of Interpretations*. Evanston, IL: Northwestern University Press.

Robertson, William J. 2017. 'The Irrelevance Narrative: Queer (In)Visibility in Medical Education and Practice', *Medical Anthropology Quarterly* 31(2): 159–76.

Roncaglia, Sara. 2013. *Feeding the City: Work and Food Culture of the Mumbai Dabbawalas*. Cambridge: Open Book Publishers.

Rosenberg, Charles E. 2002. 'The Tyranny of Diagnosis. Specific Entities and Individual Experiences', *Milbank Quarterly* 80(2): 237–60.

Rosenhan, D.L. 1973. 'On Being Sane in Insane Places', *Science* 179 (4070): 250–58.

Row Kavi, Ashok. 2007. 'Kothis versus Other MSM: Identity Versus Behaviour in the Chicken and Egg Paradox', in Brinda Bose and Subhabrata Bhattacharyya (eds), *The Phobic and the Erotic: The Politics of Sexualities in Contemporary India*. London: Seagull, pp. 390–98.

Roy, Sandip. 2007. 'Double Minorities: The Experience of the Lesbian, Gay, Bisexual and Transgender Indians in the Diaspora', in Brinda Bose and Subhabrata Bhattacharyya (eds), *The Phobic and the Erotic: The Politics of Sexualities in Contemporary India*. London: Seagull, pp. 323–38.

Ryan, J., G. Woodyatt and D. Copeland. 2010. 'Procedural Discourse in Intellectual Disability and Dual Diagnosis', *Journal of Intellectual Disability Research* 54(1): 70–80.

Sachan, Dinsa. 2013. 'Mental Health Bill Set to Revolutionise Care in India', *The Lancet* 382: 296.

Sadowsky, Jonathan Hal. 2004. 'Symptoms of Colonialism: Content and Context of Delusion in Southwest Nigeria, 1945–1960', in Janis Hunter Jenkins and Robert John Barrett (eds), *Schizophrenia, Culture, and Sub-*

jectivity: The Edge of Experience. Cambridge: Cambridge University Press, pp. 238–55.

Sakthivel, L.M., K. Rangasami and T.N. Jayaraman. 1979. 'Treatment of Homosexuality by Anticipatory Avoidance Conditioning Technique', *Indian Journal of Psychiatry* 21: 146–48.

Saris, A. Jamie. 1995. 'Telling Stories: Life Histories, Illness Narratives, and Institutional Landscape', *Culture, Medicine and Psychiatry* 19: 39–72.

Sathyanarayana Rao, T.S., and Ajit Avasthi. 2008. 'Roadmap for Sexual Medicine: Agenda for Indian Psychiatric Society', *Indian Journal of Psychiatry* 50(3): 153–54.

Sathyanarayana Rao, T.S., and K.S. Jacob. 2012. 'Homosexuality and India', *Indian Journal of Psychiatry* 54(1): 1–3.

——. 2014. 'The Reversal on Gay Rights in India', *Indian Journal of Psychiatry* 56(1): 1–2.

Sathyanarayana Rao, T.S., et al. 2016. 'Gay Rights, Psychiatric Fraternity, and India', *Indian Journal of Psychiatry* 58: 1–3.

Satyamev Jayate. 2012. *Stories of Change: Every Life is Precious: Does Healthcare Need Healing?* Star Plus. Retrieved 20 April 2019 from http://www.satyamevjayate.in/every-life-is-precious/every-life-is-precious.aspx.

Sax, William. 2014. 'Ritual Healing and Mental Health in India', *Transcultural Psychiatry* 51(6): 829–49.

SCARF. 1998. *A Study of Mentally Disabled Women*. Chennai: Schizophrenia Research Foundation.

Sebastian, Sangeeth, and Kumar Vikram. 2015. 'Mail Today Exclusive: Delhi Doctors Use Electric Shock to Treat Homosexuality', *India Today*, 27 May. Retrieved 10 April 2019 from https://www.indiatoday.in/mail-today/story/homosexuality-cure-delhi-doctors-exposed-conversion-therapy-254849-2015-05-27.

Shamgar-Handelman, Lea, and Don Handelman. 1991. 'Celebrations of Bureaucracy: Birthday Parties in Israeli Kindergartens', *Ethnology* 30(4): 293–312.

Sharma, Maya. 2005. 'She Came from the World of the Spirits', in Arvind Narrain and Gautam Bhan (eds), *Because I Have a Voice: Queer Politics in India*. New Delhi: Yoda Press, pp. 234–43.

Sharma, S. D. 2004. 'Mental Health: The Pre-Independence Scenario', in S. P. Agarwal (ed.), *Mental Health – An Indian Perspective 1946–2003*. New Delhi: Elsevier, pp. 25–29.

Sieler, Roman. 2014. 'Patient Agency Revisited: "Healing the Hidden" in South India', *Medical Anthropology Quarterly* 28(3): 323–41.

Skultans, Vieda. 1991. 'Women and Affliction in Maharashtra: A Hydraulic Model of Health and Illness', *Culture, Medicine and Psychiatry* (15): 321–59.

——. 2000. 'Remembering and Forgetting: Anthropology and Psychiatry: The Changing Relationship', in John Lee Cox and Vieda Skultans (eds), *Anthropological Approaches to Psychological Medicine*. London: Jessica Kingsley, pp. 94–104.

——. 2003. 'Culture and Dialogue in Medical Psychiatric Narratives', *Anthropology & Medicine* 10(2): 155–65.

——. 2007. *Empathy and Healing: Essays in Medical and Narrative Anthropology*. New York: Berghahn.

Skultans, Vieda, and John Cox. 2000. 'Introduction', in John Lee Cox and Vieda Skultans (eds), *Anthropological Approaches to Psychological Medicine: Crossing Bridges*. London: Jessica Kingsley, pp. 7–40.

Smith, Lindsay, and Arthur Kleinman. 2010. 'Emotional Engagements: Acknowledgement, Advocacy, and Direct Action', in James Davies and Dimitrina Spencer (eds), *Emotions in the Field: The Psychology and Anthropology of Fieldwork Experience*. Stanford, CA: Stanford University Press, pp. 171–87.

Smith-Morris, Carolyn. 2016. 'Introduction: Diagnosis as the Threshold to 21st Century Health', in Carolyn Smith-Morris (ed.), *Diagnostic Controversy: Cultural Perspectives on Competing Knowledge in Healthcare*. New York: Routledge, pp. 1–24.

Solomon, Harris. 2015. '"The Taste No Chef Can Give": Processing Street Food in Mumbai', *Cultural Anthropology* 30(1): 65–90.

Spencer, Dimitrina. 2010. 'Introduction: Emotional Labour and Relational Observation in Anthropological Fieldwork', in Dimitrina Spencer and James Davies (eds), *Anthropological Fieldwork: A Relational Process*. Newcastle: Cambridge Scholars, pp. 1–47.

——. 2011. 'Emotions and the Transformative Potential of Fieldwork: Some Implications for Teaching and Learning Anthropology', *Teaching Anthropology* 1(2): 68–97.

Srivastava, Sanjay. 2004. 'Non-Ghandian Sexuality, Commodity Cultures and a "Happy Married Life": Masculine and Sexual Cultures in the Metropolis', in Sanjay Srivastava (ed.), *Sexual Sites, Seminal Attitudes: Sexualities, Masculinities and Culture in South Asia*. New Delhi: SAGE, pp. 342–90.

Stege, Alyssa M. Ramírez, and Kristin Elizabeth Yarris. 2017. 'Culture in la Clínica: Evaluating the Utility of the Cultural Formulation Interview (CFI) in a Mexican Outpatient Setting', *Transcultural Psychiatry* 54(4): 466–87.

Stodulka, Thomas. 2015. 'Emotion Work, Ethnography, and Survival Strategies on the Streets of Yokyakarta', *Medical Anthropology* 34(1): 84–97.

Strand, Michael. 2011. 'Where Do Classifications Come From? The DSM-III, the Transformation of American Psychiatry, and the Problem of Origins in the Sociology of Knowledge', *Theory & Sociology* 40: 273–313.

Strauss, Annika. 2011. *Ethnographie eines Rehabilitationsprojektes für psychisch kranke Obdachlose im westlichen Indien: Die heimatlosen Verrückten* (FERN/SEHEN: Perspektiven der Sozialanthropologie 5). Hamburg: Verlag Dr Kovac.

——. 2015. 'Beyond the Black Box and Therapy Culture: Verstörende Feldforschungserfahrungen als Zugang zu lokalem Wissen verstehen lernen', *Curare* 38(1 + 2): 87–102.

——. 2019. '"How Did it Feel for You?" - Teaching and Learning (by) Emotional Reflexivity in Undergraduate Fieldwork Training', in Thomas Stodulka, Samia Dinkelaker and Ferdiansyah Thajib (ed.), *Affective Dimensions of Fieldwork*. New York: Springer, pp. 305–23.
——. 2022. '"Identified as Gay"—Making up Queer Communities and Sexual Selves in Mumbai', *cultura & psyché*.
Strauss, Annika, and Helmar Kurz. 2018. 'Framing Experiences. Diagnosing and Explaining Dissociative Phenomena in Indian and Brazilian Mental Health-Care Institutions', *Curare* 41(3+4): 159–68.
Strauss, Anselm Leonard, et al. 1963. 'The Hospital and Its Negotiated Order', in Eliot Friedson (ed.), *The Hospital in Modern Society*. New York: Macmillan, pp. 147–69.
Sukthankar, Ashwini. 2005. 'Complicating Gender: Rights of Transsexuals in India', in Arvind Narrain and Gautam Bhan (eds), *Because I Have a Voice: Queer Politics in India*. New Delhi: Yoda Press, pp. 164–74.
Suresh, Mayur. 2011a. '"I am Only Here to Do Masti": Sodomy Law and the Limits of Subjectivation', in Arvind Narrain and Alok Gupta (eds), *Law like Love: Queer Perspectives on Law*. New Delhi: Yoda Press, pp. 466–80.
——. 2011b. 'Possession is 9/10ths of the Body: Law, Land and Hijra Identity', in Arvind Narrain and Alok Gupta (eds), *Law like Love: Queer Perspectives on Law*. New Delhi: Yoda Press, pp. 378–92.
Swartz, Sally. 1994. 'Issues in the Analysis of Psychotic Speech', *Journal of Psycholinguistic Research* 23(1): 29–44.
'Tarasha'. no year. Tata Institute of Social Sciences website. Retrieved 26 May 2019 from https://www.tiss.edu/view/11/projects/all-projects/tarasha/.
Taylor, E.W. 1998. *The Theory and Practice of Transformative Learning: A Critical Review* (Information Series No. 374). Columbus, OH: ERIC Clearinghouse on Adult, Career and Vocational Education.
Tedlock, Barbara. 1991. 'From Participant Observation to the Observation of Participation: The Emergence of Narrative Ethnography', *Journal of Anthropological Research* 47(1): 69–94.
Tessier, Laurence Anne. 2016. 'A Flavour of Alzheimer's', *Journal of the Royal Anthropological Institute* 23: 249–66.
Thara, R., and T.N. Srinivasan. 1997. 'Marriage and Gender in Schizophrenia', *Indian Journal of Psychiatry* 1(39): 64–69.
The Hamsafar Trust. 2016. 'Queers against Quacks', launched on 4 May. Retrieved 15 July 2017 from https://www.facebook.com/pg/queersaga instquacks/about/?ref=page_internal.
Tribhuwan, Robin D. 1998. *Medical World of the Tribals: Explorations in Illness Ideology, Body Symbolism and Ritual Healing*. New Delhi: Discovery.
Turner, Sarah. 2010. 'Research Note: The Silenced Assistant. Reflections of Invisible Interpreters and Research Assistants', Asia Pacific Viewpoint 51(2): 206–19.
Ulrich, Helen E. 1987. 'A Study of Change and Depression among Havik Brahmin Women in a South Indian Village', *Culture, Medicine and Psychiatry* 2(11): 261–87.

Valentine, David. 2007. *Imagining Transgender: An Ethnography of a Category*. Durham, NC: Duke University Press.

Van Dijk, Rob. 1998. 'Culture as Excuse: The Failures of Health Care to Migrants in the Netherlands', in Sjaak van der Geest and Adri Rienks (eds), *The Art of Medical Anthropology: Readings*. Amsterdam: Het Spinhuis, pp. 243–51.

Van Dongen, Els. 2000. 'Anthropology and Psychiatry: Two of a Kind but Where is the Other?', in John Lee Cox and Vieda Skultans (eds), *Anthropological Approaches to Psychological Medicine*. London: Jessica Kingsley, pp. 123–42.

——. 2002. *Walking Stories: An Oddnography of Mad People's Work with Culture*. West Lafayette, IN: Purdue University Press.

——. 2003. 'Walking Stories: Narratives of Mental Patients as Magic', *Anthropology & Medicine* 10(2): 207–22.

——. 2004. *Worlds of Psychotic People: Wanderers, 'Bricoleurs' and Strategists*. London: Routledge.

Van Maanen, John. 1995. 'An End to Innocence: The Ethnography of Ethnography', in John van Maanen (ed.), *Representation in Ethnography*. Thousand Oaks: Sage, pp. 1–35.

Vanita, Ruth. 2002. *Queering India: Same-Sex Love and Eroticism in Indian Culture and Society*. New York and London: Routledge.

——. 2005. *Gandhi's Tiger and Sita's Smile: Essays on Gender, Sexuality, and Culture*. New Delhi: Yoda Press.

Vanita, Ruth, and Saleem Kidwai. 2001. *Same-Sex Love in India: Readings from Literature and History*. New York: Palgrave.

Verghese, Abraham. 2014. 'Letters to Editor: A Fresh Look at Homosexuality', *Indian Journal of Psychiatry* 56(2): 209–10.

Vidhya, U., Kiranmayi, A. and V. Vijayalakshmi. 2012. 'Women: Evidence from A Hospital-based Study', in Dalal, Ajit K. and Girishwar Misra (eds.), *New Directions in Health Psychology*. New Delhi: Sage, pp. 155–78.

Weiss, Mitchell G., et al. 1988. 'Humoral Concepts of Mental Illness in India', *Social Science & Medicine* 27(5): 471–77.

Weiss, Mitchell G., et al. 2001. 'Global, National, and Local Approaches to Mental Health: Examples from India', *Tropical Medicine and International Health* 1: 4–23.

Wengle, John L. 1987. 'Death and Rebirth in Fieldwork: A Case Study', *Culture, Medicine and Psychiatry* 11: 357–85.

Wig, N.N., and Ajit Awasthi. 2004. 'Origin and Growth of General Hospital Psychiatry', in S.P. Agarwal (ed.), *Mental Health: An Indian Perspective 1946–2003*. New Delhi: Elsevier, pp. 101–7.

Wilce, James M. 1995. '"I Can't Tell You All My Troubles": Conflict, Resistance, and Metacommunication in Bangladeshi Illness Interactions', *American Ethnologist* 22(4): 927–52.

——. 1998. 'The Pragmatics of "Madness": Performance Analysis of a Bangladeshi Woman's "Aberrant" Lament', *Culture, Medicine and Psychiatry* 1(22): 1–54.

Williams, Donna. 2005. *The Jumbled Jigsaw: An Insider's Approach to the Treatment of Autistic Spectrum 'Fruit Salads'*. London: Jessica Kingsley.

Wind, Gitte. 2008. 'Negotiated Interactive Observation. Doing Fieldwork in Hospital Settings', *Anthropology & Medicine* 15(2): 79–89.

Windzio, Alina Charlotte. 2014. *Doing Transgender?: Praktiken des Geschlechts in Indien*. Unveröffentlichte Bachelorarbeit. Münster: Institut für Ethnologie, Westfälische Wilhelms-Universität.

World Health Organisation (WHO). 2004. *Gender in Mental Health Research*. Geneva: WHO Library Cataloguing-in-Publication Data.

Yaron, Hadas. 2009. '"Your Papers or Your Life": The Significance of Documents in the Life Experiences of African Refugees in Israel', *New Proposals: Journal of Marxism and Interdisciplinary Inquiry* 3(1): 7–14.

Yergeau, Melanie. 2013. 'Clinically Significant Disturbance: On Theorists Who Theorize Theory of Mind', *Disability Studies Quarterly* 33(4). Retrieved 23 February 2019 from http://dsq-sds.org/article/view/3876/3405.

Young, Allan. 1993. 'A Description of How Ideology Shapes Knowledge of a Mental Disorder (Posttraumatic Stress Disorder)', in Shirley Lindenbaum and Margaret Lock (eds), *Knowledge, Power, and Practice: The Anthropology of Medicine and Everyday Life*. Berkeley, CA: University of California Press, pp. 108–28.

Zaman, Shahaduz. 2005. *Broken Limbs, Broken Lives: Ethnography of a Hospital Ward in Bangladesh*. Amsterdam: Het Spinhuis.

INDEX

www.ingramcontent.com/pod-product-compliance
Ingram Content Group UK Ltd.
Pitfield, Milton Keynes, MK11 3LW, UK
UKHW021836100926
8556IPUK00004B/374

9 781805 390688